# Clinical Practice in Urology

# Clinical Practice in Urology

Editor: Ezra Martin

AMERICAN
MEDICAL PUBLISHERS
www.americanmedicalpublishers.com

AMERICAN
MEDICAL PUBLISHERS
www.americanmedicalpublishers.com

**Cataloging-in-Publication Data**

Clinical practice in urology / edited by Ezra Martin.
p. cm.
Includes bibliographical references and index.
ISBN 979-8-88740-006-8
1. Urology. 2. Urinary organs--Diseases. 3. Urinary organs--Diseases--Treatment.
4. Urinary organs--Diseases--Diagnosis. I. Martin, Ezra.
RC900 .C55 2023
616.6--dc23



American Medical Publishers,
41 Flatbush Avenue,
1st Floor, New York,
NY 11217, USA

ISBN 979-8-88740-006-8 (Hardback)

# Contents

# Preface

The world is advancing at a fast pace like never before. Therefore, the need is to keep up with the latest developments. This book was an idea that came to fruition when the specialists in the area realized the need to coordinate together and document essential themes in the subject. That's when I was requested to be the editor. Editing this book has been an honour as it brings together diverse authors researching on different streams of the field. The book collates essential materials contributed by veterans in the area which can be utilized by students and researchers alike.

Urology is a discipline of medical science that deals with diseases of the urinary and the reproductive tracts. The different sub-disciplines under the domain of urology are andrology, pediatric urology, urologic oncology, endourology, female urology, and reconstructive urology. Urological diseases and conditions can be dealt by medical and surgical methods. Some common urologic diseases are enlarged prostate, nocturia, microscopic hematuria, urinary tract infection, vasectomy, kidney stones and urethral cancer. This area of medicine involves the diagnosis of the patient by physical examination followed by tests such as blood test, urinalysis, and prostate-specific antigen test. This book is a valuable compilation of topics that present a detailed explanation of clinical practice in urology. A number of latest researches have been included to keep the readers up-to-date with the global concepts in this area of study. This book will prove to be immensely beneficial to students and researchers involved in the field of urology.

Each chapter is a sole-standing publication that reflects each author´s interpretation. Thus, the book displays a multi-facetted picture of our current understanding of application, resources and aspects of the field. I would like to thank the contributors of this book and my family for their endless support.

**Editor**

# 1

# A rare case of herniated duplex collecting system causing obstructive uropathy

Christopher El Mouhayyar[1,2*], Haoyang Wang[1,2], Laith Hattar[1,2], Fang-Yu Liu[1,2], Karen Feghali[1,2] and Vaidyanathapuram Balakrishnan[1,2]

**Abstract**

**Background:** An inguinal hernia is the protrusion of intraabdominal organs through an opening in the abdominal wall. Structures such as small and large intestines are commonly contained within inguinal hernias. However, uretero-inguinal hernia of the native collecting system is an extremely rarely reported entity. If unrecognized, acute kidney injury due to obstructive uropathy or serious intraprocedural ureteral injuries during hernia repair can occur. A duplex collecting system is a congenital kidney anomaly with an incidence of 0.8%. A uretero-inguinal hernia involving duplicated ureters has not been previously described in literature. Here we report a case of obstructive uropathy secondary to uretero-inguinal hernia involving duplicated ureters.

**Case presentation:** A 78-year-old male known to have a left sided inguinal hernia presented to the Emergency department with two weeks of intermittent suprapubic tenderness, dysuria, frequency, urgency, frothy urine as well as nausea and vomiting. Workup on admission revealed an elevated creatinine of 2.8 mg/dl. CT imaging revealed duplicated left sided ureters with left inguinal hernia containing the ureters. There was cystic ureteral dilation within the herniation sac as well as moderate left hydroureteronephrosis. Patient had an elective inguinal hernia repair with left ureteral stent placement. Following the surgery, he had recovery of kidney function to the previous baseline serum creatinine of 1.5 mg/dl.

**Conclusion:** A duplex collecting system arises when two ureteral buds are formed during fetal development. However, diagnosis can be made in rare instances during adulthood when duplex collecting systems are usually found incidentally. Uretero-inguinal hernias have been reported as a common complication of renal transplant. However, uretero-inguinal hernias in native kidneys are considered an uncommon finding, especially with a duplex collecting system. When patients present with herniation and acute kidney injury, it is important to rule out the possibility of uretero-inguinal hernia to minimize complications such as obstructive uropathy and kidney failure. CT scan providing cross-sectional imaging is the ideal modality for identification of the site and etiology of urinary tract obstruction and site of herniation. If during imaging, an obstructive uropathy is observed, a nephroureteral stent or nephrostomy tube can be inserted to protect the ureter as well as relieve the obstruction, respectively.

**Keywords:** Uretero-inguinal hernia, Duplex collecting system, Acute kidney injury

* Correspondence: christopher.elmouhayyar@steward.org
[1]Department of Medicine, St. Elizabeth's Medical Center, Boston, MA, USA
[2]Department of Medicine, Tufts University School of Medicine, Boston, MA, USA

## Background

An inguinal hernia is the protrusion of intraabdominal or extraperitoneal organs through an opening in the abdominal wall that is widely prevalent amongst male population [1, 2]. A wide range of structures such as small bowel, large bowel and bladder are commonly contained within inguinal hernias. However, uretero-inguinal hernia is a rarely reported entity that is more frequently seen following a kidney transplant. Even further, uretero-inguinal hernias of the native kidneys have rarely been reported. This phenomenon is potentially associated with acute kidney injury due to obstructive uropathy or serious ureteral injuries if unrecognized prior to surgical hernia repair. A duplex collecting system is a common congenital kidney anomaly, with an incidence of 0.8% [3]. A uretero-inguinal hernia involving duplicated ureters has not been previously described in literature (Table 1). Here we report a case of obstructive uropathy secondary to uretero-inguinal hernia involving duplicated ureters.

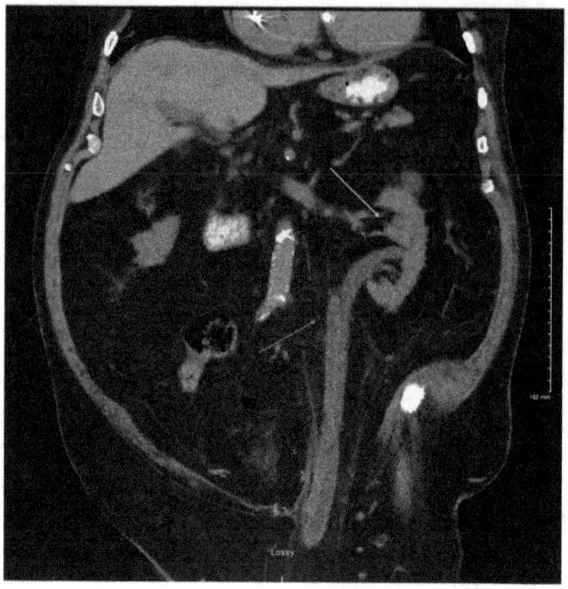

**Fig. 1** CT scan of the abdomen and pelvis showing the hydroureternephrosis. (Green arrow: Hydronephrosis, Red arrow: ureteronephrosis)

## Case presentation

A 78-year-old male with past medical history significant for CKD stage 3 known to have a left sided inguinal hernia presented to the Emergency department with two weeks of intermittent suprapubic tenderness, dysuria, frequency, urgency, frothy urine as well as nausea and vomiting. Workup on admission revealed an elevated creatinine of 2.8 mg/dl from a baseline of 1.5 mg/dl, with leukocytosis of 7000. Urine analysis was performed that revealed large leukocyte esterase, urine WBC greater 180, and white blood cell clumps. The patient was diagnosed with acute kidney injury as well as a urinary tract infection. Computed tomography of the abdomen and pelvis revealed duplicated left sided pelvis and ureters with the left inguinal hernia containing the ureters with cystic ureteral dilation within the herniation sac as well as moderate left hydroureteronephrosis (Figs. 1 and 2). The patient was managed with volume repletion and

**Table 1** Table showing Case reports in literature describing ureteroinguinal hernia in transplant vs native kidneys with a single or double collecting system, findings on imaging as well as the modality of management

| Authors | Collecting System | Kidney | Imaging Finding | Management |
|---|---|---|---|---|
| He et al. [4] | Single | Native | Left Hydrourertero-nephrosis | Nephro-ureteral stent |
| Hong et al. [5] | Single | Native | Left Hydrourertero-nephrosis | Conservative |
| Lu et al. [6] | Single | Native | Right Hydrourertero-nephrosis | Conservative |
| Eilber et al. [7] | Single | Native | Right Hydrourertero-nephrosis | Conservative |
| Sidqi et al. [8] | Single | Native | Left Uretero-nephrosis | Lichtenstein repair |
| Yahya et al. [9] | Single | Native | Right Hydrourertero-nephrosis | Lichtenstein repair<br>Nephro-ureteral stent |
| Otani et al. [10] | Single | Transplant | Right hydronephrosis | Nephro-ureteral stent |
| Furtado et al. [11] | Single | Transplant | Left Hydrourertero-nephrosis | Hernia Repair |
| Weingarten et al. [12] | Single | Transplant | Left Hydronephrosis | Nephro-ureteral catheter<br>Hernia Repair |
| Osman et al. [13] | Single | Transplant | Right Hydrourertero-nephrosis | Hernioplasty<br>Nephrostomy tube |
| Abu-areda et al. [14] | Single | Transplant | Right Hydrourertero-nephrosis | Nephrostomy tube |
| Won et al. [15] | Single | Native | Pelvic–ureteric junction obstruction | Conservative |
| Malde et al. [16] | Single | Native | Left Hydrourertero-nephrosis | Mesh Hernia Repair |
| Sanchez et al. [17] | Single | Transplant | Right Hydrourertero-nephrosis | Hernioplasty |

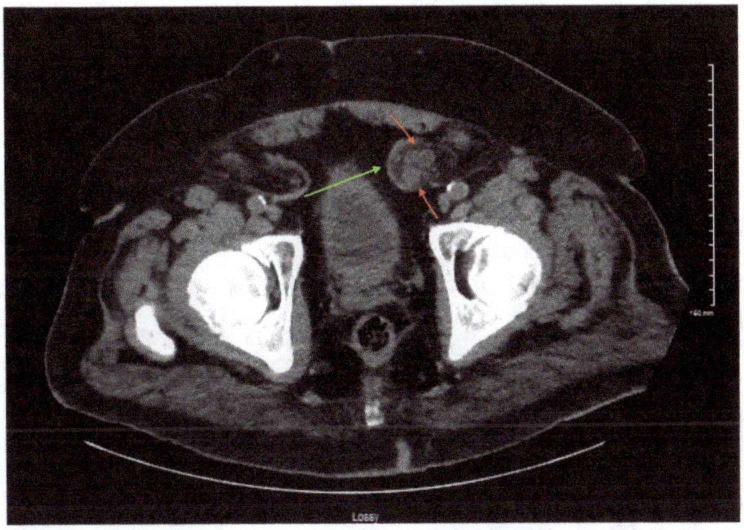

**Fig. 2** CT scan of the abdomen and pelvis showing the uretero-inguinal hernia involving duplicated ureters (Green arrow: Hernia, Red arrow: Two ureters)

antibiotics for his urinary tract infection. There was some improvement in kidney function although not to his previous baseline. He was discharged with an outpatient urology follow up and was subsequently readmitted for an elective paraperitoneal inguinal hernia repair with a Kumpe catheter placement up to the left kidney externalizing through the urethral meatus.

When it comes to the inguinal hernia repair, a large portion of the herniated extraperitoneal fat was freed from its incarcerated position in the scrotum and then dissected back to the internal ring. A typical mesh repair was not done in order to avoid placing the mesh in direct contact with the ureter causing erosions as well as ureteral structuring further down the line. Thus, the internal ring was primarily closed first to maintain the ureter in a reduced position deep to the ring then a Lichtenstein repair was done using a polypropelene patch that was sutured to the tissues overlying the pubic tubercle medially to the shelving edge of the inguinal ligament inferiorly and to the conjoined tendon superiorly, laterally the arms of the patch were passed around the spermatic cord at the internal ring and sutured together and to the tissue lateral to the internal ring.

Following the surgery, he had recovery of kidney function to the previous baseline serum creatinine of 1.5 mg/dl. (Table 2) (Fig. 3).

**Table 2** Table showing Creatinine (Cr: mg/dL) as an indication of kidney function over time (prior to the operation and post operation) POD: post-operative day. PrOD: Pre-operative day

| Days | PrOD | POD1 | POD2 | POD3 | POD4 | POD5 |
|---|---|---|---|---|---|---|
| Cr (mg/dL) | 2.8 | 2.2 | 1.75 | 1.65 | 1.5 | 1.43 |

## Discussion and conclusion

Ureteral development begins in fetus at the age of four weeks with the ureteral bud branching from the mesonephric duct [18]. The ureteric bud is responsible for the formation of the collecting system. If two ureteral buds arise, the caudal ureter drains the lower pole and the cephalic ureter drains the upper pole [19]. Patients usually present in childhood with recurrent UTIs, flank pain, incontinence and hematuria [20]. However, diagnosis can be made in rare instances during adulthood when duplex collecting systems are usually found incidentally on abdominal imaging or during surgery [21–23].

Uretral herniation can occur at different sites including inguinal, femoral, sciatic, thoracic and parailiac [24, 25]. Uretero-inguinal hernias have been reported as a

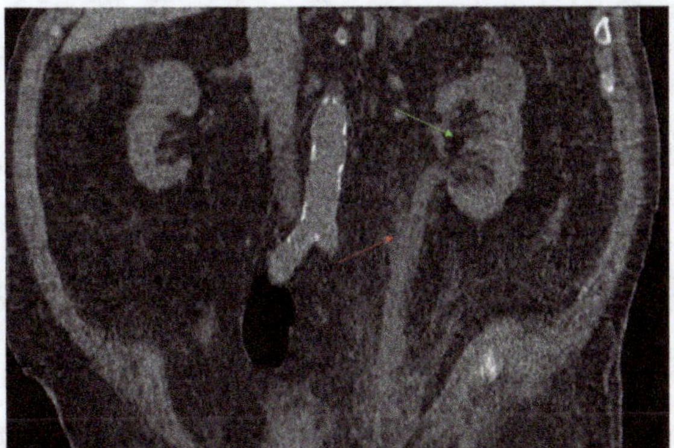

**Fig. 3** CT scan of the abdomen and pelvis post-operation day 20 showing improvement in hydroureternephrosis. (Green arrow: Hydronephrosis, Red arrow: ureteronephrosis)

common complication of renal transplant [26].However, uretero-inguinal hernias in native kidneys are considered an uncommon finding. They are divided into two types: the paraperitoneal or extraperitoneal with paraperitoneal accounting for majority of cases [6, 27].

A paraperitoneal hernia occurs when the ureter is adherent to the posterior peritoneum and is herniated alongside the peritoneal sac into the inguinal canal. It is a sliding type of hernia thought to be caused by traction of the underlying structures or adhesions that attach the ureter to the posterior peritoneum. This type of herniation is often accompanied by herniation of other organs such as the colon [15].

On the other hand, extraperitoneal herniation is herniation of the ureter without the peritoneal sac. It is theorized to be due to a congenital embryonic defect that resulted in the fusion of the ureter and the genitoinguinal ligament due to the failure of separation of the ureteric bud from the wolffian duct [26, 28]. However, one case report attributed the formation of extraperitoneal ureteral hernia to adhesions from a previous hernia repair [29].

Uretero-inguinal hernias can potentially cause obstructive uropathy and in some cases lead to kidney failure if left undiagnosed. Further, if undiagnosed, iatrogenic ureteral injury can occur during hernia repair [30].

Obesity as well as deficiency in collagen synthesis are risk factors for ureteral hernias. These hernias are more frequent on the right side compared to the left due to differences in fascia of Toldt morphology [30].

Ultrasound is the ideal first line imaging modality to assess the upper urinary tract as it can identify hydronephrosis as well as the integrity of the proximal ureter. However, ultrasound of the urinary tract does not routinely include assessment of the inguinal orifices making the tracking of the ureter in the retroperitoneal space a challenge. Cross-sectional imaging (CT scan or MRI) are more reliable for identification of the site and etiology of urinary tract obstruction and can allow identification of the site of herniation as well as anatomical classification with CT remaining more easily accessible between the two modalities.

Herniorrhaphy is considered the treatment modality for uretero-inguinal hernias causing obstructive symptoms [7]. If during imaging, an obstructive uropathy is observed, a nephroureteral stent or nephrostomy tube can be inserted to protect the ureter as well as relieve the obstruction, respectively [4].

A uretero-inguinal hernia is a rare condition that can potentially lead to obstructive uropathy. CT is currently the modality of choice for identification, diagnosis as well as anatomical classification of the hernia and its possible complications. In this case report, we describe a unique uretero-inguinal hernia involving a duplicated ureter causing obstructive uropathy. Recognizing such an entity is important in identifying causes of acute kidney injury and preventing surgical complications.

**Abbreviations**

CT scan: Computerized Tomography scan; MRI: Magnetic Resonance Imaging; POD: post-operative day; PrOD: Pre-operative day; Cr: Creatinine

**Acknowledgments**

Not applicable.

**Authors' contributions**

CEM and HW were the primary team taking care of the patient and contributed in writing this article. LH reviewed the literature and contributed in writing the manuscript. FYL and KF followed up on the patient post operation and contributed in writing as well. VB is the attending physician who supervised, contributed to and guided us while writing this manuscript. All authors approved the final version of the submitted manuscript.

**Competing interests**

The authors declare that they have no competing interests.

**References**

1. Dabbas N, Adams K, Pearson K, Royle G. Frequency of abdominal wall hernias: is classical teaching out of date?. JRSM Short Rep. 2011;2(1):5. https://doi.org/10.1258/shorts.2010.010071.
2. Kark AE, Kurzer M. Groin hernias in women. Hernia. 2008;12(3):267–270. https://doi.org/10.1007/s10029-007-0330-4.
3. Malek RS, Kelalis PP, Stickler GB, Burke EC. Observations on ureteral ectopy in children. J Urol. 1972;107(2):308–313. https://doi.org/10.1016/s0022-5347(17)61012-7.
4. He L, Herts BR, Wang W. Paraperitoneal ureteroinguinal hernia. J Urol. 2013; 190(5):1903–1904. https://doi.org/10.1016/j.juro.2013.08.005.
5. Hong LE, Tan C, Li J. Obstructive Uropathy Secondary to Uretero-inguinal Hernia. J Clin Imaging Sci. 2015;5:33. https://doi.org/10.4103/2156-7514.159448.
6. Lu A, Burstein J. Paraperitoneal inguinal hernia of ureter. J Radiol Case Rep. 2012;6:22–6.
7. Eilber KS, Freedland SJ, Rajfer J. Obstructive Uropathy secondary to Ureteroinguinal herniation. Rev Urol. 2001;3:207–8.
8. Sidiqi MM, Menezes G. Asymptomatic herniation of ureter in the routine inguinal hernia: A dangerous trap for general surgeons. Int J Surg Case Rep. 2018;49:244–246. https://doi.org/10.1016/j.ijscr.2018.07.013.
9. Yahya Z, Al-habbal Y, Hassen S. Ureteral inguinal hernia: an uncommon trap for general surgeons. Case Reports. 2017;2017:bcr2017219288.
10. Otani LH, et al. Sonographic diagnosis of a ureteral inguinal hernia in a renal transplant. J Ultrasound Med. 2008;27(12):1759–65.
11. Furtado CD, Sirlin C, Precht A, et al. Unusual cause of ureteral obstruction in transplant kidney. Abdom Imaging. 2006;31:379–82.
12. Weingarten KE, et al. Obturator herniation of the ureter in a renal transplant recipient causing hydronephrosis: perioperative percutaneous management. J Vasc Interv Radiol. 1996;7(6):939–41.
13. Osman Y, et al. Sliding hernia containing the ureter—a rare cause of graft hydroureteronephrosis: a case report. Transplant Proceed. 2004;36:5.
14. Areda MA, Bailey CR, O'Mara D, Weiss CR. Transplant uretero-inguinal hernia resulting in urosepsis. Radiol Case Rep. 2018;14(1):14–7.
15. Won ACM, Testa G. Chronic obstructive uropathy due to uretero-inguinal hernia: a case report. Int J Surg Case Rep. 2012;3:379–81.
16. Malde S, Bilagi P, Marsh H. Obstructive uropathy due to uretero-inguinal hernia: an uncommon occurrence. Indian J Urol. 2013;29(4):355–6.
17. Sánchez ASS, Tebar JC, Martín MS, Bachs JMG, Moreno MJD, Navarro HP, Rodríguez JAV. Obstructive Uropathy secondary to ureteral herniation in a pediatric *En Bloc* renal graft. Am J Transplant. 2005;5:2074–7.
18. Brehmer B, Makris A, Jakse G. Laparoscopic heminephrectomy and resection of ectopic ureter in an adult. Urol Int. 2007;79:280–3.
19. Lavallée G, et al. Obstructed duplex kidney in an adult: ultrasonic evaluation. J Clin Ultrasound JCU. 1985;13:281–3.
20. Gao Z, Wu J, Lin C, Men C. Transperitoneal laparoscopic heminephrectomy in duplex kidney: our initial experience. Urology. 2011;77:231–6.

21. Balén EM, Pardo F, Lecumberri FJ, Longo J. Giant megalo-ureter and duplex kidney in an asymptomatic adult. Scand J Urol Nephrol. 1997;31:413–6.
22. Mahajan NN, Sahay S, Kale A, Nasre M. Unilateral upper-pole giant hydroureter in a duplex renal system: an incidental finding in cesarean section. Arch Gynecol Obstet. 2008;278:149–51.
23. Zissin R, et al. Renal duplication with associated complications in adults: CT findings in 26 cases. Clin Radiol. 2001;56:58–63.
24. Hwang CM, Miller FH, Dalton DP, Hartz WH. Accidental ureteral ligation during an inguinal hernia repair of patient with crossed fused renal ectopia. Clin Imaging. 2002;26:306–8.
25. Giglio M, et al. Scrotal extraperitoneal hernia of the ureter: case report and literature review. Urol Int. 2001;66:166–8.
26. Odisho AY, Freise CE, Tomlanovich SJ, Vagefi PA. Inguinal herniation of a transplant ureter. Kidney Int. 2010;78:115.
27. Bertolaccini L, Giacomelli G, Bozzo R, Gastaldi L, Moroni M. Inguino-scrotal hernia of a double district ureter: case report and literature review. Hernia. 2005;9:291–3.
28. Peters CA, Schlussel RN, Mendelsohn C. Ectopic ureter, ureterocele, and ureteral anomalies. In: Wein A.J., editor. Campbell-Walsh Urology. 10th ed. Philadelphia: Saunders Elsevier. Chap 117; 2012.
29. Golgor E, Stroszczynski C, Froehner M. Extraperitoneal inguinoscrotal herniation of the ureter: a rare case of recurrence after hernia repair. Urol Int. 2009;83:113–5.
30. Giuly J, François GF, Giuly D, Leroux C, Nguyen-Cat RR. Intrascrotal hernia of the ureter and fatty hernia. Hernia. 2003;7:47–9.

# 2

# Prognostic value of systemic inflammatory factors NLR, LMR, PLR and LDH in penile cancer

Chen Hu, Yu Bai*, Jun Li, Guoyin Zhang, Libo Yang, Chengwei Bi, Bin Zhao, Yong Yang, Ruiqian Li, Hongyi Wu, Qilin Wang and Yang Qin

## Abstract

**Background:** Penile squamous cell carcinoma (PSCC) represents an important public health problem for developing countries. The major prognostic factors in PSCC are pathological subtype, perineural invasion, lymphovascular invasion, depth of invasion and grade, which are hard to obtain precisely before the operation. Besides, micro-metastases will be detected in about 30% of intermediate-risk patients with clinically non-palpable inguinal lymph nodes after inguinal lymph node dissection (ILND). It means approximately 70% of patients are unable to benefit from ILND who might suffered from the complications of surgery. We hope some biomarkers could be found which are able to predict the outcome before surgery and reflect the inguinal lymph nodes metastasis.

**Methods:** A total of 349 consecutive patients of penile cancer in Yunnan cancer hospital in China between October 2002 and December2017. Two hundred twenty-five was succeed to follow-up. The association between NLR, LMR, PLR, LDH and Overall survival (OS), progression free survival (PFS), inguinal lymph node (N stage) was analyzed with K-M analysis, univariable, multivariable logistic regression and Kendall's tau-b correlation coefficient.

**Results:** Multivariable analysis reveal that only PLR was significant independent factor which is associated with inferior OS and PFS; Age and LDH was associated with inferior OS; Lymph node and metastatic status remained significant for OS and PFS as NCCN and EAU Guidelines indicated; the tumor type, initial treatment and NLR LMR were not significant in predicting both OS and PFS. NLR, LMR and PLR were corresponded to N stage, while LDH was not associated with the N stage based on logistic regression model analysis. NLR, LMR and PLR were found weakly related to N stage through an application of Kendall's tau-b correlation coefficient.

**Conclusions:** PLR was significant independent factors for OS and PFS, Age and LDH was significant independent factors for OS. NLR, LMR, PLR was corresponded to N stage.

**Keywords:** Penile cancer, NLR, LMR, PLR, LDH

## Background

Penile squamous cell carcinoma has a low incidence among all cancers, according to the report there are 26, 000 new cases occurring worldwide annually [1]. However, in developing countries such as Africa, Asia, South America, etc. penile cancer is still a difficult problem, where its incidence varies from 3 to 8.3 cases per 100, 000 [2], especially in southwestern of China. The management of the regional lymph nodes is extremely important for long-term survival of the patient according to the National Comprehensive Cancer Network (NCCN) and the European Association of Urology (EAU) clinical practice guidelines. Both guidelines

* Correspondence: 2447519483@qq.com
Department of Urology, Yunnan Cancer Hospital, The Third Affiliated Hospital of Kunming Medical University, Kunming 650118, Yunnan, China

subdivide penile cancer into three groups of low risk, intermediate risk and high risk. Low-risk patients with non-palpable inguinal lymph node (cN0) can be managed by surveillance or dynamic sentinel node biopsy (DSNB), however, due to earlier Inguinal Lymph Node Dissection (ILND) surgery has a better prognosis than ILND after local lymph node recurrence, the indications for ILND recommended by the guidelines are do the operation as long as the inguinal lymph node are palpable, whether it is low-risk, moderate or high risk [3]. However intermediate-risk patients with clinically non-palpable inguinal lymph nodes, only about 30% of them are able to detect micro-metastases after ILND. That means the rest of patients approximately 70% have no benefit from ILND and suffered from the complications of surgery. So it is crucial to selected the patients who are really benefits from ILND before surgery. Because prognosis of PSCC is highly correlated with lymph nodes stage, plenty of articles have select patients through the prognostic role of biomarkers. The major prognostic factors in PSCC are perineural invasion, pathological subtype, depth of invasion, grade and lymphovascular invasion [4, 5]. These factors are hard to precisely obtain before the operation. Besides some articles used biomarkers such as p53 and squamous cell carcinoma antigen to predict inguinal lymph node positive rate and prognosis of penile cancer, but they were not applied to clinical practice [6, 7]. So we hope to find some markers that is associated with inguinal lymph nodes metastatic or can predict the outcomes.

As we known that systemic inflammatory factors play an significant role in cancer progression [8, 9]. The tumor micro-environment regulated by inflammatory cells is clearly related to cancer progression [8]. Systemic inflammatory factors are obviously reflected by changes of peripheral leukocyte, lymphocytes,neutrophils, monocytes and platelets. These factors above mentioned can reflect the tumor micro environment indirectly [8], so we collected the data of peripheral blood parameters including the neutrophil-to-lymphocyte ratio (NLR), lymphocyte-to-monocyte ratio (LMR), platelet-to-lymphocyte ratio (PLR) which have been reported to be independent prognostic factors in various of cancers [8, 10–14]. Besides, high lactate dehydrogenase (LDH) has also shown that associated with poor OS in urologic cancer [15].

Recently it has been reported that cancer patients with high NLR is associated with worse OS [16] and worse RFS and CSS [17, 18]. However, there has been no study evaluating the PLR associated with outcomes of penile cancer. In this retrospective study, we investigated the role of NLR, LMR, PLR and LDH before surgery to predicting whether micro-metastases of inguinal lymph node exist and assessed the prognostic value in penile cancer.

## Methods

We reviewed our electronic medical records system to identify men treated for penile SCC at Yunnan cancer hospital in China between October 2002 and December 2017. Experimental procedures were approved by the Human Ethics Committee of Yunnan Cancer Hospital.A total of 349 consecutive patients treated with ILND in PSCC, 225 was succeed to follow-up, Epidemiological and clinical data, including age, preoperative full blood count results NLR, LMR, PLR LDH and TNM clinical staging, tumor pathology, treatment history and oncological outcome (OS, PFS). Survival analysis was performed by the Kaplan–Meier method for univariable analysis and Cox regression method for multivariable analysis. The NLR was calculated by neutrophil-to-lymphocyte ratio, LMR was lymphocyte-to-monocyte ratio and PLR was platelet-to lymphocyte ratio which were obtained through peripheral complete blood count and blood biochemistry before the surgery. We calculate the cut-off point of the Ages, NLR, LMR, PLR and LDH according to the area under curve (AUC) given consideration to sensitivity and specificity levels.

The primary end point were overall survival (OS) and progression free survival (PFS) which defined as the time from the dates of pathological diagnosis to death and tumor progression. Univariable analysis (K-M analysis) was performed to compare the higher and lower groups of NLR, LMR, PLR and LDH. Multivariable analysis (COX logistic regression) were used to verify the individual factors respectively. *P* values less than 0.05 were considered statistical significance.

We also analyse the relation between the NLR, LMR, PLR, LDH and N stage through the logistic regression, meantime we use method of Kendall's tau-b correlation coefficient to determine the correlation.

## Results

### NLR, LMR, PLR, LDH vs OS/PFS

A total of 225 patients had collected peripheral complete blood count and blood biochemistry before surgery. The mean (±SD) ages were 50.6 ± 13.4. The detailed data of patients are summarized in Table 1. We performed AUC curve to determine the Age, NLR, LMR, PLR and LDH cut-off value which were 53,2.94,4.74,133.5 and 188.5 respectively. The median interquartile range follow-up was 30 (16.0–63.5) months. Among the 225 patients, 171 was survival which the median interquartile range follow-up was 34 (18.0–84.0) months; 150 was disease free which the median interquartile range follow-up was 33

**Table 1** Patients' characteristics

| Variable | | NLR | | | LMR | | | PLR | | | LDH | | |
|---|---|---|---|---|---|---|---|---|---|---|---|---|---|
| | All *n*= 225 | NLR≤2.94 | NLR>2.94 | p | LMR≤4.74 | LMR>4.74 | p | PLR≤133.5 | PLR>133.5 | p | LDH≤188.5 | LDH>188.5 | p |
| Age, y | | | | 0.296 | | | 0.169 | | | 0.566 | | | 0.184 |
| <53 | 140 | 103 | 37 | | 55 | 85 | | 105 | 35 | | 115 | 25 | |
| ≥53 | 85 | 54 | 31 | | 45 | 40 | | 55 | 30 | | 65 | 20 | |
| Tumor type | | | | 0.026 | | | 0.091 | | | 0.131 | | | 0.943 |
| benign | 44 | 35 | 9 | | 17 | 27 | | 38 | 6 | | 35 | 9 | |
| well | 96 | 69 | 27 | | 39 | 57 | | 62 | 34 | | 79 | 17 | |
| moderate | 74 | 49 | 25 | | 35 | 39 | | 52 | 22 | | 59 | 15 | |
| poor | 8 | 4 | 4 | | 7 | 1 | | 6 | 2 | | 6 | 2 | |
| others | 3 | 0 | 3 | | 2 | 1 | | 2 | 1 | | 2 | 1 | |
| Anatomic stage | | | | 0.002 | | | 0.063 | | | 0.005 | | | 0.076 |
| 0 | 44 | 33 | 9 | | 17 | 25 | | 36 | 6 | | 33 | 9 | |
| I | 67 | 51 | 16 | | 23 | 44 | | 48 | 19 | | 57 | 10 | |
| II | 39 | 28 | 11 | | 18 | 21 | | 31 | 8 | | 33 | 6 | |
| III | 62 | 41 | 21 | | 31 | 31 | | 39 | 22 | | 50 | 12 | |
| IV | 15 | 4 | 11 | | 11 | 4 | | 6 | 9 | | 8 | 7 | |
| N stage | | | | 0.001 | | | 0.024 | | | 0.009 | | | 0.053 |
| 0 | 148 | 112 | 36 | | 58 | 90 | | 115 | 33 | | 123 | 25 | |
| 1 | 28 | 15 | 13 | | 18 | 10 | | 15 | 13 | | 24 | 4 | |
| 2 | 36 | 26 | 10 | | 15 | 21 | | 24 | 12 | | 27 | 9 | |
| 3 | 13 | 4 | 9 | | 9 | 4 | | 6 | 7 | | 7 | 6 | |
| M | | | | 0.008 | | | 0.051 | | | 0.146 | | | 0.545 |
| 0 | 222 | 157 | 65 | | 97 | 125 | | 159 | 63 | | 179 | 43 | |
| 1 | 3 | 0 | 3 | | 3 | 0 | | 1 | 2 | | 2 | 1 | |
| Initial treatment | | | | 0.004 | | | 0.094 | | | 0.863 | | | 0.052 |
| surveillance | 23 | 10 | 13 | | 14 | 9 | | 16 | 7 | | 15 | 8 | |
| surgery | 225 | 147 | 55 | | 85 | 116 | | 144 | 59 | | 166 | 36 | |
| Recurrence | | | | 0.01 | | | 0.635 | | | 0.004 | | | 0.235 |
| no | 150 | 113 | 37 | | 65 | 85 | | 116 | 34 | | 124 | 26 | |
| yes | 75 | 44 | 31 | | 35 | 40 | | 44 | 31 | | 57 | 18 | |
| Vital status | | | | 0.000 | | | 0.001 | | | 0 | | | 0.003 |
| Alive | 171 | 131 | 40 | | 65 | 106 | | 134 | 37 | | 145 | 26 | |
| Dead | 54 | 26 | 28 | | 35 | 19 | | 26 | 28 | | 36 | 18 | |

(18.0–85.25) months; 29 was alive with disease progression,8 was dead of other causes.

On Kaplan-Meier analysis, NLR > 2.94 was associated with inferior OS (log-rank $p = 0.001$), and inferior PFS (log-rank $p = 0.004$) in Figs. 1 and 2; LMR > 4.74 was associated with inferior OS (log-rank $p = 0.001$), but not associated with PFS (log-rank $p = 0.547$) in Figs. 3 and 4; PLR > 133.5 was associated with inferior OS (log-rank $p < 0.001$) and inferior PFS (log-rank $p = 0.001$) in Figs. 5 and 6. LDH < 188.5 was associated with inferior OS (log-rank $p = 0.004$), but not associated with PFS (log-rank $p = 0.155$) in Figs. 7 and 8.

In univariable analyses, NLR > 2.94 was associated with inferior OS (HR = 2.967; 95% CI: 1.739–5.064, $p < 0.001$) and inferior PFS (HR = 1.944; 95% CI: 1.226–3.081,$p =$ 0.005); LMR > 4.74 was associated with inferior OS

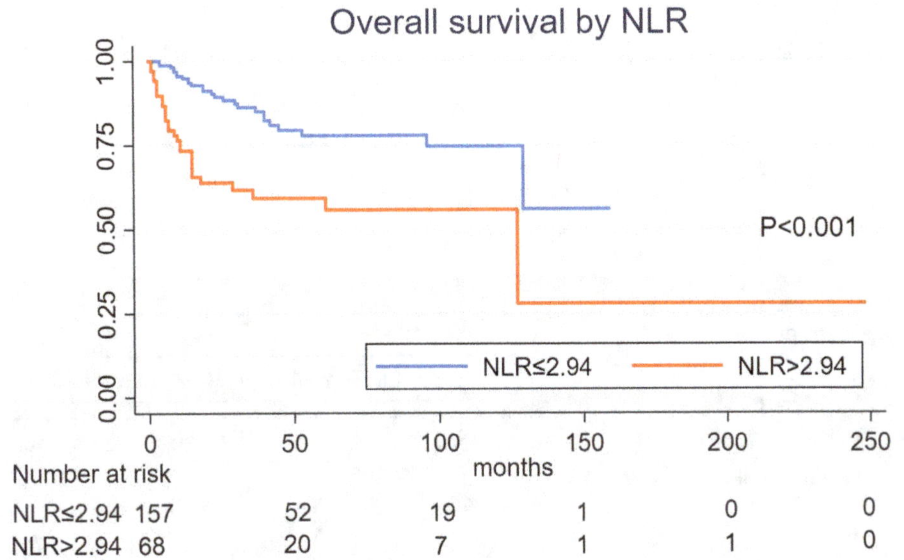


**Fig. 1** KaplanMeier curve of NLR for overall survival (OS)

(HR = 0.394; 95% CI: 0.225–0.689, $p = 0.001$) and not associated with inferior PFS (HR = 0.871; 95% CI: 0.553–1.372,$p = 0.551$); PLR > 133.5 was associated with inferior OS (HR = 3.439; 95% CI: 2.011–5.881, $p < 0.001$) and inferior PFS (HR = 2.194; 95% CI: 1.384–3.478,$p =$ 0.001); LDH > 188.5 was associated with inferior OS (HR = 2.252; 95% CI: 1.267–4.002, $p = 0.006$) and not associated with inferior PFS (HR = 1.462; 95% CI: 0.859–2.487,$p = 0.162$).

We performed a multivariate analysis which reveal NLR was not significant independent factors for OS($p =$ 0.516) and PFS($p = 0.594$); LMR was not associated with OS($p = 0.97$) and PFS; PLR was significant independent factors for both OS($p = 0.001$) and PFS($p = 0.02$); LDH was significant independent factors for OS($P = 0.035$) but not for PFS. At multivariate analysis, lymph node status ($P = 0.03$) and metastasis status remained significant for OS and PFS as NCCN or EAU Guidelines

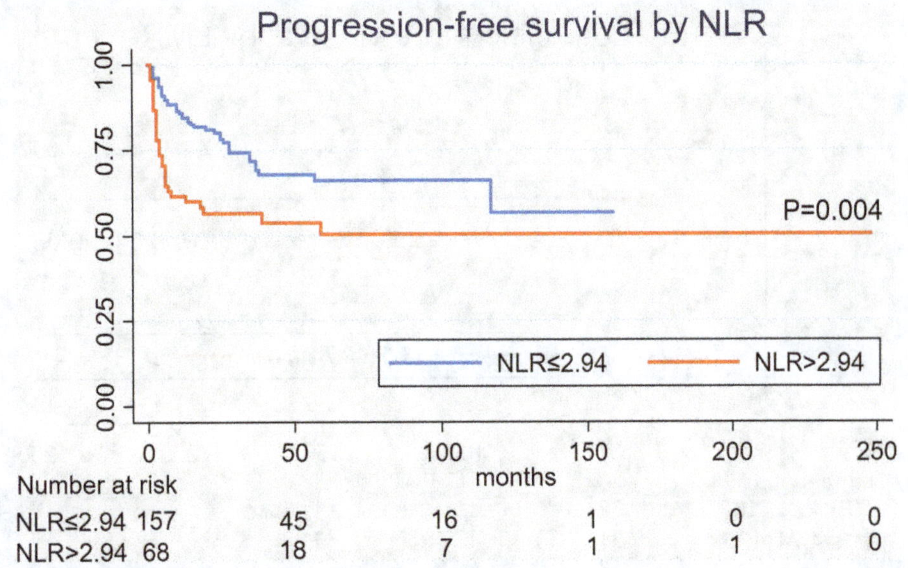


**Fig. 2** KaplanMeier curve of NLR for progression free survival (PFS)

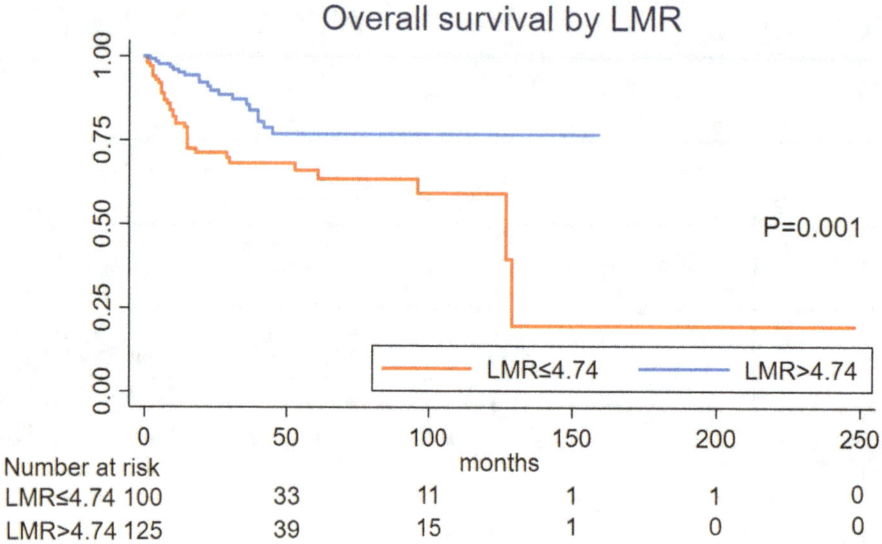


**Fig. 3** KaplanMeier curve of LMR for overall survival (OS) and 4

indicated; However, ages, the tumor type and initial treatment was not significant for OS and PFS in multivariable analyses (Table 2).

### NLR LMR PLR LDH vs inguinal lymph node-negative/ positive

In logistic regression analyses, NLR (HR = 2.212; 95% CI: 1.228–3.985,$p$ = 0.008), LMR (HR = 0.537; 95% CI: 0.308–0.937,$p$ = 0.029), PLR (HR = 2.478; 95% CI:1.365–4.497,$p$ = 0.003) was significant corresponded to N stage which divided into the Node-negative group and Node-positive groups, however the LDH ($p$ = 0.165) was not associated with the N stage. Meantime we also use Kendall's tau-b method to evaluated the correlations, NLR (Kendall's tau-b = 0.131, $P$ = 0.017) LMR (Kendall's tau-b = – 0.109, $P$ = 0.046) PLR (Kendall's tau-b = 0.161, $P$ = 0.003) were weakly correlated to the N stage. In other words, higher NLR, PLR and lower LMR was more likely to detected pathologically positive inguinal lymph node after ILND. The

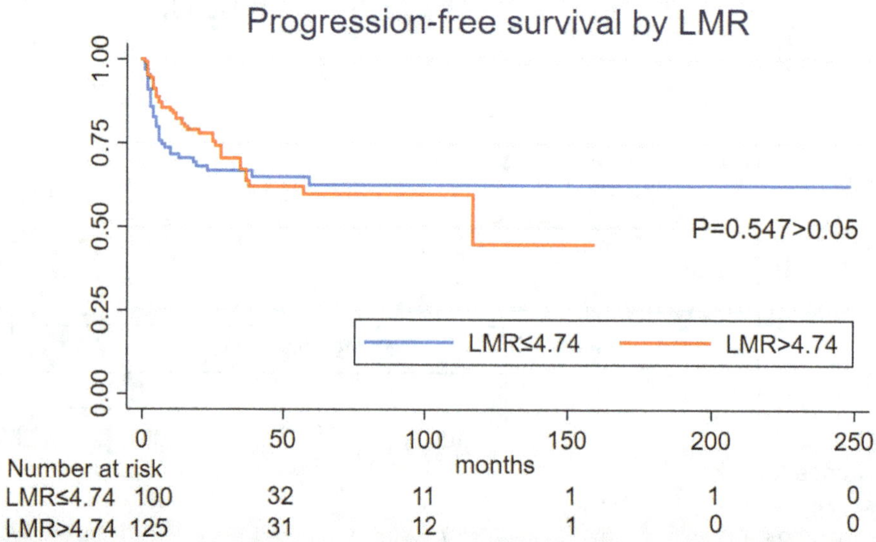


**Fig. 4** KaplanMeier curve of LMR for progression free survival (PFS)

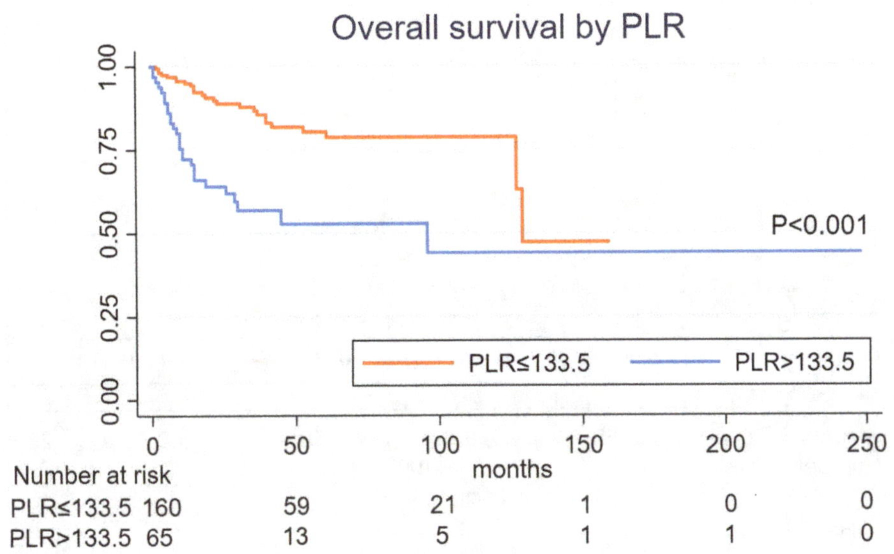


**Fig. 5** KaplanMeier curve of PLR for overall survival (OS)

biomarkers of NLR LMR and PLR could predict the pathological outcomes of ILND.

## Discussion

In recent years, the role of inflammatory factors in cancer development and progression has received more attention. The tumor micro-environment may be associated with systemic inflammation. Several types of cancer have been adopt inflammatory factors in prognostic scores for predict the outcome [19] and IMDC scores of advanced renal cell carcinoma also added those factors.

Recently, an elevated ratio of peripheral neutrophils-to-lymphocytes (NLR) has been recognized as a poor prognostic indicator in penile cancer, Patients with a high NLR had significantly worse CSS [17, 18] and OS [16];Patients with a low LMR had significantly worse RFS and CSS than those with a high LMR [18].

However, there is no date about the PLR and LDH in penile cancer, this paper aims to collect data from China

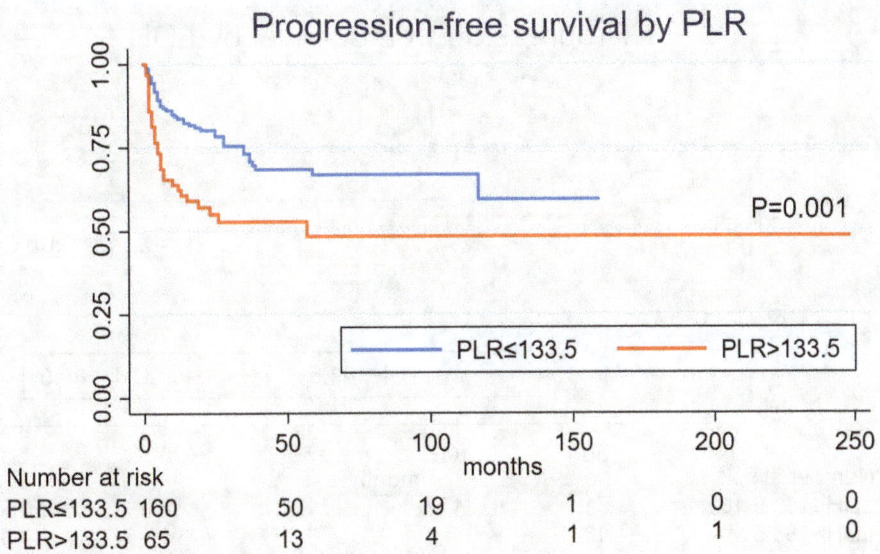


**Fig. 6** KaplanMeier curve of PLR for progression free survival (PFS)

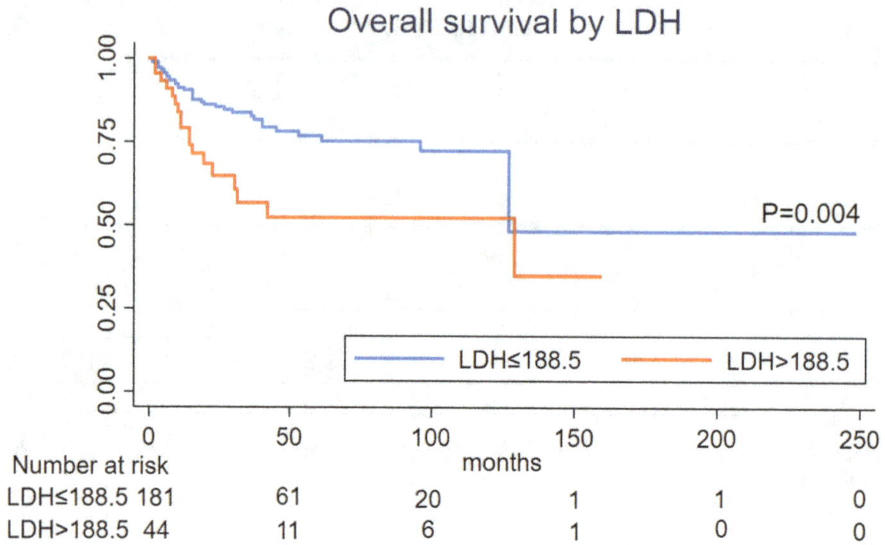


**Fig. 7** KaplanMeier curve of LDH for overall survival (OS)

and conduct comparative analysis of NLR, LMR, PLR and LDH, these bio-markers are critical in guiding clinical management decisions and follow-up strategies.

The incidence of penile cancer itself is very low, so it is difficult to analyze with a large sample size. The incidence of penile cancer is relatively high in China, especially in Yunnan Province, so the sample size of this paper is relatively large.

In addition, it is difficult to judge whether there is lymph node metastasis before ILND, therefore, we also hope to assist in judgment whether there is lymph node metastasis from these indicators, so that we can choose the different surgical approach.

We acknowledge the several limitations to this study including inherent biases associated with its retrospective design, insufficient time to follow-up and population heterogeneity. Besides, more than 20% of the patients were lost to follow-up which may affect the statistical results.

We originally wanted to analyze C-reactive protein (CRP) at the same time. Since the early patients failed to perform CRP testing uniformly, the indicator failed to enter the analysis.

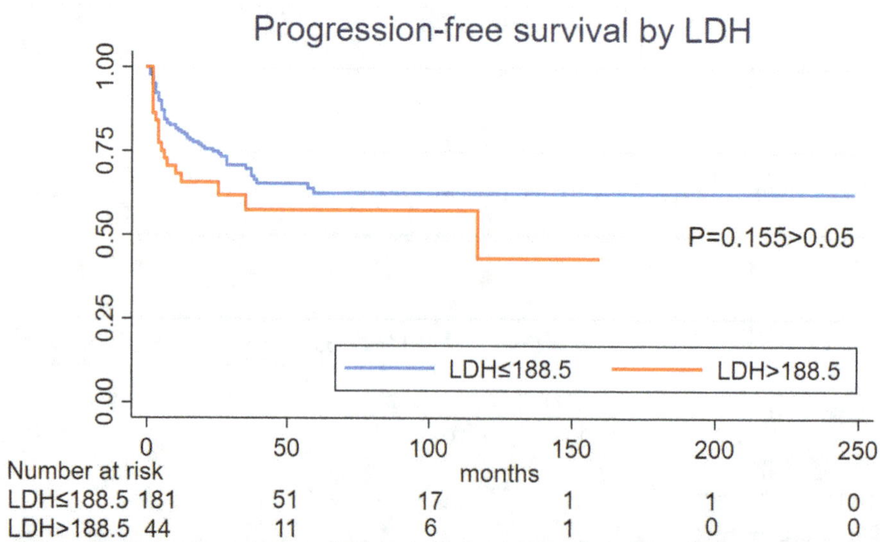


**Fig. 8** KaplanMeier curve of LDH for progression free survival (PFS)

**Table 2** Cox regression model for OS and PFS

| Variables | OS | | | | | | PFS | | | | | |
|---|---|---|---|---|---|---|---|---|---|---|---|---|
| | Univariable | | | Multivariable | | | Univariable | | | Multivariable | | |
| | HR | 95%CI | p | HR | 95%CI | p | HR | 95%CI | p | HR | 95%CI | p |
| **Ages** | | | | | | | | | | | | |
| <53 | reference | 1.077-3.174 | 0.026 | reference | 1.055-3.983 | 0.035 | reference | 0.785-1.974 | 0.352 | | | |
| ≥53 | 1.849 | | | 1.961 | | | 1.245 | | | | | |
| **Tumor type** | | | | | | | | | | | | |
| benign tumor | reference | | 0.002 | reference | | 0.205 | reference | | 0.006 | reference | | 0.135 |
| Well | 0.97 | 0.021-0.448 | | 0.305 | 0.054-1.715 | | 0.046 | 0.039-0.970 | | 0.405 | 0.075-2.186 | |
| moderate | 0.211 | 0.060-0.737 | | 0.22 | 0.052-0.938 | | 0.332 | 0.116-2.070 | | 0.51 | 0.111-2.336 | |
| poor | 0.447 | 0.130-1.541 | | 0.419 | 0.106-1.655 | | 0.868 | 0.211-3.716 | | 0.895 | 0.201-3.982 | |
| others | 0.594 | 0.130-2.719 | | 0.265 | 0.051-1.378 | | 0.646 | 0.109-3.944 | | 0.301 | 0.043-2.112 | |
| **Inguinal lymph node** | | | | | | | | | | | | |
| negigitve | reference | 5.243-20.918 | 0.000 | reference | 3.224-15.784 | 0.000 | reference | 3.096-8.080 | 0.000 | reference | 2.198-6.250 | 0.000 |
| positive | 10.472 | | | 7.133 | | | 5.002 | | | 3.706 | | |
| **Metastasis** | | | | | | | | | | | | |
| 0 | reference | 6.637-85.927 | 0.000 | reference | 2.223-40.238 | 0.002 | reference | 2.484-26.505 | 0.001 | reference | 1.184-18.072 | 0.028 |
| 1 | 23.881 | | | 9.458 | | | 8.114 | | | 4.626 | | |
| **Initial treatment** | | | | | | | | | | | | |
| surveillance | reference | 0.222-0.937 | 0.033 | reference | 0.18-1.006 | 0.052 | reference | 0.345-1.307 | 0.241 | | | |
| surgery | 0.456 | | | 0.425 | | | 0.671 | | | | | |
| **NLR** | | | | | | | | | | | | |
| low NLR | reference | 1.739-5.064 | 0.000 | reference | 0.605-2.718 | 0.516 | reference | 1.226-3.081 | 0.005 | reference | 0.679-1.966 | 0.594 |
| high NLR | 2.967 | | | 1.283 | | | 1.944 | | | 1.115 | | |
| **LMR** | | | | | | | | | | | | |
| low LMR | reference | 0.025-0.689 | 0.001 | reference | 0.448-2.164 | 0.97 | reference | 0.553-1.372 | 0.871 | | | |
| high LMR | 0.394 | | | 0.985 | | | 0.551 | | | | | |
| **PLR** | | | | | | | | | | | | |
| low PLR | reference | 2.011-5.881 | 0.000 | reference | 1.644-6.171 | 0.001 | reference | 1.384-3.478 | 0.001 | reference | 1.104-3.242 | 0.02 |
| high PLR | 3.439 | | | 3.186 | | | 2.194 | | | 1.892 | | |
| **LDH** | | | | | | | | | | | | |
| low LDH | reference | 1.267-4.002 | 0.006 | reference | 1.051-3.808 | 0.035 | reference | 0.859-2.487 | 0.162 | | | |
| high LDH | 2.252 | | | 2 | | | 1.462 | | | | | |

## Conclusion

PLR was significant independent factors for OS and PFS, Ages and LDH was significant independent factors for OS. NLR, LMR, PLR was corresponded to N stage.

**Abbreviations**

NLR: Neutrophil-to-lymphocyte ratio; LMR: Lymphocyte-to-monocyte ratio; PLR: Platelet-to-lymphocyte ratio; LDH: Lactate dehydrogenase

**Acknowledgments**

Not applicable.

**Authors' contributions**

YB, CH were participated in the conception and initial design. JL, LBY, CWB performed the clinical treatment of the penile cancer, CH, YB was a major contributor in writing the manuscript. CH, BZ, YY, RQL were participate in articles search, review, data extract, statistical analysis. CH, HYW, GYZ were participate in project development and pictures processing. QLW, YQ were participating in manuscript writing and revising. All authors have read and approved the manuscript.

**Competing interests**

The authors declare that they have no competing interests.

**References**


1. de Martel C, Plummer M, Vignat J, et al. Worldwide burden of cancer attributable to HPV by site, country and HPV type. Int J Cancer. 2017;141(4): 664–70.
2. Wanick FB, Teichner TC, Silva R, et al. Squamous cell carcinoma of the penis: clinicopathologic study of 34 cases. An Bras Dermatol. 2011;86(6):1082–91.
3. Kroon BK, Horenblas S, Lont AP, et al. Patients with penile carcinoma benefit from immediate resection of clinically occult lymph node metastases. J Urol. 2005;173(3):816–9.
4. Cubilla AL. The role of pathologic prognostic factors in squamous cell carcinoma of the penis. World J Urol. 2009;27(2):169.
5. Winters BR, Mossanen M, Holt SK, et al. Predictors of nodal upstaging in clinical node negative patients with penile carcinoma: a national cancer database analysis. Urology. 2016;96:29–34.
6. Zhu Y, Zhou XY, Yao XD, et al. The prognostic significance of p53, Ki-67, epithelial cadherin and matrix metalloproteinase-9 in penile squamous cell carcinoma treated with surgery. BJU Int. 2007;100(1):204–8.
7. Zhu Y, Ye DW, Yao XD, et al. The value of squamous cell carcinoma antigen in the prognostic evaluation, treatment monitoring and followup of patients with penile cancer. J Urol. 2008;180(5):2019–23.
8. Coussens LM, ZJN W. Inflammation and cancer. Nature.2002;420(6917):860.
9. Sandler RS, Halabi S, Baron JA, et al. A randomized trial of aspirin to prevent colorectal adenomas in patients with previous colorectal cancer. N Engl J Med. 2003;348(10):883–90.
10. Wang D, Yang JX, Cao DY, et al. Preoperative neutrophil-lymphocyte and platelet-lymphocyte ratios as independent predictors of cervical stromal involvement in surgically treated endometrioid adenocarcinoma. OncoTargets and therapy. 2013;6:211.
11. Wei X, Huang F, Wei Y, et al. Low lymphocyte-to-monocyte ratio predicts unfavorable prognosis in non-germinal center type diffuse large B-cell lymphoma. Leuk Res. 2014;38(6):694–8.
12. Takeuchi H, Fukuyama S, Kubo N, et al. The prognostic significance of the preoperative platelet-lymphocyte ratio in Japanese patients with localized breast cancer. Adv Breast Cancer Res. 2016;5(02):49.
13. Asher V, Lee J, Innamaa A, et al. Preoperative platelet lymphocyte ratio as an independent prognostic marker in ovarian cancer. Clin Transl Oncol. 2011;13(7):499.
14. Kwon HC, Kim SH, Oh SY, et al. Clinical significance of preoperative neutrophil-lymphocyte versus platelet-lymphocyte ratio in patients with operable colorectal cancer. Biomarkers. 2012;17(3):216–22.
15. Zhang Y, Xu T, Wang Y, et al. . Prognostic role of lactate dehydrogenase expression in urologic cancers: a systematic review and meta-analysis. Oncol Res Treat. 2016;39(10):592–604.
16. Azizi M, Peyton CC, Boulware DC, et al. Prognostic value of neutrophil-to-lymphocyte ratio in penile squamous cell carcinoma patients undergoing inguinal lymph node dissection. Eur Urol Focus. 2019;5(6):1085–1090.
17. Tan T W, Chia S J, Chong K T. Management of penile cancer in a Singapore tertiary hospital. Arab J Urol. 2017;15(2):123–30.
18. Kasuga J, Kawahara T, Takamoto D, et al. Increased neutrophil-to-lymphocyte ratio is associated with disease-specific mortality in patients with penile cancer. BMC Cancer. 2016;16(1):396.
19. McMillan DC. The systemic inflammation-based Glasgow Prognostic Score: a decade of experience in patients with cancer. Cancer Treat Rev. 2013;39(5): 534–40.

# 3

# Prognostic significance of the albumin-to-globulin ratio for upper tract urothelial carcinoma

Shota Omura[1], Satoru Taguchi[1*], Shogo Miyagawa[1], Ryuki Matsumoto[1], Mio Samejima[1], Naoki Ninomiya[1], Kazuki Masuda[1], Yu Nakamura[1], Tsuyoshi Yamaguchi[1], Manami Kinjo[1], Mitsuhiro Tambo[1], Takatsugu Okegawa[1], Eiji Higashihara[2] and Hiroshi Fukuhara[1]

**Abstract**

**Background:** Although the albumin-to-globulin ratio (AGR) is a promising biomarker for various malignancies, few studies have investigated its prognostic significance for upper tract urothelial carcinoma (UTUC).

**Methods:** This retrospective study conformed to the REporting recommendations for tumour MARKer prognostic studies (REMARK) guideline. We reviewed 179 patients with UTUC who underwent radical nephroureterectomy at our institution between 2008 and 2018. Associations of preoperative clinicopathological factors, including the AGR, with cancer-specific survival (CSS) and overall survival (OS) were assessed. The Cox proportional hazards model was used for univariate and multivariable analyses. AGR was dichotomized as $< 1.25$ and $\geq 1.25$, according to the most discriminatory cutoff determined from the receiver operating characteristic curve analysis.

**Results:** During a median follow-up of 34 months after surgery, 37 patients died from UTUC and 13 died of other causes. The preoperative AGR significantly correlated with pathological T stage, pathological N stage, and adjuvant chemotherapy. Multivariate analyses demonstrated that a decreased ($< 1.25$) preoperative AGR was an independent poor prognostic factor for both CSS (hazard ratio [HR] = 2.81, $P < 0.01$) and OS (HR = 2.09, $P < 0.05$).

**Conclusions:** Preoperative AGR $< 1.25$ might serve as a useful prognostic marker for patients with UTUC undergoing radical nephroureterectomy.

**Keywords:** AGR, Albumin-to-globulin ratio, Biomarker, Radical nephroureterectomy, REMARK, Upper tract urothelial carcinoma

## Background

Upper tract urothelial carcinoma (UTUC) is a relatively rare malignancy that accounts for 5–10% of urothelial carcinomas and generally has a poor prognosis [1, 2]. Radical nephroureterectomy with bladder cuff excision is the gold standard treatment for nonmetastatic UTUC [3], whereas up to 19% of patients with UTUC have metastasis upon initial presentation [4].

Clinicopathological factors [5–15] including laboratory markers [11–15] serve as prognostic markers for UTUC. In contrast, the significance of the albumin-to-globulin ratio (AGR), which serves as a useful biomarker for various malignancies [16–26], has not been fully investigated in UTUC [23–26]. Therefore, the present study assessed the significance of the association of preoperative AGR on oncological outcomes of patients with UTUC undergoing radical nephroureterectomy.

* Correspondence: satorutaguchi33@gmail.com
[1]Department of Urology, Kyorin University School of Medicine, 6-20-2 Shinkawa, Mitaka, Tokyo 181-8611, Japan

## Methods

This retrospective study conformed to the REporting recommendations for tumour MARKer prognostic studies (REMARK) guideline [27] (Supplementary Table 1 shows the REMARK checklist of the present study). This study was approved by the internal institutional review board of Kyorin University School of Medicine (approval number: 1154).

### Patients

We retrospectively reviewed 185 consecutive patients who underwent radical nephroureterectomy with curative intent at Kyorin University Hospital between 2008 and 2018. We excluded six patients because of pathological diagnoses of urothelial dysplasia ($n = 3$), renal cell carcinoma ($n = 2$), and squamous cell carcinoma ($n = 1$), which left 179 available for analysis.

### Preoperative AGR

Routine preoperative blood tests including serum total protein and albumin levels (g/dl) were performed within 1 month before surgery. The AGR was calculated using the following formula: AGR = [albumin / (total protein − albumin)]. No patient had active infectious disorders during the blood tests.

### Endpoints and follow-up

We assessed the associations of preoperative clinicopathological factors, including the AGR, with cancer-specific survival (CSS) and overall survival (OS). The follow-up period started on the day of surgery. Follow-up information was obtained as of October 2018.

### Statistical analysis

Receiver operating characteristic (ROC) curve analysis was used to determine the optimal cutoff value of the AGR. Sensitivity, specificity and area under the curve (AUC) were calculated using a 2 × 2 contingency table for different cutoff values of the AGR. The optimal cutoff value of the AGR was determined by maximization of the Youden's index [Sensitivity − (1 − Specificity)]. Relations of the AGR to other variables were evaluated using the $\chi^2$ test or Spearman's rank correlation coefficient. Survival curves were generated using the Kaplan–Meier method and compared using log-rank tests. The Cox proportional hazard regression model was used for univariate and multivariate analyses. All statistical analyses were performed using JMP Pro version 14.0.0 (SAS Institute, Cary, NC, USA). $P < 0.05$ was considered to indicate a significant difference.

## Results

Patients' baseline characteristics are summarized in Table 1. The median follow-up was 34 months (interquartile range [IQR], 17–63) months. Thirty-seven patients died from UTUC and 13 died of other causes. ROC curve analysis identified 1.25 as the most discriminatory cutoff value of AGR by maximization of the Youden's index [Sensitivity − (1 − Specificity)] for both endpoints of CSS and OS (Fig. 1).

**Table 1** Patient characteristics ($n = 179$)

| Parameter | Value |
|---|---|
| Age at surgery, years, median (IQR) | 75 (66–79) |
| Sex, no. (%): | |
| Male | 132 (73.7) |
| Female | 47 (26.3) |
| Surgical technique, no. (%): | |
| Open | 16 (8.9) |
| Laparoscopic | 163 (91.1) |
| Tumor location, no. (%): | |
| Renal pelvis | 96 (53.6) |
| Ureter | 81 (45.3) |
| Both | 2 (1.1) |
| Tumor grade, no. (%): | |
| G1 | 10 (5.6) |
| G2 | 94 (52.5) |
| G3 | 75 (41.9) |
| Pathological T stage, no. (%): | |
| Ta/1/is | 91 (50.8) |
| T2 | 13 (7.3) |
| T3 | 70 (39.1) |
| T4 | 5 (2.8) |
| Pathological N stage, no. (%): | |
| N0/x | 157 (87.7) |
| N1 | 16 (8.9) |
| N2 | 6 (3.4) |
| N3 | 0 (0) |
| Adjuvant chemotherapy, no. (%): | |
| Yes | 39 (21.8) |
| No | 140 (78.2) |
| Bladder cancer status, no. (%): | |
| No | 145 (81.0) |
| Previous | 19 (10.6) |
| Synchronous | 15 (8.4) |
| AGR, median (IQR) | 1.41 (1.18–1.63) |
| Follow-up duration, months, median (IQR) | 35 (17–63) |

Abbreviations: *AGR* albumin-to-globulin ratio, *IQR* interquartile range

$\chi^2$ test revealed pathological T stage (≥T3, $P < 0.01$), pathological N stage (N1–3, $P < 0.01$), and adjuvant chemotherapy (yes, $P < 0.05$) to be significantly associated with AGR < 1.25, while the other variables (sex,

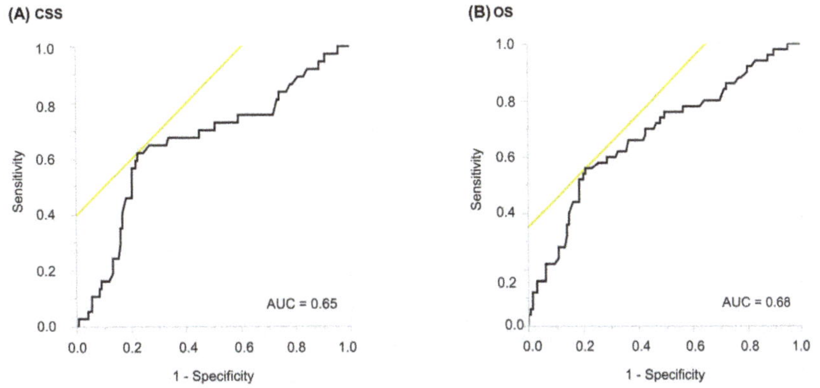


| Cutoffs of AGR | Sensitivity | Specificity | Sensitivity - (1 - Specificity) | AUC |
|---|---|---|---|---|
| <1.10 | 30% | 84% | 14% | 0.57 |
| <1.15 | 41% | 83% | 24% | 0.62 |
| <1.20 | 46% | 80% | 26% | 0.63 |
| **<1.25** | **62%** | **78%** | **40% (maximized)** | **0.70** |
| <1.30 | 65% | 70% | 35% | 0.67 |
| <1.35 | 68% | 63% | 31% | 0.65 |
| <1.40 | 68% | 55% | 23% | 0.61 |
| <1.45 | 70% | 51% | 21% | 0.60 |
| <1.50 | 73% | 46% | 19% | 0.59 |
| <1.55 | 76% | 38% | 14% | 0.57 |
| <1.60 | 76% | 30% | 6% | 0.53 |

| Cutoffs of AGR | Sensitivity | Specificity | Sensitivity - (1 - Specificity) | AUC |
|---|---|---|---|---|
| <1.10 | 32% | 86% | 18% | 0.59 |
| <1.15 | 40% | 85% | 25% | 0.63 |
| <1.20 | 44% | 81% | 25% | 0.63 |
| **<1.25** | **56%** | **79%** | **35% (maximized)** | **0.68** |
| <1.30 | 60% | 71% | 31% | 0.66 |
| <1.35 | 62% | 64% | 26% | 0.63 |
| <1.40 | 68% | 57% | 25% | 0.63 |
| <1.45 | 72% | 53% | 25% | 0.63 |
| <1.50 | 76% | 49% | 25% | 0.62 |
| <1.55 | 78% | 40% | 18% | 0.59 |
| <1.60 | 80% | 32% | 12% | 0.56 |

**Fig. 1** ROC curve analyses for (**a**) CSS and (**b**) OS. The optimal cutoff value of AGR was estimated as < 1.25 by maximizing the Youden's index [Sensitivity – (1 – Specificity)] for both endpoints of CSS and OS. Abbreviations: AGR = albumin-to-globulin ratio; CSS = cancer-specific survival; OS = overall survival; ROC = receiver operating characteristic

surgical technique, tumor location, tumor grade and previous or synchronous bladder cancer) were not. Spearman's rank correlation coefficient showed a weakly significant negative correlation between age at surgery and the AGR ($\rho = -0.25$, $P < 0.01$).

Kaplan–Meier curves with log-rank tests showed significant associations of preoperative AGR < 1.25 with shorter CSS (Fig. 2) and OS (Fig. 3). Multivariate Cox proportional hazard regression analyses identified preoperative AGR < 1.25 as an independent poor prognostic factor for both CSS (hazard ratio [HR] = 2.81, $P < 0.01$) (Table 2) and OS (HR = 2.09, $P < 0.05$; Table 3).

## Discussion

The present study demonstrates that a decreased (< 1.25) preoperative AGR was an independent indicator of poor prognosis for CSS and OS of patients with UTUC treated with radical nephroureterectomy.

Clinicopathological factors that serve as prognostic factors for UTUC [5–15] include sex [5], age [6], tumor size [7, 8], ureteral involvement [9], and body mass index [10], as well as laboratory markers [11–15] such as the neutrophil-to-lymphocyte ratio [11, 12], albumin [13], hemoglobin [14], and the prognostic nutritional index [15]. On the other hand, the AGR has been reported as a useful biomarker in various malignancies [16–26], including urological cancers [20–26]. However, the significance of the AGR as a prognostic marker for UTUC has not been fully investigated [23–26]. For example, a study of a Chinese cohort of 187 operable patients with UTUC [23] demonstrated that AGR < 1.45 is an independent risk factor for poorer CSS and OS. Another study of a Chinese cohort of 620 patients with UTUC treated with radical nephroureterectomy found that AGR < 1.45 is an independent predictor of adverse pathologic features, recurrence-free survival, CSS, and OS [24]. Similarly, analysis of a Japanese cohort of 124 patients with UTUC undergoing radical nephroureterectomy identified AGR < 1.40 as an independent prognostic factor for recurrence-free survival, CSS, and OS [25]. Finally, another Japanese study comprising 105 patients with UTUC undergoing radical nephroureterectomy reported that AGR < 1.24 was an independent predictor for both worse disease-free and overall survivals [26]. Our results are consistent with those of these previous reports and add further evidence in this field.

The association between a low AGR and poor outcome of patients with cancer requires further research. However, the available data show that poor nutritional status or hypoalbuminemia is a negative prognostic factor for certain malignancies [13, 15, 16]. Chronic inflammation involving serum globulins plays a crucial

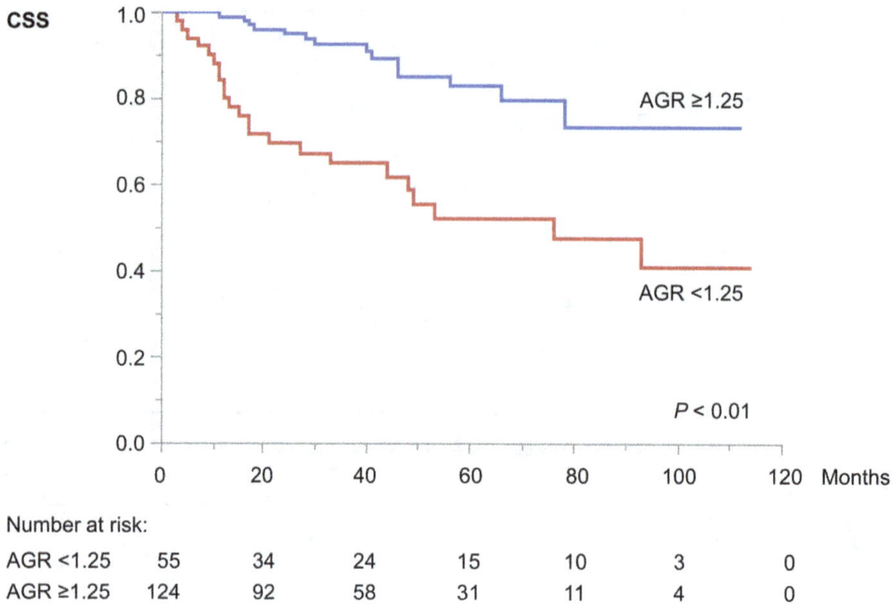


**Fig. 2** Kaplan–Meier curves depicting CSS in patients with AGR < 1.25 versus ≥1.25 ($P < 0.01$, log-rank test). Abbreviations: AGR = albumin-to-globulin ratio; CSS = cancer-specific survival

role in tumor proliferation, immune evasion, and metastasis. These serum globulins secreted by tumor-related cells reportedly promote tumor development, immunosuppression, and metastasis [16]. A low AGR may thus reflect the degree of poor nutritional status (hypoalbuminemia) and tumor progression (hyperglobulinemia) in a more sensitive manner than either measure alone and may therefore serve as a highly significant prognostic biomarker. Based on a similar concept as AGR (i.e. use of a ratio), several systemic inflammatory markers, such as the neutrophil-to-lymphocyte ratio [11, 12, 28], platelet-to-lymphocyte ratio [28], and lymphocyte-to-

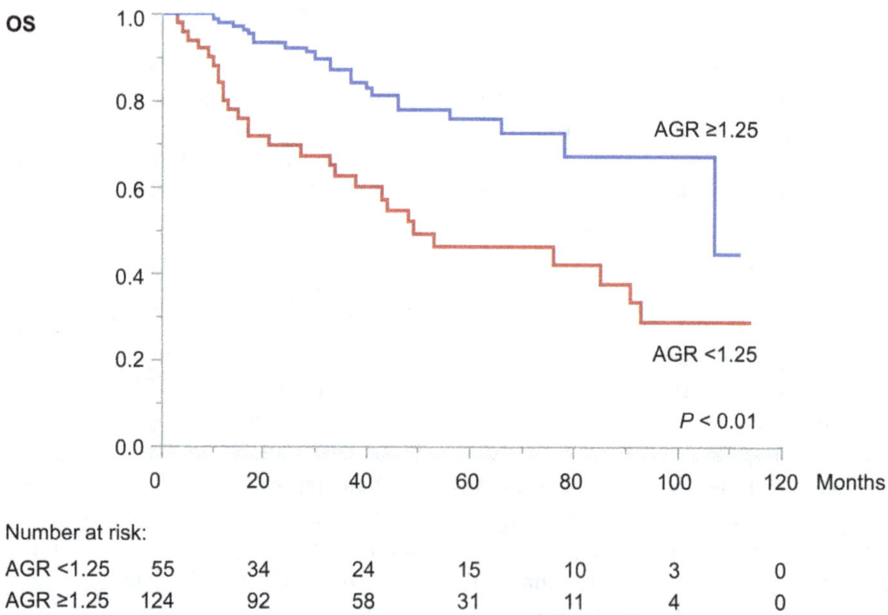


**Fig. 3** Kaplan–Meier curves depicting OS a in patients with AGR < 1.25 versus ≥1.25 ($P < 0.01$, log-rank test). Abbreviations: AGR = albumin-to-globulin ratio; OS = overall survival

**Table 2** Univariate and multivariate Cox proportional hazard regression analyses of CSS

| Parameter | Cutoff | Univariate | | Multivariate | |
|---|---|---|---|---|---|
| | | HR (95% CI) | *P* | HR (95% CI) | *P* |
| Age at surgery | Continuous | 1.03 (0.99 to 1.07) per score | 0.07 | 1.03 (0.99 to 1.08) per score | 0.18 |
| Sex | Male | Reference | < 0.05* | Reference | 0.14 |
| | Female | 2.15 (1.09 to 4.13) | | 1.73 (0.83 to 3.51) | |
| Surgical technique | Open | Reference | 0.16 | Reference | 0.21 |
| | Laparoscopic | 0.50 (0.23 to 1.34) | | 2.26 (0.63 to 8.93) | |
| Tumor location | Renal pelvis or both | Reference | 0.56 | Reference | 0.72 |
| | Ureter | 1.21 (0.63 to 2.33) | | 1.14 (0.55 to 2.42) | |
| Tumor grade | G1/2 | Reference | < 0.01* | Reference | < 0.05* |
| | G3 | 4.10 (2.07 to 8.66) | | 2.56 (1.07 to 6.50) | |
| Pathological T stage | ≤T2 | Reference | < 0.01* | Reference | 0.06 |
| | ≥T3 | 3.67 (1.88 to 7.59) | | 2.51 (0.96 to 6.70) | |
| Pathological N stage | N0/x | Reference | < 0.01* | Reference | 0.20 |
| | N1–3 | 4.82 (2.20 to 9.77) | | 2.21 (0.65 to 7.00) | |
| Adjuvant chemotherapy | Yes | Reference | < 0.05* | Reference | 0.51 |
| | No | 0.49 (0.25 to 0.97) | | 1.36 (0.55 to 3.37) | |
| Previous or synchronous bladder cancer | No | Reference | < 0.01* | Reference | < 0.01* |
| | Yes | 3.61 (1.83 to 6.92) | | 3.49 (1.66 to 7.19) | |
| AGR | ≥1.25 | Reference | < 0.01* | Reference | < 0.01* |
| | < 1.25 | 3.90 (2.02 to 7.79) | | 2.81 (1.34 to 6.10) | |

Abbreviations: *HR* hazard ratio, *CI* confidence interval, *AGR* albumin-to-globulin ratio
*Statistically significant

**Table 3** Univariate and multivariate Cox proportional hazard regression analyses of OS

| Parameter | Cutoff | Univariate | | Multivariate | |
|---|---|---|---|---|---|
| | | HR (95% CI) | *P* | HR (95% CI) | *P* |
| Age at surgery | Continuous | 1.03 (1.00 to 1.07) per score | < 0.05* | 1.03 (0.99 to 1.07) per score | 0.07 |
| Sex | Male | Reference | 0.08 | Reference | 0.23 |
| | Female | 1.72 (0.93 to 3.07) | | 1.48 (0.77 to 2.76) | |
| Surgical technique | Open | Reference | < 0.05* | Reference | 0.60 |
| | Laparoscopic | 0.44 (0.23 to 0.98) | | 1.33 (0.47 to 4.03) | |
| Tumor location | Renal pelvis or both | Reference | 0.92 | Reference | 0.88 |
| | Ureter | 1.03 (0.58 to 1.80) | | 1.05 (0.57 to 1.94) | |
| Tumor grade | G1/2 | Reference | < 0.01* | Reference | < 0.05* |
| | G3 | 2.61 (1.49 to 4.67) | | 2.15 (1.03 to 4.52) | |
| Pathological T stage | ≤T2 | Reference | < 0.01* | Reference | 0.27 |
| | ≥T3 | 2.30 (1.32 to 4.08) | | 1.54 (0.71 to 3.35) | |
| Pathological N stage | N0/x | Reference | < 0.01* | Reference | 0.09 |
| | N1–3 | 4.32 (2.14 to 8.12) | | 2.56 (0.87 to 7.09) | |
| Adjuvant chemotherapy | Yes | Reference | 0.33 | Reference | 0.23 |
| | No | 1.36 (0.73 to 2.43) | | 1.62 (0.74 to 3.61) | |
| Previous or synchronous bladder cancer | No | Reference | < 0.01* | Reference | < 0.05* |
| | Yes | 2.43 (1.28 to 4.39) | | 1.99 (1.01 to 3.75) | |
| AGR | ≥1.25 | Reference | < 0.01* | Reference | < 0.05* |
| | < 1.25 | 2.90 (1.66 to 5.15) | | 2.09 (1.12 to 3.92) | |

Abbreviations: *HR* hazard ratio, *CI* confidence interval, *AGR* albumin-to-globulin ratio
*Statistically significant

monocyte ratio [28], have been established and well-investigated in the field of oncology, including urothelial carcinoma.

The major limitations of this study are its retrospective, single-institutional design and the limited number of patients. Further studies with larger populations are needed to confirm our results.

## Conclusions

Given the significant prognostic associations of the AGR with CSS and OS, AGRs are easy to determine in routine clinical practice, and a preoperative AGR < 1.25 might serve as a useful prognostic biomarker of patients with UTUC treated with radical nephroureterectomy.

#### Abbreviations

AGR: Albumin-to-globulin ratio; AUC: Area under the curve; CSS: Cancer-specific survival; IQR: Interquartile range; OS: Overall survival; ROC: Receiver operating characteristic; UTUC: Upper tract urothelial carcinoma

#### Acknowledgements

We thank Dr. Alla Bradley from Edanz Group for editing a draft of this manuscript.

#### Authors' contributions

SO and ST contributed to the conception, study design, analysis, interpretation of data, and drafted the first manuscript. SM, RM, MS, NN, KM, YN, TY, MK, and MT contributed to acquisition of data. TO, EH, and HF supervised the study, helped to draft the manuscript, and were involved in revising it critically for important intellectual content. All authors read and approved the final manuscript.

#### Competing interests

The authors declare that they have no competing interests.

#### Author details

[1]Department of Urology, Kyorin University School of Medicine, 6-20-2 Shinkawa, Mitaka, Tokyo 181-8611, Japan. [2]Department of ADPKD Research, Kyorin University School of Medicine, 6-20-2 Shinkawa, Mitaka, Tokyo 181-8611, Japan.

#### References

1. Siegel RL, Miller KD, Jemal A. Cancer statistics, 2019. CA Cancer J Clin. 2019; 69:7–34.
2. Munoz J, Ellison L. Upper tract urothelial neoplasms: incidence and survival during the last 2 decades. J Urol. 2000;164:1523–5.
3. Margulis V, Shariat SF, Matin SF, Kamat AM, Zigeuner R, Kikuchi E, Lotan Y, Weizer A, Raman JD. Wood CG; upper tract Urothelial carcinoma collaboration. The upper tract Urothelial carcinoma collaboration. Outcomes of radical nephroureterectomy: a series from the upper tract Urothelial carcinoma collaboration. Cancer. 2009;115:1224–33.
4. Akaza H, Koiso K, Niijima T. Clinical evaluation of urothelial tumors of the renal pelvis and ureter based on a new classification system. Cancer. 1987; 59:1369–75.
5. Fernández MI, Shariat SF, Margulis V, Bolenz C, Montorsi F, Suardi N, Remzi M, Wood CG, Roscigno M, Kikuchi E, Oya M, Zigeuner R, Langner C, Weizer A, Lotan Y, Koppie TM, Raman JD, Karakiewicz P, Bensalah K, Schultz M, Bernier P. Evidence-based sex-related outcomes after radical nephroureterectomy for upper tract urothelial carcinoma: results of large multicenter study. Urology. 2009;73:142–6.
6. Kobayashi H, Kikuchi E, Tanaka N, Shirotake S, Miyazaki Y, Ide H, Obata J, Hoshino K, Matsumoto K, Kaneko G, Hagiwara M, Kosaka T, Oyama M, Nakajima Y, Oya M. Patient age was an independent predictor of cancer-specific survival in male patients with upper tract urothelial carcinoma treated by radical nephroureterectomy. Jpn J Clin Oncol. 2016;46:554–9.
7. Shibing Y, Liangren L, Qiang W, Hong L, Turun S, Junhao L, Lu Y, Zhengyong Y, Yonghao J, Guangqing F, Yunxiang L, Dehong C. Impact of tumour size on prognosis of upper urinary tract urothelial carcinoma after radical nephroureterectomy: a multi-institutional analysis of 795 cases. BJU Int. 2016;118:902–10.
8. Su X, Fang D, Li X, Xiong G, Zhang L, Hao H, Gong Y, Zhang Z, Zhou L. The influence of tumor size on oncologic outcomes for patients with upper tract Urothelial carcinoma after radical Nephroureterectomy. Biomed Res Int. 2016;2016:4368943.
9. Waseda Y, Saito K, Ishioka J, Matsuoka Y, Numao N, Fujii Y, Sakai Y, Koga F, Okuno T, Arisawa C, Kamata S, Nagahama K, Masuda H, Yonese J, Kageyama Y, Noro A, Tsujii T, Morimoto S, Gotoh S, Kihara K. Ureteral involvement is associated with poor prognosis in upper urinary tract Urothelial carcinoma patients treated by Nephroureterectomy: a multicenter database study. Eur Urol Focus. 2016;2:296–302.
10. Dabi Y, El Mrini M, Duquesnes I, Delongchamps NB, Sibony M, Zerbib M, Xylinas E. Impact of body mass index on the oncological outcomes of patients treated with radical nephroureterectomy for upper tract urothelial carcinoma. World J Urol. 2018;36:65–71.
11. Azuma T, Matayoshi Y, Odani K, Sato Y, Sato Y, Nagase Y, Oshi M. Preoperative neutrophil-lymphocyte ratio as an independent prognostic marker for patients with upper urinary tract urothelial carcinoma. Clin Genitourin Cancer. 2013;11:337–41.
12. Vartolomei MD, Kimura S, Ferro M, Vartolomei L, Foerster B, Abufaraj M, Shariat SF. Is neutrophil-to-lymphocytes ratio a clinical relevant preoperative biomarker in upper tract urothelial carcinoma? A meta-analysis of 4385 patients. World J Urol. 2018;36:1019–29.
13. Ku JH, Kim M, Choi WS, Kwak C, Kim HH. Preoperative serum albumin as a prognostic factor in patients with upper urinary tract urothelial carcinoma. Int Braz J Urol. 2014;40:753–62.
14. Yeh HC, Chien TM, Wu WJ, Li CC, Li WM, Ke HL, Chou YH, Wang CJ, Huang SP, Li CF, Liang PI, Huang CN. Is preoperative anemia a risk factor for upper tract urothelial carcinoma following radical nephroureterectomy? Urol Oncol. 2016;34:337.e1–9.
15. Huang J, Yuan Y, Wang Y, Chen Y, Kong W, Xue W, Chen H, Zhang J, Huang Y. Preoperative prognostic nutritional index is a significant predictor of survival in patients with localized upper tract urothelial carcinoma after radical nephroureterectomy. Urol Oncol. 2017;35:671.e1–9.
16. He J, Pan H, Liang W, Xiao D, Chen X, Guo M, He J. Prognostic effect of albumin-to-globulin ratio in patients with solid tumors: a systematic review and meta-analysis. J Cancer. 2017;8:4002–10.
17. Azab BN, Bhatt VR, Vonfrolio S, Bachir R, Rubinshteyn V, Alkaied H, Habeshy A, Patel J, Picon AI, Bloom SW. Value of the pretreatment albumin to globulin ratio in predicting long-term mortality in breast cancer patients. Am J Surg. 2013;206:764–70.
18. Shibutani M, Maeda K, Nagahara H, Ohtani H, Iseki Y, Ikeya T, Sugano K, Hirakawa K. The pretreatment albumin to globulin ratio predicts chemotherapeutic outcomes in patients with unresectable metastatic colorectal cancer. BMC Cancer. 2015;15:347.
19. Yoshino Y, Taguchi A, Shimizuguchi T, Nakajima Y, Takao M, Kashiyama T, Furusawa A, Kino N, Yasugi T. A low albumin to globulin ratio with a high serum globulin level is a prognostic marker for poor survival in cervical cancer patients treated with radiation based therapy. Int J Gynecol Cancer. 2019;29:17–22.
20. Liu J, Dai Y, Zhou F, Long Z, Li Y, Liu B, Xie D, Tang J, Tan J, Yao K, Zhang Y, Tang Y, He L. The prognostic role of preoperative serum albumin/globulin ratio in patients with bladder urothelial carcinoma undergoing radical cystectomy. Urol Oncol. 2016;34:484.e1–8.
21. Niwa N, Matsumoto K, Ide H, Nagata H, Oya M. Prognostic value of pretreatment albumin-to-globulin ratio in patients with non-muscle-invasive bladder Cancer. Clin Genitourin Cancer. 2018;16:e655 61.
22. Koparal MY, Polat F, Çetin S, Bulut EC, Sözen TS. Prognostic role of preoperative albumin to globulin ratio in predicting survival of clear cell renal cell carcinoma. Int Braz J Urol. 2018;44:933–46.
23. Zhang B, Yu W, Zhou LQ, He ZS, Shen C, He Q, Li J, Liu LB, Wang C, Chen XY, Fan Y, Hu S, Zhang L, Han WK, Jin J. Prognostic significance of preoperative albumin-globulin ratio in patients with upper tract Urothelial carcinoma. PLoS One. 2015;10:e0144961.

24. Xu H, Tan P, Ai J, Huang Y, Lin T, Yang L, Wei Q. Prognostic impact of preoperative albumin-globulin ratio on oncologic outcomes in upper tract Urothelial carcinoma treated with radical Nephroureterectomy. Clin Genitourin Cancer. 2018;16:e1059–68.
25. Otsuka M, Kamasako T, Uemura T, Takeshita N, Shinozaki T, Kobayashi M, Komaru A, Fukasawa S. Prognostic role of the preoperative serum albumin : globulin ratio after radical nephroureterectomy for upper tract urothelial carcinoma. Int J Urol. 2018;25:871–8.
26. Fukushima H, Kobayashi M, Kawano K, Morimoto S. Prognostic value of albumin/globulin ratio in patients with upper tract Urothelial carcinoma patients treated with radical Nephroureterectomy. Anticancer Res. 2018; 38:2329–34.
27. McShane LM, Altman DG, Sauerbrei W, Taube SE, Gion M, Clark GM. Statistics Subcommittee of the NCI-EORTC Working Group on Cancer Diagnostics. REporting recommendations for tumour MARKer prognostic studies (REMARK). Eur J Cancer. 2005;41:1690–6.
28. Cantiello F, Russo GI, Vartolomei MD, ARA F, Terracciano D, Musi G, Lucarelli G, Di Stasi SM, Hurle R, Serretta V, Busetto GM, Scafuro C, Perdonà S, Borghesi M, Schiavina R, Cioffi A, De Berardinis E, Almeida GL, Bove P, Lima E, Ucciero G, Matei DV, Crisan N, Verze P, Battaglia M, Guazzoni G, Autorino R, Morgia G, Damiano R, de Cobelli O, Mirone V, Shariat SF, Ferro M. Systemic Inflammatory Markers and Oncologic Outcomes in Patients with High-risk Non-muscle-invasive Urothelial Bladder Cancer. Eur Urol Oncol. 2018;1:403–10.

# 4

# Circulating sex hormone levels in relation to male sperm quality

Wei Zhao[1†], Jun Jing[1†], Yong Shao[1], Rong Zeng[1], Cencen Wang[1], Bing Yao[1,2*] and Dong Hang[3*]

**Abstract**

**Background:** Although sex hormones play critical roles in spermatogenesis and sperm maturation, it remains inconclusive whether circulating sex hormones can serve as non-invasive biomarkers to improve the assessment of sperm quality.

**Methods:** We systematically evaluated the association of various sex hormones in serum with sperm quality among 338 men in subfertile couples. Concentrations of luteinizing hormone (LH), follicle-stimulating hormone (FSH), total testosterone (TT), total estradiol (E2), and sex hormone-binding globulin (SHBG) were detected by chemiluminescent immunoassay. Free testosterone and estradiol were calculated using a validated algorithm. A generalized liner regression model controlling for lifestyle factors was used to evaluate the associations with sperm count, concentration, motility, and morphology.

**Results:** After adjusting for age, body mass index, current smoking and alcohol drinking, LH, FSH, and TT levels were all inversely associated with sperm motility (all $P$ for trend < 0.05); however, in mutual adjustment analysis, only LH remained an inverse association with sperm motility after adjusting for FSH and TT levels ($P$ for trend = 0.04). Higher concentrations of LH were also associated with lower sperm progressive motility ($P$ for trend = 0.04). Moreover, LH and FSH levels were both inversely associated with normal sperm morphology ($P$ for trend = 0.04 and 0.02, respectively).

**Conclusions:** Increased levels of LH are associated with poor sperm motility and morphology, suggesting that LH may play a central role in sperm maturation. Future studies are warranted to assess potential clinical utility of LH for risk stratification and tailed prevention of male infertility.

**Keywords:** Sex hormone, Luteinizing hormone, Sperm quality, Sperm motility, Sperm morphology

## Background

Over the past decades, infertility has become a serious health problem worldwide. Nearly 10–15% of couples at optimal reproductive age suffer from infertility [1], and 50% of cases are attributable to impaired sperm quality [2, 3]. In 2010, the WHO proposed a new manual for the laboratory examination of human semen, in which new reference values for semen characteristics were markedly lower than those reported in previous versions [4]. In addition to semen analysis, a blood test is commonly conducted to examine sex hormone concentrations for the males seeking fertility evaluation or treatment. Nevertheless, due to limited and inconsistent results from population-based studies, it is not well understood how variability in the levels of circulating sex hormones impact semen quality.

Sex hormones, such as luteinizing hormone (LH), follicle-stimulating hormone (FSH), estradiol (E2), testosterone, and sex hormone-binding hormone (SHBG),

* Correspondence: yaobing@nju.edu.cn; hangdong@njmu.edu.cn
†Wei Zhao and Jun Jing contributed equally to this work.
[1]Reproductive Medical Center, Jinling Hospital Affiliated Medical School of Nanjing University, Nanjing, China
[3]Department of Epidemiology and Biostatistics, School of Public Health, Nanjing Medical University, Nanjing 211166, China

are demonstrated to play vital roles in spermatogenesis and sperm maturation [5, 6]. Several population-based studies, but not others [7–9], reported that circulating levels of sex hormones were associated with sperm concentration, motility, or morphology [10–12]. The exact reasons for this inconsistency remain unknown, but most of the studies were limited by small sample sizes and inadequate control for potential confounding (e.g., age, body mass index [BMI], smoking, and alcohol consumption). Moreover, because various sex hormones tend to be correlated with each other, statistical analysis is required to separate their independent effects. Therefore, current data are far from conclusive to guide clinical evaluation of semen quality. Further investigations are warranted to address the relationship between circulating sex hormones and sperm quality, which may provide a non-invasive tool to improve early detection and treatment of male infertility.

In this study, we systematically evaluated the association of various sex hormones in serum with sperm quality among 338 men in subfertile couples. We not only adjusted for the factors including age, BMI, smoking, and alcohol consumption, but also performed mutual adjustment for sex hormones. The results could reveal the independent association of aforementioned hormones, and provide the clues about the specific effect of each hormone on semen quality.

## Method

### Study population

This study included a cohort of men in subfertile couples who sought evaluation and treatment at Nanjing Jinling Hospital between August 2012 and June 2015. They were aged 18 to 50 years, and their partners had not conceived within 12 months after stopping use of contraception. All participants were asked to complete a questionnaire about occupation, lifestyle factors (e.g., alcohol consumption and smoking history), and medical and reproductive history. After undergoing physical examination, they provided semen specimens and fasting venous blood. Exclusion criteria included azoospermia or current use of exogenous hormones. Among 338 eligible participants, 305 (90.2%) had normal semen concentrations, 189 (55.9%) had normal sperm total motility, and 229 (67.8%) had normal sperm morphology, according to the 2010 WHO reference values. A total of 165 (48.8%) men had one or more parameter below the reference value. This study was approved by the Human Subject Committees of Nanjing Jinling Hospital, and written informed consent was obtained from each participant.

### Analysis of semen parameters

Semen specimens were collected through masturbation after 2–7 days of sexual abstinence according to the 2010 WHO guidelines. After liquefaction at 37 °C, total sperm count, sperm concentration, total motility, and progressive motility were analyzed using a computer-aided sperm analysis system (CFT-9201; Jiangsu Rich Life Science Instrument Co., Ltd., Nanjing, China). Sperm morphology was evaluated using Diff-Quik staining according to the manufacture's protocol (Nanjing Xindi Biological Pharmaceutical Engineering Co., Ltd. Nanjing, China). At least 200 spermatozoa were counted for each specimen, and the experiments were performed at least twice.

### Determinations of serum sex hormones

Serum was isolated from blood samples by centrifugation at 3000 g for 5 min. Concentrations of LH, FSH, TT, E2, and SHBG were determined by chemiluminescent immunoassay with commercially available kits (Beckman Coulter, Inc., USA) and an automated Unicel Dxl 800 Access Immunoassay System (Beckman Coulter, Inc., USA). The lower detection limits were 0.2 IU/L for LH, 0.2 IU/L for FSH, 0.35 nmol/L for TT, 18 pmol/L for E2, and 0.33 nmol/L for SHBG. The intra-assay coefficients of variation (CV) for LH, FSH, TT, E2 and SHBG were all less than 5%, and the inter-assay CVs were all less than 8%.Free testosterone and estradiol were calculated using a validated method based on total testosterone or estradiol, SHBG, an assumed constant representing the normal albumin concentration, and the association constants for the binding of testosterone and estradiol to SHBG and albumin [13]. Calculated values for free testosterone and estradiol was shown to be highly correlated ($r \geq 0.85$) with direct measurements of free hormone levels [14], and this method was commonly used in previous studies [15, 16].

### Statistical analysis

We calculated the partial Spearman correlation coefficients between each two of the hormones after adjusting for age at blood collection. Adjusted least-squares means (LSM) of semen parameters by tertiles of hormone concentrations were calculated using a generalized liner regression model controlling for age, BMI, current smoking and alcohol drinking status. In mutual adjustment analysis, all hormones associated with sperm quality were included in the multivariate models. We tested for linear trend across hormone categories by treating them as ordinal prediction in multivariate linear regression models. All data analyses were conducted using SAS version 9.4 (SAS Institute, Cary, NC). *P*-value $< 0.05$ was considered statistically significant.

## Result

### Study population

Table 1 shows the characteristics of 338 male participants and the concentrations of serum sex hormones.

**Table 1** Basic characteristics of study participants[a]

| Variable | $N = 338$ |
|---|---|
| Age at blood draw (year) | 28.8 ± 5.1 |
| BMI (kg/m$^2$) | 24.0 ± 3.1 |
| Married, % | 81.1 |
| Current smoking, % | 47.9 |
| Current alcohol drinking, % | 63.3 |
| Serum sex hormone | |
| Luteinizing hormone (IU/L) | 4.6(2.8) |
| Follicle-stimulating hormone (IU/L) | 4.5(2.3) |
| Total testosterone (nmol/L) | 14.0(6.1) |
| Free testosterone (nmol/L) | 0.3(0.1) |
| Total estradiol (pmol/L) | 98.5(57.0) |
| Free estradiol (pmol/L) | 1.7(1.1) |
| Sex hormone-binding hormone (nmol/L) | 27.9(17.8) |

[a]Mean ± SD is presented for continuous variables, percentage for categorical variables, and median value (interquartile range) for sex hormones

The mean age of participants was 28.8 years, and most of them had been married (81%). The proportions of current smoking and alcohol drinking were 48 and 63%, respectively.

### Correlation between serum sex hormone

Before analyzing the association between sex hormones and sperm parameters, we evaluated the correlation between sex hormones (Table 2). According to age-adjusted Spearman correlation coefficients, moderate positive correlations ($r = 0.22–0.55$, all $P < 0.001$) were observed for LH and FSH, LH and total testosterone, total/free testosterone and total estradiol, total testosterone and SHBG. We also found moderate inverse associations of SHBG with free testosterone ($r = -0.32$, $P < 0.001$) and free estradiol ($r = -0.24$, $P < 0.001$), supporting the known role of SHBG in lowering free testosterone and estradiol.

### LH and FSH are associated with sperm motility and morphology

Table 3 shows the association between sex hormone levels and sperm total motility.. The adjusted LSM (95% CI) of sperm motility was calculated according to the tertiles of each sex hormone. We found that LH, FSH, and TT levels were all inversely associated with sperm motility (all $P$ for trend < 0.05). In mutual adjustment analysis, only LH remained a statistically significant association with sperm total motility after further adjusting for FSH and TT ($P$ for trend = 0.01). Compared to the lowest tertile of LH (adjusted LSM = 47.1%), the highest tertile group had decreased sperm total motility (adjusted LSM = 40.5%, $P = 0.04$).

We further analyzed the association between sex hormone levels and sperm progressive motility, i.e. swimming in a straight line or in a large circle, which is necessary for fertilization. In Table 4, serum LH levels were inversely associated with sperm progressive motility. Compared to the lowest tertile of LH (adjusted LSM = 30.0%), the highest tertile group showed decreased progressive motility (adjusted LSM = 26.5%, $P = 0.04$).

In Table 5, we observed that LH and FSH were both inversely associated with the proportion of normal sperm morphology. Compared with the lowest tertile of LH (adjusted LSM = 6.8%), the highest tertile group had a lower proportion of normal sperm morphology (adjusted LSM = 6.0%, $P = 0.01$). Moreover, the highest tertile of FSH showed a lower proportion of normal sperm morphology (adjusted LSM = 6.0%, $P = 0.01$) than the lowest tertile (adjusted LSM = 7.0%). The associations for LH and FSH remained statistically significant in mutual adjustment analysis.

We also analyzed the association between sex hormone levels and total sperm count and sperm concentrations. We found that none of sex hormones was associated with total sperm count (All $P$ for trend > 0.05) (Supplementary Table 1). Higher levels of LH and

**Table 2** Age-adjusted Spearman correlation coefficient between serum sex hormones

| Sex hormone | Luteinizing hormone | Follicle-stimulating hormone | Total testosterone | Free testosterone | Total estradiol | Free estradiol | Sex hormone-binding hormone |
|---|---|---|---|---|---|---|---|
| Luteinizing hormone | – | | | | | | |
| Follicle-stimulating hormone | 0.28[c] | – | | | | | |
| Total testosterone | 0.24[c] | 0.18[b] | – | | | | |
| Free testosterone | 0.16[b] | 0.08 | 0.55[c] | – | | | |
| Total estradiol | 0.02 | −0.08 | 0.28[c] | 0.22[c] | – | | |
| Free estradiol | −0.03 | − 0.13[a] | 0.09 | 0.32[c] | 0.94[c] | – | |
| Sex hormone-binding hormone | 0.12[a] | 0.11[a] | 0.55[c] | −0.32[c] | 0.08 | −0.24[c] | – |

[a]$P < 0.05$; [b]$P < 0.01$; [c]$P < 0.001$

**Table 3** Association between serum sex hormone levels and sperm total motility[a]

| Sex hormone | n | Sperm total motility (%) | | |
|---|---|---|---|---|
| | | Least-squares mean (95% CI) | *P* | *P* for trend |
| Luteinizing hormone | | | | |
| Tertile 1 | 112 | 48.4(44.4, 52.3) | Ref | 0.002 |
| Tertile 2 | 114 | 43.9(40.1, 47.8) | 0.12 | |
| Tertile 3 | 112 | 39.4(35.4, 43.3) | 0.002 | |
| Luteinizing hormone[b] | | | | |
| Tertile 1 | 101 | 47.1(42.9, 51.3) | Ref | 0.04 |
| Tertile 2 | 98 | 44.3(40.2, 48.5) | 0.36 | |
| Tertile 3 | 91 | 40.5(36.0, 44.9) | 0.04 | |
| Follicle-stimulating hormone | | | | |
| Tertile 1 | 112 | 46.6(42.6, 50.5) | Ref | 0.01 |
| Tertile 2 | 114 | 45.5(41.6, 49.4) | 0.71 | |
| Tertile 3 | 112 | 39.6(35.6, 43.5) | 0.01 | |
| Follicle-stimulating hormone[b] | | | | |
| Tertile 1 | 93 | 44.3(39.9, 48.6) | Ref | 0.54 |
| Tertile 2 | 97 | 45.7(41.5, 49.9) | 0.65 | |
| Tertile 3 | 100 | 42.4(38.1, 46.6) | 0.54 | |
| Total testosterone | | | | |
| Tertile 1 | 96 | 48.2(43.8, 52.6) | Ref | 0.03 |
| Tertile 2 | 97 | 43.0(38.8, 47.2) | 0.09 | |
| Tertile 3 | 97 | 41.1(367, 45.5) | 0.03 | |
| Total testosterone[b] | | | | |
| Tertile 1 | 96 | 47.3(42.9, 51.7) | Ref | 0.14 |
| Tertile 2 | 97 | 42.7(38.5, 46.9) | 0.14 | |
| Tertile 3 | 97 | 42.3(37.9, 46.8) | 0.14 | |
| Free testosterone | | | | |
| Tertile 1 | 96 | 46.7(42.3, 51.0) | Ref | 0.06 |
| Tertile 2 | 97 | 44.9(40.7, 49.1) | 0.56 | |
| Tertile 3 | 97 | 40.7(36.5, 45.0) | 0.06 | |
| Total estradiol | | | | |
| Tertile 1 | 113 | 44.2(40.3, 48.2) | Ref | 0.60 |
| Tertile 2 | 115 | 44.7(40.8, 48.6) | 0.87 | |
| Tertile 3 | 110 | 42.7(38.7, 46.7) | 0.59 | |
| Free estradiol | | | | |
| Tertile 1 | 96 | 43.5(39.3, 47.7) | Ref | 0.339 |
| Tertile 2 | 97 | 48.3(44.0, 52.5) | 0.12 | |
| Tertile 3 | 97 | 40.5(36.3, 44.7) | 0.32 | |
| Sex hormone-binding hormone | | | | |
| Tertile 1 | 112 | 45.4(41.2, 49.6) | Ref | 0.95 |
| Tertile 2 | 113 | 41.3(37.4, 45.3) | 0.18 | |
| Tertile 3 | 113 | 44.9(40.9, 49.0) | 0.88 | |

[a]General linear models were adjusted for age at sample collection, BMI (continuous), current smoking (yes or no), and current alcohol consumption (yes or no). *P* for trend was calculated by treating hormone categories as ordinal predictors in multivariate linear regression models
[b]Mutual adjustment for hormones associated with sperm motility in multivariate linear regression models

**Table 4** Association between serum sex hormone levels and sperm progressive motility[a]

| Sex hormone | n | Progressive motility (%) | | |
|---|---|---|---|---|
| | | Least-squares mean (95% CI) | *P* | *P* for trend |
| Luteinizing hormone | | | | |
| Tertile 1 | 112 | 30.0(27.6, 32.4) | Ref | 0.04 |
| Tertile 2 | 114 | 27.8(25.5, 30.2) | 0.20 | |
| Tertile 3 | 112 | 26.5(24.1, 28.9) | 0.04 | |
| Follicle-stimulating hormone | | | | |
| Tertile 1 | 112 | 28.9(26.5, 31.3) | Ref | 0.14 |
| Tertile 2 | 114 | 29.1(26.7, 31.4) | 0.94 | |
| Tertile 3 | 112 | 26.4(24.0, 28.8) | 0.14 | |
| Total testosterone | | | | |
| Tertile 1 | 96 | 29.6(26.9, 32.3) | Ref | 0.22 |
| Tertile 2 | 97 | 28.3(25.7, 30.8) | 0.48 | |
| Tertile 3 | 97 | 27.1(24.4, 29.9) | 0.23 | |
| Free testosterone | | | | |
| Tertile 1 | 96 | 30.3(27.6, 32.9) | Ref | 0.05 |
| Tertile 2 | 97 | 28.2(25.7, 30.8) | 0.28 | |
| Tertile 3 | 97 | 26.5(23.9, 29.2) | 0.06 | |
| Total estradiol | | | | |
| Tertile 1 | 113 | 28.4(26.0, 30.7) | Ref | 0.69 |
| Tertile 2 | 115 | 28.3(26.0, 30.7) | 0.98 | |
| Tertile 3 | 110 | 27.7(25.2, 30.1) | 0.69 | |
| Free estradiol | | | | |
| Tertile 1 | 96 | 28.16(25.6, 30.7) | Ref | 0.35 |
| Tertile 2 | 97 | 30.5(27.9, 33.1) | 0.21 | |
| Tertile 3 | 97 | 26.4(23.8, 28.9) | 0.34 | |
| Sex hormone-binding hormone | | | | |
| Tertile 1 | 112 | 27.6(25.0, 30.1) | Ref | 0.26 |
| Tertile 2 | 113 | 27.2(24.8, 29.6) | 0.85 | |
| Tertile 3 | 113 | 29.6(27.1, 32.0) | 0.29 | |

[a]General linear models were adjusted for age at sample collection, BMI (continuous), current smoking (yes or no), and current alcohol consumption (yes or no). *P* for trend was calculated by treating hormone categories as ordinal predictors in multivariate linear regression models

FSH appeared to be associated with lower sperm concentrations, but the trend tests were statistically non-significant (Supplementary Table 2).

In a sensitivity analysis by excluding participants with semen concentrations at the top and bottom 5%, the above results were essentially unchanged (data not shown).

## Discussion

This study showed that serum concentrations of LH were inversely associated with sperm motility and normal morphology, after adjusting for various lifestyle factors and other sex hormone levels. In addition, higher

**Table 5** Association between serum sex hormone levels and the proportion of normal sperm morphology[a]

| Sperm parameters | n | Normal sperm morphology (%) | | |
|---|---|---|---|---|
| | | Least-squares mean (95% CI) | *P* | *P* for trend |
| Luteinizing hormone | | | | |
| Tertile 1 | 112 | 6.8(6.5, 7.5) | Ref | 0.01 |
| Tertile 2 | 114 | 6.9(6.4, 7.3) | 0.74 | |
| Tertile 3 | 112 | 6.0(5.5, 6.5) | 0.01 | |
| Luteinizing hormone[b] | | | | |
| Tertile 1 | 111 | 6.9(6.4, 7.4) | Ref | 0.04 |
| Tertile 2 | 111 | 6.8(6.4, 7.3) | 0.87 | |
| Tertile 3 | 109 | 6.1(5.6, 6.6) | 0.04 | |
| Follicle-stimulating hormone | | | | |
| Tertile 1 | 112 | 7.0(6.5, 7.5) | Ref | 0.01 |
| Tertile 2 | 114 | 6.8(6.3, 7.3) | 0.46 | |
| Tertile 3 | 112 | 6.0(5.5, 6.5) | 0.01 | |
| Follicle-stimulating hormone[b] | | | | |
| Tertile 1 | 109 | 7.0(6.5, 7.5) | Ref | 0.02 |
| Tertile 2 | 114 | 6.8(6.3, 7.2) | 0.54 | |
| Tertile 3 | 108 | 6.1(5.6, 6.6) | 0.02 | |
| Total testosterone | | | | |
| Tertile 1 | 96 | 7.1(6.5, 7.6) | Ref | 0.06 |
| Tertile 2 | 97 | 6.8(6.2, 7.3) | 0.41 | |
| Tertile 3 | 97 | 6.3(5.7, 6.9) | 0.06 | |
| Free testosterone | | | | |
| Tertile 1 | 96 | 6.7(6.1, 7.2) | Ref | 0.94 |
| Tertile 2 | 97 | 6.7(6.2, 7.2) | 0.99 | |
| Tertile 3 | 97 | 6.7(6.2, 7.3) | 0.94 | |
| Total estradiol | | | | |
| Tertile 1 | 113 | 6.5(6.0, 7.0) | Ref | 0.91 |
| Tertile 2 | 115 | 6.8(6.3, 7.3) | 0.50 | |
| Tertile 3 | 110 | 6.6(6.1, 7.1) | 0.92 | |
| Free estradiol | | | | |
| Tertile 1 | 96 | 6.5(5.9, 7.0) | Ref | 0.49 |
| Tertile 2 | 97 | 6.9(6.4, 7.4) | 0.27 | |
| Tertile 3 | 97 | 6.7(6.2, 7.3) | 0.50 | |
| Sex hormone-binding hormone | | | | |
| Tertile 1 | 112 | 7.0(6.5, 7.6) | Ref | 0.06 |
| Tertile 2 | 113 | 6.5(6.0, 7.0) | 0.14 | |
| Tertile 3 | 113 | 6.3(5.8, 6.8) | 0.06 | |

[a]General linear models were adjusted for age at sample collection, BMI (continuous), current smoking (yes or no), and current alcohol consumption (yes or no). *P* for trend was calculated by treating hormone categories as ordinal predictors in multivariate linear regression models
[b]Mutual adjustment for hormones associated with the proportion of normal sperm morphology in multivariate linear regression models

levels of FSH showed an independent association with a lower proportion of normal sperm morphology. No statistically significant association was observed between sex hormones and total sperm count or sperm concentrations. Our findings suggested that LH might play a central role in the sperm motility and morphology, supporting the utility of circulating LH levels as a biomarker for assessing sperm quality.

A few studies have investigated the relationship between circulating sex hormones and sperm parameters. *Kumanov* et al. found that serum concentrations of LH and FSH were inversely correlated with sperm count, motility, and morphology, while testosterone was not correlated [10]. Similarly, another study by *Meeker* et al. reported significant negative correlations of LH and FSH with sperm concentration, motility, and morphology; however, testosterone levels were significantly positively correlated with motility [11]. In contrast, two small studies reported that only FSH levels had a negative correlation with semen parameters, while LH and testosterone levels did not [7, 8]. Compared with those studies, the current study had relatively large sample size, included various sex hormones, adjusted for lifestyle factors, and performed mutual adjustment analysis. We found that LH, FSH, and TT were all inversely associated with sperm total motility; however, only LH had an independent association after adjusting for FSH and TT, supporting the central role of LH in sperm motility. Consistently, only LH levels were found to be inversely associated with sperm progressive motility. We also observed that LH and FSH were inversely associated with sperm morphology after mutual adjustment, suggesting that both of them are important for sperm to maintain normal morphology. To our knowledge, the current study represents a first attempt to disentangle independent effects of various sex hormones on sperm quality.

The primary role of LH in the male is to stimulate the production of testosterone by the Leydig cells which then, together with FSH, control spermatogonial cell formation and spermatogenesis in the Sertoli cells [17]. Early studies indicated that gonadal failure, a cause of infertility, was characterized by increased levels of LH and FSH [18]. Male patients with idiopathic oligozoospermia were also found to have a higher mean LH pulse frequency than the controls [19]. The increase in LH or FSH concentrations may reflect that the testicles have insufficient capacity for normal spermatogenesis. In the current study, we observed a suggestive association between LH/FSH and sperm concentration. On the other hand, LH may affect fructose utilization, glucose oxidation, and adenyl cyclase activity in sperm, which are important means by which spermatozoa derive energy for motility [20]. The acquisition of sperm motility occurs during sperm maturation in the epididymis, and LH receptors have been detected in epididymal epithelium [21, 22]. Moreover, in the absence of LH, addition of TT and FSH can only partly rescue the phenotype of abnormal sperm [23]. These evidences are in support of our findings, suggesting a critical role of LH in sperm motility. Although recent studies support that LH may be also implicated in sperm morphology [24, 25], specific mechanisms remain unknown. More functional research is warranted to clarify the current results.

This study has several strengths, including relatively large sample size, inclusion of various sex hormones, adjustment for potential confounding, and mutual adjustment analysis to determine independent effects. However, our analysis was cross-sectional, which limited the ability to make causal inference. Additionally, only a single measurement of circulating hormones was available that may not represent long-term levels. Prospective studies with repeated assessment of circulating hormones are necessary to validate our findings. Finally, semen parameters are variable within individuals over time and one semen sample may not well reflect a man's long-term values. However, prior studies have reported no significant differences between the first semen sample and the remaining replicates, suggesting one semen sample may suffice to identify average differences in semen quality between individuals [26, 27].

## Conclusions

In summary, our study demonstrates that circulating LH is inversely associated with sperm motility and morphology, suggesting that LH might act as a major regulator in sperm maturation. Further studies are needed to confirm our findings and assess the clinical utility of LH as a non-invasive biomarker for risk stratification and tailed prevention of male infertility.

#### Abbreviations

LH: Luteinizing hormone; FSH: Follicle-stimulating hormone; TT: Total testosterone; E2: Estradiol; SHBG: Sex hormone-binding hormone; BMI: Body mass index; LSM: Least-squares means; CV: Coefficients of variation

#### Acknowledgements

Not applicable.

#### Authors' contributions

WZ and JJ performed statistical analysis and drafted the manuscript. YS, RZ, and CW were involved in the acquisition, analysis, and interpretations of data. DH and BY were responsible for study design. All authors critically assessed, edited, and approved the final manuscript.

#### Competing interests

None declared.

#### Author details

[1]Reproductive Medical Center, Jinling Hospital Affiliated Medical School of Nanjing University, Nanjing, China. [2]Reproductive Medical Centre, Nanjing Jinling Hospital, Nanjing University School of Medicine, 305 Zhongshan East

Road, Nanjing 210002, Jiangsu, China. [3]Department of Epidemiology and Biostatistics, School of Public Health, Nanjing Medical University, Nanjing 211166, China.

## References

1. Sharlip ID, Jarow JP, Belker AM, Lipshultz LI, Sigman M, Thomas AJ, Schlegel PN, Howards SS, Nehra A, Damewood MD, et al. Best practice policies for male infertility. Fertil Steril. 2002;77(5):873–82.
2. Ross C, Morriss A, Khairy M, Khalaf Y, Braude P, Coomarasamy A, El-Toukhy T. A systematic review of the effect of oral antioxidants on male infertility. Reprod BioMed Online. 2010;20(6):711–23.
3. Skakkebaek NE, Rajpert-De Meyts E, Buck Louis GM, Toppari J, Andersson AM, Eisenberg ML, Jensen TK, Jorgensen N, Swan SH, Sapra KJ, et al. Male reproductive disorders and fertility trends: influences of environment and genetic susceptibility. Physiol Rev. 2016;96(1):55–97.
4. Organization WH. WHO Laboratory manual for the examination and processing of human semen. 5th ed; 2010.
5. Weinbauer GF, Nieschlag E. Gonadotrophin control of testicular germ cell development. Adv Exp Med Biol. 1995;377:55–65.
6. Patel DP, Chandrapal JC, Hotaling JM. Hormone-based treatments in subfertile males. Current Urol Rep. 2016;17(8):56.
7. Subhan F, Tahir F, Ahmad R, Khan ZD. Oligospermia and its relation with hormonal profile. JPMA The Journal of the Pakistan Medical Association. 1995;45(9):246–7.
8. Uhler ML, Zinaman MJ, Brown CC, Clegg ED. Relationship between sperm characteristics and hormonal parameters in normal couples. Fertil Steril. 2003;79(Suppl 3):1535–42.
9. Keskin MZ, Budak S, Zeyrek T, Celik O, Mertoglu O, Yoldas M, Ilbey YO. The relationship between serum hormone levels (follicle-stimulating hormone, luteinizing hormone, total testosterone) and semen parameters. Archivio italiano di urologia, andrologia : organo ufficiale [di] Societa italiana di ecografia urologica e nefrologica. 2015;87(3):194–7.
10. Kumanov P, Nandipati K, Tomova A, Agarwal A. Inhibin B is a better marker of spermatogenesis than other hormones in the evaluation of male factor infertility. Fertil Steril. 2006;86(2):332–8.
11. Meeker JD, Godfrey-Bailey L, Hauser R. Relationships between serum hormone levels and semen quality among men from an infertility clinic. J Androl. 2007;28(3):397–406.
12. Bhongade MB, Prasad S, Jiloha RC, Ray PC, Mohapatra S, Koner BC. Effect of psychological stress on fertility hormones and seminal quality in male partners of infertile couples. Andrologia. 2015;47(3):336–42.
13. Sodergard R, Backstrom T, Shanbhag V, Carstensen H. Calculation of free and bound fractions of testosterone and estradiol-17 beta to human plasma proteins at body temperature. J Steroid Biochem. 1982;16(6):801–10.
14. Rinaldi S, Geay A, Dechaud H, Biessy C, Zeleniuch-Jacquotte A, Akhmedkhanov A, Shore RE, Riboli E, Toniolo P, Kaaks R. Validity of free testosterone and free estradiol determinations in serum samples from postmenopausal women by theoretical calculations. Cancer Epidemiol Biomarkers Prev. 2002;11(10 Pt 1):1065–71.
15. Farhat GN, Cummings SR, Chlebowski RT, Parimi N, Cauley JA, Rohan TE, Huang AJ, Vitolins M, Hubbell FA, Manson JE, et al. Sex hormone levels and risks of estrogen receptor-negative and estrogen receptor-positive breast cancers. J Natl Cancer Inst. 2011;103(7):562–70.
16. Lin JH, Zhang SM, Rexrode KM, Manson JE, Chan AT, Wu K, Tworoger SS, Hankinson SE, Fuchs C, Gaziano JM, et al. Association between sex hormones and colorectal cancer risk in men and women. Clin Gastroenterol Hepatol. 2013;11(4):419–24 e411.
17. Jarow JP. Endocrine causes of male infertility. Urologic Clinics North America. 2003;30(1):83–90.
18. Beastall GH, Ferguson KM, O'Reilly DS, Seth J, Sheridan B. Assays for follicle stimulating hormone and luteinising hormone: guidelines for the provision of a clinical biochemistry service. Ann Clin Biochem. 1987;24(Pt 3):246–62.
19. Bennet A, Bujan L, Plantavid M, Barbe P, Caron P, Louvet JP. Luteinizing hormone pulse frequency and in vitro bioactivity in male idiopathic infertility. Fertil Steril. 1991;55(3):612–8.
20. Sheth AR, Shah GV, Mugatwala PP. Levels of luteinizing hormone in semen of fertile and infertile men and possible significance of luteinizing hormone in sperm metabolism. Fertil Steril. 1976;27(8):933–6.
21. Sun LP, Du QZ, Song YP, Yu JN, Wang SJ, Sang L, Song LW, Yue YM, Lian YZ, Zhang SL, et al. Polymorphisms in luteinizing hormone receptor and hypothalamic gonadotropin-releasing hormone genes and their effects on sperm quality traits in Chinese Holstein bulls. Mol Biol Rep. 2012;39(6):7117–23.
22. Sun LP, Song YP, Liu JJ, Liu XR, Guo AZ, Yang LG. Differential expression of luteinizing hormone receptor, androgen receptor and heat-shock protein 70 in the testis of long-distance transported mice. Genetics Mol Res. 2015;14(3): 9985–93.
23. Pakarainen T, Zhang FP, Makela S, Poutanen M, Huhtaniemi I. Testosterone replacement therapy induces spermatogenesis and partially restores fertility in luteinizing hormone receptor knockout mice. Endocrinology. 2005;146(2): 596–606.
24. Liu Z, Shi X, Wang L, Yang Y, Fu Q, Tao M. Associations between male reproductive characteristics and the outcome of assisted reproductive technology (ART). Biosci Rep. 2017;37(3):BSR20170095.
25. Kovac JR, Smith RP, Cajipe M, Lamb DJ, Lipshultz LI. Men with a complete absence of normal sperm morphology exhibit high rates of success without assisted reproduction. Asian J Androl. 2017;19(1):39–42.
26. Chiu YH, Edifor R, Rosner BA, Nassan FL, Gaskins AJ, Minguez-Alarcon L, Williams PL, Tanrikut C, Hauser R, Chavarro JE, et al. What does a single semen sample tell you? Implications for male factor infertility research. Am J Epidemiol. 2017;186(8):918–26.
27. Stokes-Riner A, Thurston SW, Brazil C, Guzick D, Liu F, Overstreet JW, Wang C, Sparks A, Redmon JB, Swan SH. One semen sample or 2? Insights from a study of fertile men. J Androl. 2007;28(5):638–43.

# 5

# A meta-ethnography to understand the experience of living with urinary incontinence: 'Is it just part and parcel of life?'

Francine Toye[1,2*] and Karen L. Barker[1,2]

**Abstract**

**Background:** Urinary incontinence (UI) is highly prevalent and affects the lives of many men and women. We aimed to conduct a qualitative evidence synthesis (QES) to explore the experience of living with UI and to develop a conceptual model that can help us to understand this experience, and the potential barriers to appropriate healthcare.

**Methods:** We used the methods of meta-ethnography developed by Noblit and Hare and recently refined for larger studies. Meta-ethnography involves identifying concepts from the studies and abstracting these concepts into a line of argument. We searched for studies that explored the experience of adults with UI. We used the GRADE-CERQual framework to assess confidence in review findings.

**Results:** We screened 2307 titles, 429 abstracts, 107 full texts and included 41 studies (36 unique samples) in the synthesis. We organised the concepts into 26 conceptual categories, which we further abstracted into 6 themes: (1) Am I ill or is this normal? (2) It effects who I am and how I feel; (3) I feel stigmatised, ashamed and guilty; (4) talking can be difficult but it can help; (5) keeping incontinence under control; (6) have I got to the point that I need help? Our model conceptualises living with UI as navigating antagonists: Is UI normal or am I ill? Do I need help or am I managing? Do I keep UI to myself (and manage alone) or do I tell other people (and get the support that I need)? Do I use control strategies that focus on concealing (avoid risky situations, wear pads) versus, I use strategies that focus on improving the bodily function to improve continence. Our model highlights the experience of stigma, shame and guilt which exert a pull towards concealment.

**Conclusions:** The culture of secrecy and profound sense of shame is barrier to seeking help. An environment which reduces the shame and stigma of UI may help people to switch the focus to strategies that will improve continence, rather than conceal incontinence.

**Keywords:** Incontinence, Qualitative research, Qualitative evidence synthesis, Meta-ethnography

* Correspondence: Francine.toye@ouh.nhs.uk
[1]Nuffield Orthopaedic Centre, Oxford University Hospitals NHS Foundation Trust, Windmill Road, Oxford OX3 7HE, UK
[2]Nuffield Department of Orthopaedics, Rheumatology and Musculoskeletal Sciences (NDORMS), University of Oxford, Oxford, UK

## Background

Urinary incontinence (UI) is defined by the International Continence Society as 'the complaint of any involuntary leakage of urine'. UI is highly prevalent and experienced by approximately one quarter of women [1] and potentially half as many men [2]. UI is a very broad term and may include stress, urgency, and mixed UI as well as UI of other types; for example, UI with a neurological diagnosis. Interventions for UI are chosen based on diagnosis and adults (in the absence of a neurological diagnosis) may be offered some type of voiding programme, frequency and urgency strategies, in combination with pelvic floor muscle training (PFMT). However, even though interventions such as PFMT can improve UI [3] it may be that only a minority of people with UI seek help [4]. Those that seek help, they will tend to consult a primary health care clinician, and some will never be referred to a clinician with training in continence management.

The Cochrane Qualitative Research Methods Group acknowledges the importance of including qualitative findings within evidence based healthcare [5]. Qualitative evidence synthesis (QES) can bring together qualitative research findings to make them accessible for public, policy, practice and education. We wanted to explore people's experience of living with UI in order to further understand its impact on the lives of men and women, and to understand some of the barriers to seeking help. We aimed to conduct a qualitative evidence synthesis (QES) and to develop a conceptual model that can help us to understand some of the barriers to appropriate healthcare [6]. There are likely to be differences in the experience of UI for men and women of different ages with diverse pathophysiology, we wanted to explore themes that cut across this experience and to identify areas for further research.

## Methods

We used the 7 stages of Meta-ethnography developed, refined and reported by Toye and colleagues [7, 8] and the recent eMERGe meta-ethnography reporting guidelines as a guide for our report [9].

### Selecting meta-ethnography and getting started (stage 1)

This phase incorporates the rationale and aims of the study. Meta-ethnography, first developed by Noblit and Hare [6] has provided insight into a range of healthcare experiences including chronic musculoskeletal pain [10], rheumatoid arthritis [11], fibromyalgia [12], osteoporosis [13] and chronic pelvic pain [14]. There are various methods for QES [15–19]. Some focus on amalgamating and describing findings: other, such as meta-ethnography, aim to develop conceptual understandings through a process of constant comparison and abstraction [6]. We planned to develop a line of argument synthesis, and thus make 'a whole into something more than the parts alone imply' [6] (page 28). We first identified any existing QES, using search terms developed for this purpose [20, 21]. We identified three QES that explored specific areas of UI: French and colleagues explored the uptake and delivery of behavioural interventions for UI (6 studies) [22]; Hay-Smith and colleagues explore the adherence to PFMT (13 studies) [23]; Avery and colleagues explored the psychosocial aspects of living with UI (10 studies) [24]. We also found two QES that explored the global experience of UI: Siddiqui and colleagues explored ethnic and racial differences [25] ($n = 23$ studies); Mendes and colleagues explored women's experience of living with UI ($n = 30$ studies) using the Joanna Briggs Institute Qualitative Appraisal and Review Instrument (JBI-QARI) [26]. JBI-QARI is a descriptive method for QES. The innovation of our study is: (1) to undertake a conceptual synthesis using the methods of meta-ethnography; (2) to incorporate the experience of men from published qualitative findings.

### Deciding what is relevant (stage 2)

We included primary qualitative studies that explored the experience of men and women with UI. UI is a broad term and we intended to be broad in our inclusion. We used subject headings and free text terms for qualitative research, combined with subject heading and free text terms for incontinence (Table 1). Our search terms were adapted from the InterTASC Information Specialists' Sub-Group (ISSG) Search Filter Resources [27–30] and have been used in other meta-ethnographies [7, 31, 32] We excluded studies that exclusively explored: peri-partum, neurological, faecal, long-term care, acute hospitalisation, pelvic organ prolapse and incontinence surgery. In their original text, Noblit and Hare do not advocate an exhaustive search [6] and the number of studies included in meta-ethnographies ranges [16, 18, 33]. We took a selective approach to searching in order to be purposeful, yet also comprehensive enough to develop rich ideas. Similarly, some qualitative reviewers suggest a more targeted approach to searching. For example, you could stop searching when collecting additional data adds no more insight (theoretical saturation) [34]. This approach is more comparable with the sampling strategies for qualitative research. One option might be to start your search with a single data base and expand as analysis proceeds [17]. Our previous QES indicate that Medline retrieves the majority of studies [7, 13, 14, 35]. We therefore limited our initial search to one bibliographic database (Medline) from inception to January 2017 and subsequently updated the search to include studies to February 2019. Campbell and colleagues suggest that 38

**Table 1** Starlite Report

| STARLITE CATEGORY | DESCRIPTION |
|---|---|
| Sampling Strategy | Selective |
| Type of studies | Qualitative research, fully reported |
| Approaches | Single electronic medical database (medline) |
| Range of years | 1990 to January 2017; updated Feb 2019 |
| Limits | [Human age groups Young adult OR Adult OR Middle aged OR Aged Or Aged, 80 and over] [Languages English] |
| Inclusion and exclusions | Incontinence Excluded: peri-partum, neurological, faecal, long-term care and acute hospitalisation, pelvic organ prolapse, incontinence surgery |
| Terms used | ((exp "FOCUS GROUPS"/ OR exp. "ANTHROPOLOGY, CULTURAL"/ OR exp. "QUALITATIVE RESEARCH"/ OR exp. "INTERVIEWS AS TOPIC"/ OR exp. "ATTITUDE TO HEALTH"/ OR exp. "NURSING METHODOLOGY RESEARCH"/ OR (Qualitative ADJ5 (theor* OR study OR studies OR research OR analysis)).ti,ab OR (ethno*).ti,ab OR (emic OR etic).ti,ab OR (phenomenolog*).ti,ab OR (hermeneutic*).ti,ab OR (heidegger* OR husserl* OR colaizzi* OR giorgi* OR glaser OR strauss OR (van AND kaam*) OR (van AND manen) OR ricoeur OR spiegelberg* OR merleau).ti,ab OR (constant ADJ3 compar*).ti,ab OR (focus ADJ3 group*).ti,ab OR (grounded ADJ3 (theor* OR study OR studies OR research OR analysis)).ti,ab OR (narrative ADJ3 analysis).ti,ab OR (discourse ADJ3 analysis).ti,ab OR ((lived OR life) ADJ3 experience*).ti,ab OR ((theoretical OR purposive) ADJ3 sampl*).ti,ab OR (field ADJ (note* OR (field ADJ record*) OR fieldnote*)).ti,ab OR (participant* ADJ3 observ*).ti,ab OR (action ADJ research).ti,ab OR ((co AND operative) AND inquir*).ti,ab OR (co-operative AND inquir*).ti,ab OR (cooperative AND inquir*).ti,ab OR ((semi-structured OR semistructured OR unstructured OR structured) ADJ3 interview*).ti,ab OR ((informal OR in-depth OR indepth OR "in depth") ADJ3 interview*).ti,ab OR (("face-to-face" OR "face to face") ADJ3 interview*).ti,ab OR ("IPA" OR "interpretive phenomenological analysis").ti,ab OR ("appreciative inquiry").ti,ab OR (social AND construct*).ti,ab OR (poststructural* OR post structural* OR post-structural*).ti,ab OR (postmodern* OR post modern* OR post-modern*).ti,ab OR (feminis*).ti,ab OR (humanistic OR existential OR experiential).ti,ab) AND (exp ENURESIS/ OR exp. ENCOPRESIS/ OR exp. "FECAL INCONTINENCE"/ OR exp. "ABSORBENT PADS"/ OR exp. "URINARY INCONTINENCE"/ OR exp. "NOCTURNAL ENURESIS"/ OR exp. "DIURNAL ENURESIS"/ OR exp. "URINARY INCONTINENCE, STRESS"/ OR exp. "URINARY INCONTINENCE, URGE"/ OR exp. "URINARY BLADDER, OVERACTIVE"/ OR (incontinence).ti, ab OR (enuresis).ti,ab OR (encopresis).ti,ab OR ((overactiv* OR "over active" OR over-activ*) ADJ5 bladder).ti,ab)) |
| Electronic sources | Medline |

studies is adequate for meta-ethnography [33] . Our plan was to widen our search if the initial search did not identify this many studies, or if analysis did not yield rich ideas. Table 1 reports the elements of STARLITE (sampling strategy, type of study, approaches, range of years, limits, inclusion and exclusions, terms used, electronic sources) for reporting qualitative literature searches [36].

A single reviewer screened potential articles for potential relevance. A second researcher did not verify the screening for the following reasons: (1) qualitative research methods do not hinge upon statistical analysis of an entire data set; (2) conceptual reviews such as mega-ethnography focus on conceptual analysis. We feel that, in reviews of this scale, research time is more productively spent on data extraction and analysis, rather than being exhaustive. (3) The reviewer had the experience to recognise a qualitative study. To determine if studies were *good enough* to be included in analysis, both reviewers appraised studies, as suggested by Dixon-Woods, as: 'irrelevant', 'fatally flawed', 'satisfactory', or 'key' (conceptually rich) [37]. We excluded 'irrelevant' and 'fatally flawed' studies. Fatally flawed studies included those that had very limited qualitative data. Although appraisal tools are often used in qualitative synthesis [18], QES reviewers do not always use them to determine inclusion [33] and there tends to be low agreement between reviewers [37]. Our approach to quality appraisal for QES is described fully in Toye and colleagues [38].

#### Reading included studies (stage 3)

We used NVivo 11 software for qualitative analysis to facilitate close reading of the studies and to keep track of the analytical decisions [39]. Using NVivo allows you to link originating text with your findings. We extracted contextual information about each study (location, condition, age, gender, study aim, recruitment and methods) to determine how studies were related. Once we had decided which studies to include, two reviewers closely read the full studies in alphabetical order by author, to identify the *ideas* or concepts from each primary study. Close reading is an approach which challenges the reviewer to critically appraise the intentions of the author, and ask what does this mean and what it is an example of? Schütz [33] distinguishes between (1) *first-order constructs* (the participants' 'common sense' interpretations in their own words) and (2) *second order constructs* (the researchers' interpretations of first order constructs). In meta-ethnography, the 'data' are second order constructs. These are the ideas or concepts that are further abstracted to develop *third order constructs* (reviewer's interpretations of second order constructs) which are the QES findings. We excluded data from analysis if both reviewers could not decipher a clear concept. We then rewrote the concepts in the first person. Writing in the first person facilitates the use of accessible language, and we have found it a powerful way for readers (and reviewers) to fully engage in the meaning and sentiment of the ideas.

### Determining how studies are related and translating studies (stages 4 and 5)

Once we had a list of second order concepts, two reviewers 'translated' [6] these by comparing similarities and differences and gradually organising them into *conceptual categories*. The aim of constant comparison is to distil 'the essence of an idea' [20]. This process of abstraction is integral to qualitative analysis [40]. Other meta-ethnographies [33], researchers have used themes from an 'index' paper as a template to organise the analysis [41]. We did not use an index paper as there are also issues about how to decide which paper is *index* [38], and also this can be cumbersome when translating a large number of studies. It is not uncommon to find that some concepts from primary studies do not fit or add anything to a conceptual analysis and, for transparency, these are reported. When both reviewers had agreed on a description of each conceptual category, one reviewer rewrote the descriptions in the first person and printed them on cards. Both reviewers then organised the cards collaboratively through comparison and discussion to develop the QES findings.

### Synthesising translations and expressing the synthesis (stage 6 and 7)

The final stage of meta-ethnography involves organising final themes into a storyline or conceptual model. We intended to produce a line of argument by developing 'a grounded theory that puts the similarities and differences between studies into interpretive order' [6] (page 64). A line of argument can incorporate *similar* and *contrasting* ideas from primary studies, thus allowing both reciprocal *and* refutational translation simultaneously, rather than choosing one or the other. We applied the GRADE-CERQual framework [42–49] to define our confidence in the themes entering the conceptual model as the framework was not designed to be applied to conceptual models. GRADE-CERQual suggest four domains: (1) *'Methodological limitations'*; (2) *'Relevance'*; (3) *'Adequacy of data'* (the 'degree of richness and quantity of data supporting a review finding'); *(4)* *'Coherence'* (consistency across primary studies); and finally, an overall rating of confidence (high, moderate, low, very low).

## Results

Figure 1 illustrates the results of our systematic search. We screened 2307 titles, 429 abstracts and 107 full texts. We excluded 66 out of 107: reviews [50–55]; long term care and acute hospitalisation [56–66]; faecal incontinence [67–78]; family experience [79–84]; healthcare professionals' experience [85–95] Pelvic organ prolapse [96, 97], Continence surgery [98], Post-partum pelvic floor dysfunction [99], multiple pathologies [100], not qualitative or very limited qualitative data [101–115]. We included 41 studies in the final analysis [116–156]. Our purposive search using a single database identified 41 studies in total, including 18 additional studies to Mendes and colleagues [26] and Siddiqui and colleagues [25], who identified 30 and 23 studies respectively. Siddiqui identified an additional 3 studies [157–159] and Mendes identified an additional 7 studies [110, 158, 160–164]. Table 2 shows the overlaps and additional studies found in all 3 QES. Our updated search (February 2019 identified two additional studies [168, 169].

Table 3 shows the country, condition and age of participants, number or participants (number of men), aim of the study and the data collection and methodology of included studies. These studies explore the experience of 1046 participants from a range of countries: UK (9 studies), Australia (8 studies), USA (7 studies), Sweden (4 studies), Germany (2 studies), Hong Kong (3 studies), The Netherlands (2 studies), Brazil (1 study), Canada (1 study), China (1 study), Ethiopia (1 study), Iran (1 study) and Taiwan (1 study). All reports explored women's' experience. Eleven reports (9 unique studies) explored the experience of 190 men [128, 129, 131, 132, 139, 140, 145, 146, 151, 153, 154]. However, the reports did not indicate differences in men's and women's experience and we have analysed these findings together.

We organised the concepts into 26 conceptual categories, which we further abstracted into 6 QES findings (Fig. 2): (1) Am I ill or is this normal? (2) It effects who I am and how I feel; (3) I feel stigmatised, ashamed and guilty; (4) talking can be difficult but it can help; (5) keeping incontinence under control; (6) have I got to the point that I need help? Figure 2 shows the abstraction of conceptual categories into themes. There were nine concepts that did not fit or add anything to our analysis (Fig. 3). We describe each of these themes and illustrate them with examples of concepts from the primary studies. These concepts are written in the first person and are not quotations from the primary studies.

### Am I ill or is this normal?

This theme describes the person's struggle to frame and understand UI (UI). Urination is described as a normal human function, yet also not normal. As such, some

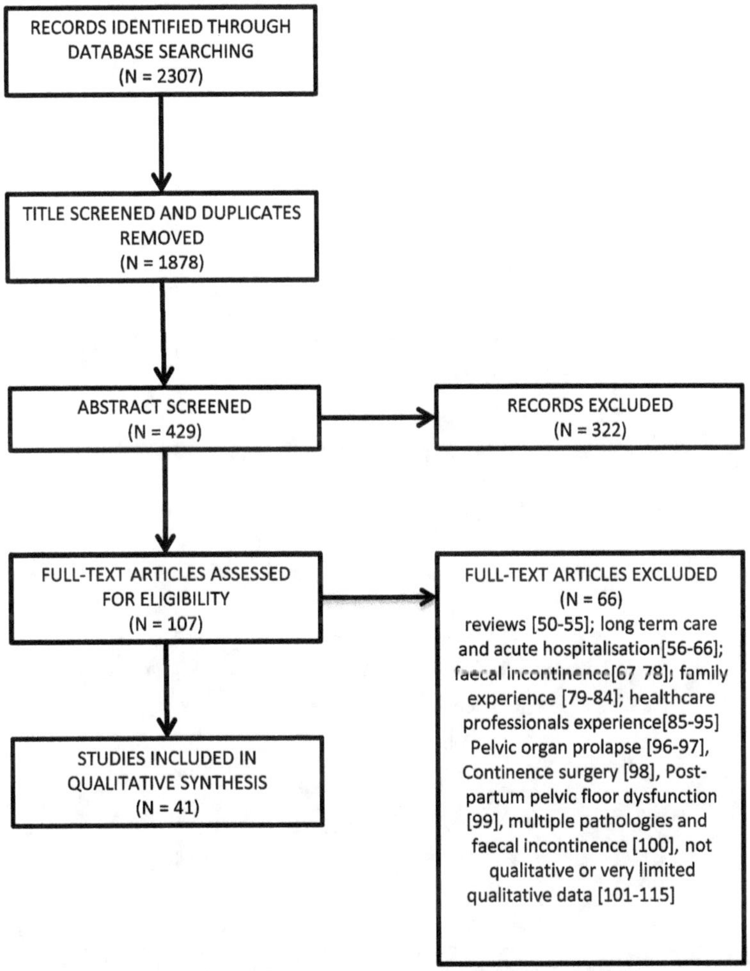


**Fig. 1** Search findings, This flowchart show the records identified through database searching, those excluded following screening and those included

described UI as 'part and parcel of my life' [142] and (female) inheritance. Accounts describe UI as part of the history of my body and who I am [142] and therefore my burden to bear. People felt that it was normal for mothers and older women to be incontinent.

> Peake, Manderson & Potts 1999 [142] - Self-control and the woman out of control: There is no single cause for my incontinence; it is part of the history of my body and who I am. My body is my inheritance. It is normal for older women and mothers to be incontinent. Others are not 'entitled' and therefore have to keep it very quiet. I expect to be incontinent because I have children. It is also normal for older women. However, this does not mean that it is socially acceptable to 'leak'. Leaking is associated with being decrepit and incompetent which makes its secrecy imperative if I am to be seen as normal. It symbolises infancy and extreme old age. It is an embarrassing anomaly.

This struggle to decide whether or not I am ill was exacerbated because UI is as an 'amorphous problem' [118]. UI is described as a condition that is not clearly defined without any particular starting point or cause; it is insidious. Accounts describe efforts to explain UI, for example; is it something I have done; is it because I have had children; is it related to another illness; is it because of heavy lifting; is it normal?

> Ashworth & Hagan 1993 [118] - Impact of incontinence on daily life: The beginning of incontinence is rarely clear. I have had a problem for a while but only realised in retrospect. There was no clear start point. A distressing accident was the spark which made me aware of the problem. Eventually I realised it was a real problem.

The struggle to understand UI was exacerbated by the thought that you were not *medically* ill. People conceptualised UI as something that was part and parcel of life:

**Table 2** studies included in QES, indicating overlap in studies identified in other QES on UI

| Author, Year | Toye & barker | Mendes & Colleagues [26] | Siddiqui & Colleagues [25] |
|---|---|---|---|
| Anger & Colleagues [107] | Excluded full text | | Y |
| Bradway & Strumpf 2008 [109] | Excluded full text | | Y |
| Bradway 2005 [111] | Excluded full text | | Y |
| Bradway & Colleagues [103] | Excluded full text | | Y |
| Brown & Colleagues 1998 [165] | Excluded on abstract | | Y |
| Chaliha & Stanton 1999 [105] | Excluded full text | | Y |
| Hatchett & Colleagues [157] | Not found | | Y |
| Klemm & Creason 1991 [166] | Excluded on abstract | | Y |
| Welch & Colleagues [158] | Not found | | Y |
| Wells and Wagg 2007 [159] | Not found | | Y |
| Bradway & Barg [110] | Not found | Y | Y |
| Elstad & Colleagues 2010 [164] | Not found | Y | Y |
| Akyuz & Colleagues 2014 [160] | Not found | Y | |
| Coyne & Colleagues 2007 [161] | Not found | Y | |
| Delarmelindo 2013 [162] | Not found | Y | |
| Higa & Colleagues [167] | Excluded on abstract | Y | |
| Macdonald & Butler [59] | Excluded full text | Y | |
| Roe & May [100] | Excluded full text | Y | |
| Siu & Lopez [163] | Not found | Y | |
| Welch & Colleagues [158] | Not found | Y | |
| Andersson et al. 2008 [116] | Y | Y | Y |
| Andersson et al. 2009 [117] | Y | Y | Y |
| Ashworth & Hagan 1993 [118] | Y | Y | |
| Cochran 1998 [119] | Y | | |
| Doshani et al. 2007 [120] | Y | Y | Y |
| Dowd 1991 [121] | Y | Y | |
| Getliffe et al. 2007 [122] | Y | | |
| Gjerde et al. 2013 [123] | Y | Y | |
| Griffiths et al. 2009 [124] | Y | | |
| Hägglund & Wadensten 2007 [125] | Y | Y | |
| Hägglund & Ahlström 2007 [126] | Y | Y | |
| Hamid et al. 2015 [127] | Y | Y | |
| Hayder & Schnepp 2010 [128] | Y | Y | Y |
| Hayder 2012 [129] | Y | | |
| Higa et al. 2011 [130] | Y | Y | |
| Horrocks et al. 2004 [131] | Y | | Y |
| Jackson et al. 2012 [132] | Y | | |
| Kao et al. 2015 [133] | Y | | |
| Komorowski & Chen 2006 [134] | Y | Y | Y |
| Li, Low & Lee 2007 [135] | Y | | Y |
| Macinnes 2008 [136] | Y | | |
| Mason et al. b2001 [138] | Y | | |
| Mason et al. 1999 [137] | Y | Y | |
| Milne 2006 [139] | Y | | |

**Table 2** studies included in QES, indicating overlap in studies identified in other QES on UI *(Continued)*

| Author, Year | Toye & barker | Mendes & Colleagues [26] | Siddiqui & Colleagues [25] |
|---|---|---|---|
| Nicolson et al. 2008 [140] | Y | Y | |
| Peake & Manderson 2003 [141] | Y | Y | Y |
| Peake, Manderson & Potts 1999 [142] | Y | | |
| Roos et al. 2014 [143] | Y | Y | |
| Sange et al. 2008 [144] | Y | Y | Y |
| Shaw, William & Assassa 2000 [147] | Y | | |
| Shaw et al. 2001 [145] | Y | | |
| Shaw et al. 2008 [146] | Y | | |
| Siu 2014 [148] | Y | | |
| Siu 2015 [149] | Y | | |
| Skoner & Haylor 1993 [150] | Y | Y | |
| St John, James & Mckenzie 2002 [151] | Y | | |
| van Den Muijsenbergh & Lagro-Janssen 2006 [152] | Y | Y | Y |
| Welch, Taubenberger & Tennstedt 2011 [154] | Y | | |
| Welch et al. 2012 [153] | Y | | |
| Wilkinson 2001 [155] | Y | | Y |
| Zeznock, Gilje & Bradway 2009 [156] | Y | Y | |

it is not a clear, medically accepted and legitimate condition. Some people with UI did not seek help because they felt that the doctor only deals with medical diseases, not 'personal matters'.

> Welch et al. 2012 [153] - Symptom Relief - no treatment as a message that their symptoms were not serious: I have not been offered treatment so it can't be serious; it must be a normal part of ageing. My tests were negative so I don't need treatment. It is not a clear, medically accepted and legitimate condition.

People described UI as a minor complaint that was not serious enough to make them go to the doctor.

> Ashworth & Hagan 1993 [118]- Incontinence is a vague condition, difficult to grasp - An illegitimate problem: It is not a clear, medically accepted and legitimate condition. It is 'just a drag' which interferes with daily life. Is the term 'incontinence' too strong to describe what I have? Having 'the odd squirt' or 'leaking' seems more accurate.

For some, UI was not a priority and other more *serious* conditions and commitments, such as family and work, took precedence.

> Hägglund & Wadensten 2007 [125] - Having personal beliefs about seeking care -Toning down their problem: It is not a top priority. Juggling home and family leaves me little time to worry about myself. I am unbearably weary at times. It is not disturbing enough to seek help. Its impact on my job has made me consider discussing it with a nurse.

#### It effects who I am and how I feel

Although UI was framed as a normal part of life, the second theme describes its profound effect on a person's life and sense of self. The constant worry about keeping incontinence under control and concealed from others curtailed peoples' lives.

> Dowd 1991 [121] - Being in Charge - Achieving a normal life means keeping in control of continence through routines: It is a constant concern as continence is unpredictable. Being prepared means I have to be acutely aware of my routine. I need to plan where, when, and with whom I do things. You can be in charge of most situations. If I am not in charge it threatens my self-esteem. If I have an accident I change my routine to increase security. At times I need to drastically alter my routine to prevent accidents and embarrassment. Sometimes I even stay at home and limit social contacts.

For some, UI threatened intimate relationships. Participants described how they no longer felt desirable, and worry about being incontinent during sex had an impact on maintaining current and future relationships.

**Table 3** Description of studies: Author, year, country, condition, age, number of participants (number of men), aim, data collection, methodology, recruitment context, assessment of relevance and quality

| Author & Year | Geography | Condition | Age | Number (male) | Aim to explore: | Data collection, methodology | Recruitment | Relevance | Assessment |
|---|---|---|---|---|---|---|---|---|---|
| 1. Andersson et al. 2008 [116] | Sweden | UI | 66–89 | 11 | Experience of UI among women who do not desire further treatment | Interviews, Phenomenology | District nurse | direct | satisfactory |
| 2. Andersson et al. 2009 [117] | Sweden | UI | 30 80+ | 14 | Experience of UI among Syrian women living in Sweden | Focus groups, Phenomenology | Snowball sample | direct | satisfactory |
| 3. Ashworth & Hagan 1993 [118] | UK | UI | 25–55 | 28 | Women's' experience of UI | Interviews, Phenomenology | newspaper | direct | key |
| 4. Cochran 1998 [119] | USA | UI | 60–88 | 19 (NK) | Experience of UI of older persons living in the community | Interviews, Not stated | Community volunteer/ doctor invite | direct | satisfactory |
| 5. Doshani et al. 2007 [120] | UK | UI | 36–82 | 24 | Experience of UI among south Asian Indian women in Leicester, UK | Focus groups, Thematic analysis | South Asian community centres | direct | satisfactory |
| 6. Dowd 1991 [121] | USA | UI | 58–79 | 7 | Experience of UI and adjustment in older women | Interviews, Grounded theory | 'convenience sample' | direct | satisfactory |
| 7. Getliffe et al. 2007 [122] | UK | UI | 29–89 | 99 | Experience of using absorbent products for 'light' UI and impact on women's quality of life | Interviews, Thematic analysis | Incontinence services, consumer organisations and adverts | indirect# | satisfactory |
| 8. Gjerde et al. 2013 [123] | Ethiopia | UI | NK | 18[1] | Experience of UI in rural and semi urban settings in Ethiopia | Interviews, Systematic text condensation | part of a Incontinence and Prolapse study. | direct | satisfactory |
| 9. Griffiths et al. 2009 [124] | UK | UI | 30–74 | 22 | Experience of physiotherapy sessions for the management of UI | Interviews, Thematic analysis | Embedded in a trial | direct | satisfactory |
| 10. Hägglund & Wadesten [125] | Sweden | UI | 34–52 | 14 | Experience of UI | Interviews, Phenomenology | Cohort study; women who had not sought help | direct | satisfactory |
| 11. Hägglund & Ahlström 2007 [126] | Sweden | UI | 37–52 | 13 | Experience of UI and health seeking in long-term UI | Interviews, Phenomenology | Cohort study; women who had sought help for UI | direct | satisfactory |
| 12. Hamid et al. 2015 [127] | Iran | UI | 52–68 | 17 | Experience of Muslim community-dwelling postmenopausal women of UI | Interviews, Phenomenology | Community snowball sample | direct | satisfactory |
| 13. Hayder & Schnepp [a] 2010 [128] | Germany | UI | 38–83 | 32 (10) | Experience of UI in daily life | Interviews, Grounded theory | Community advert | direct | key |
| 14. Hayder[a] 2012 [129] | Germany | UI | 38–83 | 32 (10) | Experience of UI and impact on sexuality and intimate relationships | Interviews, | Community advert | direct | satisfactory |
| 15. Higa et al. 2011 [130] | Brazil | UI | 30–45 | 8 | the meanings of silence for | Interviews, | Community snowball | direct | satisfactory |

**Table 3** Description of studies: Author, year, country, condition, age, number of participants (number of men), aim, data collection, methodology, recruitment context, assessment of relevance and quality *(Continued)*

| Author & Year | Geography | Condition | Age | Number (male) | Aim to explore: | Data collection, methodology | Recruitment | Relevance | Assessment |
|---|---|---|---|---|---|---|---|---|---|
| | | | | | Brazilian women with UI | Content analysis, | sample | | |
| 16. Horrocks et al. 2004 [131] | UK | UI | 66–94 | 20 (9) | Why older people living in the community do not seek help with UI | Interviews, Grounded theory | Community survey | partial* | satisfactory |
| 17. Jackson et al. 2012 [132] | USA | UI | NK | 144 (71) | How talking with others influences symptom management | Interviews, Thematic analysis | Community survey | direct | satisfactory |
| 18. Kao et al. 2015 [133] | Taiwan | UI | 44–66 | 12 | Experiences of PFMT for UI and the impact on their sexuality | Interviews, Thematic analysis | Women who had gone to a PFMT education programme | indirect | satisfactory |
| 19. Komorowski & Chen 2006 [134] | China | UI | 24–81 | 15 | Experiences of Chinese women living with UI | Interviews, IPA | Reported UK at Obstetrics and gynaecology department | direct | satisfactory |
| 20. Li, Low & Lee 2007 [135] | Hong Kong | UI | 42–77 | 9 | Community-dwelling women's experiences in coping with UI | Interviews Content analysis | Continence clinic (stress incontinence) | direct | satisfactory |
| 21. Macinnes 2008 [136] | UK | UI | 28–65 | 12 | To explore why some women with UI drop out of healthcare | Telephone interviews, Thematic analysis | Continence clinic (stress incontinence) | direct | satisfactory |
| 22. Mason et al.[b] 1999 [137] | Australia | UI | 21–45 | 52 | The effects of stress incontinence on women in their childbearing years | Interviews, Thematic analysis | One year post-partum with UI | partial | satisfactory |
| 23. Mason et al. [b]2001 [138] | Australia | UI | 21–45 | 52 | are women made aware of UI at the time of childbirth and why some do not seek help | Interviews, Thematic analysis | One year post-partum with UI | partial | satisfactory |
| 24. Milne 2006 [139] | Canada | UI | 24–86 | 38 (5) | Self-care strategies in UI and factors that influence their self-care choices | 15 interviews/3 focus groups description | Adverts in health clinics, newspapers, health education sessions, clinics | direct | satisfactory |
| 25. Nicolson et al. 2008 [140] | UK | OAB | 51–85 | 18 (8) | Experiences of overactive bladder symptoms | Interviews/focus groups, Thematic analysis | Primary care, adverts | direct | satisfactory |
| 26. Peake & Manderson[c] 2003 [141] | Australia | UI | 40–60 | 75 | Social aspects of UI in women in their middle years. | Interviews, Thematic analysis | Primary care | direct | key |
| 27. Peake, Manderson & Potts[c] 1999 [142] | Australia | UI | 40–60 | 75 | Women's discourse regarding theirown UI | Interviews, Thematic analysis | Primary care | direct | key |
| 28. Roos et al. 2014 [143] | Netherlands | POP/UI | 31–64 | 37 | Impact of pelvic organ prolapse and/or UI on sexual dysfunction | Interviews, Thematic analysis | Scheduled for corrective surgery | indirect | satisfactory |
| 29. Sange et al. 2008 [144] | UK | UI | 21–70 | 9 | Religious/cultural influences on help-seeking in south Asian Muslim women | Focus groups, Framework analysis | Language classes | direct | satisfactory |
| 30. Shaw et al. 2001 [145] | Australia | UI | 40–63 | 31 (8) | Help seeking behaviour in people with UI and barriers | Interviews Thematic analysis | Embedded in a continence service trial | indirect | satisfactory |

**Table 3** Description of studies: Author, year, country, condition, age, number of participants (number of men), aim, data collection, methodology, recruitment context, assessment of relevance and quality *(Continued)*

| Author & Year | Geography | Condition | Age | Number (male) | Aim to explore: | Data collection, methodology | Recruitment | Relevance | Assessment |
|---|---|---|---|---|---|---|---|---|---|
| | | | | | to service use | | | | |
| 31. Shaw et al. 2008 [146] | UK | UI | 41–89 | 33 (18) | help-seeking in middle and older aged people with UI | Interviews Grounded theory | Community survey | direct | satisfactory |
| 32. Shaw, William & Assassa 2000 [147] | Australia | UI | 40–62 | 23 (7) | Patients' views of a new nurse led continence service in a randomized trial | Interviews Thematic analysis | Post course led by continence nurse | direct | satisfactory |
| 33. Siu 2014 [148][d] | Hong Kong | OAB | 21–59 | 30 | Doctor-patient communication (female patients and male urologists) | Interviews Thematic analysis | OAB patient self-help group | direct | satisfactory |
| 34. Siu 2015 [149][d] | Hong Kong | OAB | 21–59 | 30 | Reasons behind doctor shopping behaviour in patients with overactive bladder | Interviews Thematic analysis | OAB patient self-help group | direct | satisfactory |
| 35. Skoner & Haylor 1993 [150] | USA | UI | 31–50 | 8 | Perceptions of UI | Interviews Grounded theory | Women's' magazines or snowball sample | direct | satisfactory |
| 36. St John, James & Mckenzie 2002 [151] | Australia | UI | 40–66 | 11 (5) | Perspectives of a service for community dwelling people with UI | Interviews Thematic analysis | Community health, continence service, home visits | direct | satisfactory |
| 37. van Den Muijsenbergh & Lagro-Janssen 2006 [152] | Netherlands | UI | 45 MEAN | 30 | The impact of UI on Moroccan and Turkish women and their treatment preferences | Interviews Thematic analysis | Primary care, pelvic floor physio, Moroccan care consultants | direct | satisfactory |
| 38. Welch et al. [e] 2012 [153] | USA | LUTS | 34–85 | 90 (49) | qualitative methods for developing patient-reported outcomes | Interviews Thematic analysis | Community survey | indirect | satisfactory |
| 39. Welch, Taubenberger & Tennstedt[e] 2011 [154] | USA | LUTS | 34–85 | 90 (49) | Treatment seeking for lower urinary tract symptoms | Interviews Thematic analysis | Community survey | indirect | satisfactory |
| 40. Wilkinson 2001 [155] | Australia | UI | 40–64 | 6 | Experiences of Pakistani women with UI | Interviews Thematic analysis | Continence service | direct | satisfactory |
| 41. Zeznock, Gilje & Bradway 2009 [156] | Alaska | UI | 33–86 | 17 | Experiences of Alaskan women living with UI in rural/urban settings | Interviews Thematic analysis | Urological, women's health and primary care | direct | satisfactory |

**_OAB_ overactive bladder, _POP_ pelvic organ prolapse, _LUTS_ lower urinary tract infection, _IPA_ interpretative phenomenological analysis**

**[1] 5/18 constant UI from obstetric fistula, others had mild to continuous leakage; [*]2 men had permanent indwelling catheters; [#] 16/99 linked to other conditions**

**[a,b,c,d,e] themes drawn from a single cohort in these studies**

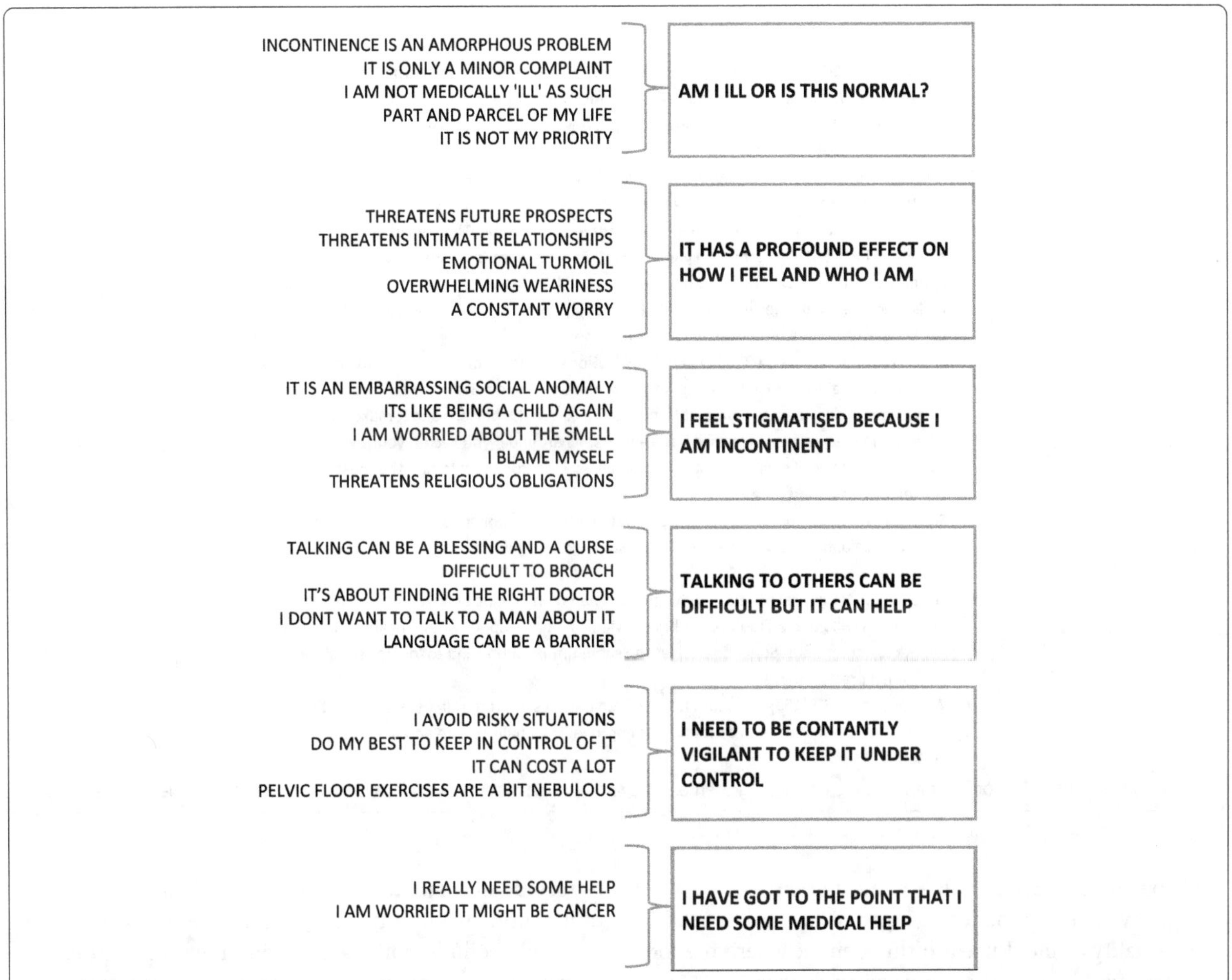


**Fig. 2** Conceptual categories abstracted into themes, This shows the conceptual categories identified and their abstraction into themes

> Peake & Manderson 2003 [141] - Intimate moments: Incontinence affects my sexuality and relationships: I 'feel guilty,' 'disgusting'; 'something no normal man should have to put up with.' It makes me anxious when pleasure and evacuation merge. Some partners see it as a strong sexual signal. It is worse to leak at times unrelated to sex. It is particularly problematic when I am trying to make new relationships.

Some felt that UI would have an impact on future prospects and framed it as the harbinger of future frailty: a 'dark threat on the horizon' [118]. Participants were afraid of becoming seriously restricted or dependent on others.

> Horrocks et al. 2004 [131] - Reactions to incontinence: I am afraid that incontinence is the harbinger of future frailty and dependence. I am worried about cleanliness and personal hygiene. I am embarrassed, ashamed, humiliated, disgusted and so I hide it because I am worried about a negative reaction from other people.

People described emotional turmoil: feeling weepy, distressed, frustrated, annoyed, sad, out of control, fed up; I have lost confidence. For some, hopelessness had made them lose the desire to go on living [127].

> Komorowski & Chen 2006 [134] - Impact of UI on quality of life - emotional isolation: I feel alone and excluded. I avoid social activity. I am embarrassed and ashamed, annoyed, frustrated, sad and depressed. It is inconvenient, uncomfortable and dirty. It makes me feel tired. People don't understand. Other people get used to it and it doesn't affect them. I am afraid, anxious and lonely. I have lost control.

Some talked about overwhelming weariness from the constant effort to keep UI under control and its effect on sleep.

Figure 3. Concepts that did not fit, or add to, the developing themes

1. Doshani et al. 2007 (120) Complementary therapy. I would consider alternative therapies, including herbal medication. Some people prefer to use prescribed medication.
2. Doshani et al. 2007 (120) Suggestions for improving services - Increasing awareness. I have not heard of continence charities.
3. Gjerde et al. 2013 (123) Seeking help: I sought advice from a HCP but did not expect a cure. I use traditional remedies, like Holy Water.
4. Griffiths et al. 2009 (124) Recommendations for Physiotherapy. This lists ideas about what should be included in information given to patients, e.g. details of what to do and what will happen on arrival, including how they will be called into the session without embarrassment. It also includes guidelines for conduct in the waiting room, e.g. avoid handing out information about incontinence in the waiting room
5. Shaw, Williams & Assassa 2000 (147): investigations and treatment investigations: My lifestyle can make it difficult to complete a 24-h pad test and a 3-day urinary diary tests so I sometimes make a best estimate. It is interesting to see the pattern and it makes me more aware of my habits. It's OK leaving pads and diaries around if you live on your own.
6. Siu 2014 (148) Social environment – Convenience: I 'doctor shop' to find the most convenient place and time
7. Siu 2014 (148) Perceptions - Lack of perceived needs: I 'doctor shop' for simple illnesses (common cold, flu, and gastroenteritis). I need a more regular doctor for more severe problems.
8. Siu 2014 (148) Cultural beliefs - Switching between biomedicine and traditional Chinese medicine: I will go to a Traditional Chinese Medicine practitioner when I have finished my biomedical treatment. Some do both at the same time. I don't tend to 'doctor shop' for a traditional practitioner.
9. WELCH et al. 2012 (153) Symptom Relief - Even partial symptom relief enhanced patient well-being: Treatment helps a bit and this improves my quality of life and makes me feel better.

**Fig. 3** Concepts that did not fit, or add to, the developing themes, This shows the concepts that were identified and not included in the analysis

Nicolson et al. 2008 [140] - The experience of urgency: The experience of urgency has an impact on my quality of life. I need to think about where the loo is. Feeling like I need to go urgency does not necessarily mean that I really need to go. It plays tricks on me. The greatest fear is when I get home and put my key in the lock. My sleep is disturbed and I am exhausted. This makes me feel more anxious and depressed.

## I feel stigmatised, ashamed and guilty

This theme describes UI as a condition that is stigmatised and hidden. As such, those with UI bore the burden of shame. Studies describe UI as an embarrassing social anomaly. Accounts described the stigma that comes from losing control; people did not want to wear the label *incontinent.* UI contravened the normal rules of social etiquette and caused shame and humiliation; it was therefore experienced as a taboo subject. People with UI felt that others would discriminate against them or pass judgement. They described feelings of dirtiness, disgust, shame, embarrassment and humiliation.

Ashworth & Hagan 1993 [118] - Incontinence is a vague condition, difficult to grasp - Incontinence is a forbidden topic: It is not 'nice' to talk about incontinence or any 'things down there'. Normally, people collude politely and don't mention it. It is a minefield of potential embarrassment. You need permission to break the taboo. Silence protects everyone from it. Even my partner has little or no inkling of the severity of the problem. I wear those panty shield things; can I mention that to you?

Loss of control symbolised infancy (and extreme old age), and some described UI as like being a child again; for example, feeling that: I am an adult and I cannot even control my own body; I have regressed to childhood; I should be responsible for controlling my own body.

Peake, Manderson & Potts 1999 [142] - The Woman in the body: When you are a child growing up, you got into trouble for wetting your pants, and now you are an adult wetting your pants. Wetting yourself is 'wilful' or 'naughty'. It contravenes important childhood messages of body control. It breaches social etiquette: 'nice' girls are supposed to 'smell nice.' Incontinence is 'part and parcel' of women's lot in life. However, at the same time it 'makes you feel not the woman you were'.

Loss of control was exacerbated by being worried about the smell:

> Griffiths et al. 2009 [124] - Embarrassment: I can tell you some terribly embarrassing stories about times I have wet myself. I worry that I smell. There is a taboo surrounding incontinences. I don't mention it to anyone, even close family. I am embarrassed to go to the doctor. Not everyone is so embarrassed.

Feeling of blame came hand in hand with the stigma of UI. Although UI was framed as natural part of life, it was a struggle to reconcile this inevitability with a sense of culpability and responsibility. Culpability came with a sense of responsibility for control.

> Peake, Manderson & Potts 1999 [142] - Controlling the boundaries of the body: I should be responsible for controlling my own body. I am failing an important social duty. Although it is 'normal,' you have a responsibility to find a solution. UI is an artefact of reproduction. It is not fair if you are incontinent and haven't had children. It makes me feel really dirty. I l have lost self-control. It is difficult to reconcile this sense of self-responsibility with inevitability.

Feelings of guilt focused on personal deficits: for example, people described how they were to blame because they did not ask for help, follow advice or do prescribed exercises.

> Ashworth & Hagan 1993 [118] - Effect of incontinence on self-image - sufferers feel that it is their fault: I blame myself because I didn't do any pelvic floor exercises. I am a bit lazy. I don't want people to see me buying pads. My health professional is going to tell me off. I am going to be categorised and stigmatised for losing control.

Shame and culpability was exacerbated if they threatened religious obligations, such as prayer. However, there were those that felt that you should not feel shame as it was created by God (Allah).

> Van den Muijsenbergh & Lagro-Janssen 2006 [152] - Consequences on daily life: Incontinence has an effect on worship. It is dirty & extremely bothersome. I wash as soon as I can. I always have a supply of pads and clean underwear. Some people talk to their families and partners about it. I am ashamed to talk about it. It has a negative effect on my intimate relationships. I wouldn't want to remarry because of the incontinence. Some say that you shouldn't be ashamed because it was created by Allah.

**Talking can be difficult (but it can help)**

Although the stigma of UI made it difficult for people to talk about it, this theme describes the recognised benefits of talking to others. Participants described talking as a blessing and a curse [132]. Talking about UI could be a positive experience and it was nice to know you weren't alone and that UI was normal. Talking could also help people to realise that there were others worse off than you. It can also mean that people can understand and support you. For some, it could help to build close relationships. Talking could also be a cathartic experience and might even help to reduce the taboo.

> Hayder & Schnepp 2010 [128] - Regain Control - forming a circle of trust: I find it difficult to talk about my incontinence because I am afraid of negative reactions. I keep it a secret from the outside world. I don't dare to confide in anyone outside of the family, not even close friends. Because I keep it quite this means I have to miss out on some leisure activities. Other people manage to be very open about it. Talking to someone else who is interested and who understands can create a bond of trust. I would only tell my closest female friends so that they can understand and appreciate my problem. I then wouldn't have to lie or hide things.

However, participants described the need to manage disclosure of their incontinence with great care.

> Ashworth & Hagan 1993 [118] - Incontinence is a vague condition, difficult to grasp - an isolating problem: No one else I know has incontinence like me and I don't want anyone to discover. I am even careful talking to someone else with a similar problem.

Participants found it difficult to broach the subject of UI with the doctor. They felt that the healthcare professional should enquire as a matter of routine, rather than wait for the patient to initiate the topic.

> Hägglund & Wadensten 2007 [125] - Having desired expectations about care - being actively asked about UI: I want my healthcare professional to ask directly about incontinence and for them to create an understanding atmosphere because I don't dare bring it up.

Some said that it was about finding the right doctor. A 'match doctor' [148] was described as more than someone who provides treatment: they hear and respect you; they create an understanding atmosphere by listening and seeing things from your perspective, they are knowledgeable and informative; they respond to individual needs; they are compassionate, empathetic and friendly. Some described how healthcare professionals could be unresponsive, rushed, disinterested, lack of empathy, or even blame you for your problem.

> St John James & McKenzie 2002 [151] - Appropriateness and acceptability: I have had negative experiences of healthcare professionals and shop around for the 'right person'. I want to see someone who is knowledgeable, empathetic, interested in my experience, compassionate, and with whom I feel at ease. I feel grateful to discuss the impact and management of incontinence but it is difficult to raise the issue. For some it is only a minor complaint with little impact.

Language could also be an additional barrier.

> Wilkinson 2001 [155] - Communicating and understanding: It is difficult to discuss it in another language and the 'unresponsiveness' from healthcare professionals makes this worse. I am too embarrassed to seek help. My healthcare professional is rushed or disinterested. I rely on family or friends to interpret. A bilingual professional would be helpful.

Some women felt that the right healthcare professional would be a woman and that it was s too embarrassing to talk to a man about it [117, 120, 131, 138, 144, 149, 154, 155]. Some were worried about a man performing physical examination. Others felt that UI was a woman's problem and that men might not be able to see it from a woman's point of view.

> Siu 2015 [149] - Feelings of not being understood: The urologist does not understand the extent of my suffering; they see things from 'a male's viewpoint'. I have other things to consider. Treatments can interfere with women's role and the urologist does not understand this.

#### I must keep incontinence under control

This theme describes the need for constant vigilance in order to keep incontinence under control. People planned their routines in advance in order to keep dry and maintain their self-esteem.

This constant worry, and feeling of vulnerability, created a need for various strategies to keep in control of it. Some described how they would rather avoid risky situations. There was a sense of dread about going to places where they didn't feel safe; they avoided places that they were not familiar with. Some stayed at home and became more and more isolated. Freedom and spontaneity was lost.

> Hayder & Schnepp 2010 [128] - A life determined by incontinence: I feel safe when I am at home but dread public areas. I feel vulnerable, ashamed, and abnormal. It affects my relationships and everything that I do. It is difficult to enter into a relationship with a new partner. It has a negative effect on my sexuality. However being able to talk openly about it can help me to build relationships. I am becoming geographically restricted. Trips or journeys into the unknown feel too risky. I feel dependent and inflexible. Over time, I am accepting these limitations and thinking of ways to overcome them.

Some restricted activities, went to the loo much more often and planned their itinerary to fit in with toileting.

> Ashworth & Hagan 1993 [118] - Impact of incontinence on daily life - special precautions become a way of life: I have to take more and more precautions. I have to be constantly aware and anticipate leakage. I go to the loo obsessively and plan toilet visits. I check there is a loo. I only do safe activities and avoid some movements. I regulate how much I drink. I choose my clothes carefully. I buy pads in bulk and carry spares. I constantly check for smells and take precautions. Sometimes I throw underwear away.

Strategies to keep UI under control were developed through trial and error and hinged on concealing bodily function, rather than improving or curing it. For example: I wear pads (preferably not incontinence pads); I always know where the loo is and limit drinks.

> Getliffe et al. 2007 [122] - Containing the problem: wearing pads doesn't make you continent, but you need to be confident that a pad will make it invisible to other people. My confidence is fragile and could easily be damaged. I am anxious about leakage. Pad discreteness and odour control is crucial to 'hiding the problem'. I need to balance absorbency and discreteness (on and in handbag). It also needs to be convenient to change my pad.

Some strategies could incur a cost. For example, pads (and clothing) were expensive.

> Milne & Moore 2006 [139] - Barriers to performance of pelvic floor muscle exercises -Financial cost:

Continence care is expensive. I am surprised and annoyed that it is not covered by the health care.

In contrast to the strategies that aimed to control through concealment, some used pelvic floor exercises as a strategy for *controlling* incontinence through physical improvement.

Kao et al. 2015 [133] - Developing awareness and gaining control - gaining control and confidence: I pay little attention to pelvic health. My first priority is to my family and I come second. I gained control over my body through pelvic floor exercises and feel more confident.

However, pelvic floor exercises were described as *nebulous* [139], meaning 'vague, indistinct, formless, ill-defined' (Oxford English Dictionary online). There was a sense that people needed feedback from the healthcare professional, firstly because it was really difficult to know if you were doing the exercises correctly; and secondly because you did not know if things were improving.

Milne & Moore 2006 [139] - Seeing enhanced believing: If the exercises work I will believe it. I want a test to show that the exercises are working; otherwise it is all a bit nebulous. Changes are very slow and insignificant. It is frustrating and I may give up. If I knew what to expect I could be more realistic about goals.

In this context, some described important competing interests that you need to balance with the effort of doing exercises that have nebulous benefits.

Milne & Moore 2006 [139] - Factors that facilitated pelvic floor muscle exercises - realistic goals and expectations: The exercise regime is very time consuming. You need to be realistic about what you can do in a day.

### Have I got to the point that I need help?

The final theme explores the question - have I got to the point that I need to tell someone about my UI and get some help? This decision was not straightforward and was underpinned by loss of control and intrusion into life. When strategies to conceal or control UI failed and UI started to interfere with life and work, it could get to the point that the need for help outweighed the embarrassment of asking for help.

Ashworth & Hagan 1993 [118] - Impact of incontinence on daily life - dreaded anticipation of worsening in the future: I know that it may sooner or later worsen. I fear being very seriously restricted. I am likely to suffer devastating embarrassment. I will find that over time my strategies will not work, and that I need medical help.

Some sought help because they were worried that UI that it might signify a serious underlying disease, such as cancer.

Shaw et al. 2008 [146] - Identification of the cause of symptoms: I try and find out what is causing this from different sources, like the media. That is how I work out when it is bad enough to seek help. If I know what the cause is, I don't worry as much. I worried that it might be cancer.

### Conceptual model – living with urinary incontinence: is it just part and parcel of life?

We developed a conceptual model (Fig. 4) which helps us to understand the challenges of living with UI and some of the barriers to seeking help and receiving appropriate care. Meta-ethnography aims to develop understanding that goes beyond conceptual categories. Our model demonstrates that UI profoundly affects a person's sense of who they are and also how they feel: it curtails life, affects relationships, and alters future; people feel hopeless and overwhelmed. Our conceptual model highlights antagonists that underpin the experience of UI. Our model illustrates the struggle to decide whether: (i) UI is a normal part of life or I am actually ill and should seek help (ii) I have got to the point that I need help or are things under control? (iii) I keep UI to myself (and manage alone) or do I tell other people (and get the support that I need)? (iv) I use control strategies that focus on *concealing* (avoid risky situations, wear pads) or strategies that focus on *improving* the bodily function to improve continence. Finally our conceptual model highlights the important place of stigma, shame and guilt which are likely to exert a pull towards not telling and concealment of UI.

### Confidence in findings

We assessed our confidence in review findings as moderate (1 finding) to high (5 findings). Details of our GRADE CERQual assessment are shown in Table 4. This assessment of confidence applies only to the 6 QES findings. GRADE-CERQUal was not designed to assess confidence in conceptual models. Two studies identified when we re ran our search did not highlight any additional concepts, suggesting saturation of conceptual categories [168, 169]. We also compared our finding to those in two descriptive QES of UI [25, 26] (Table 5) and found resonance in concepts across studies.

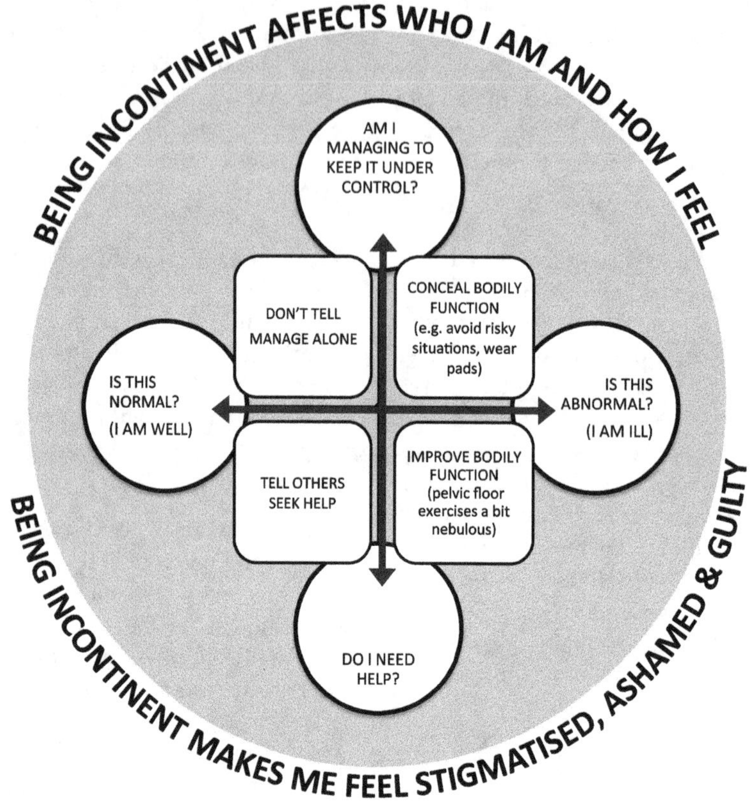


**Fig. 4** Conceptual model - Living with urinary incontinence: is it just part and parcel of life?, Our model shows that being incontinent has an effect on a person's identity and mood. It conceptualises living with UI as navigating antagonists: (i) Is UI normal or am I ill? (ii) Do I need help or am I managing? (iii) Do I keep UI to myself (and manage alone) or do I tell other people (and get the support that I need)? (iv) Do I use control strategies that focus on *concealing* (avoid risky situations, wear pads) versus, I use strategies that focus on *improving* the bodily function to improve continence. These dualities are not mutually exclusive. Our model highlights the experience of stigma, shame and guilt which exert a pull towards concealment

## Discussion

Qualitative research is interpretive and the researcher's perspectives can influence findings. FT (female, aged 51) is an anthropologist, qualitative researcher with experience in QES, and qualified physiotherapist with an interest in chronic pain. KB (female, aged 56) is clinical director of a UK, NHS musculoskeletal directorate and qualified physiotherapist. Their interest in UI comes from the desire to improve services for patients with musculoskeletal disorders who often experience UI. They also have a methodological interest in conceptual QES.

We developed six conceptual categories: (1) Am I ill or is this normal? (2) It effects who I am and how I feel; (3) I feel stigmatised, ashamed and guilty; (4) talking can be difficult but it can help; (5) keeping incontinence under control; (6) have I got to the point that I need help? These categories can help us to understand what it is like to live with UI, and also to understand the barriers to healthcare. In particular, the difficulty of deciding whether or not incontinence is a medical problem the stigma of being incontinent, finding it difficult to talk about incontinence and also the use of effective strategies to stay dry (pads, staying at home, micro-managing access to toilets) can all be barriers to seeking help and accessing strategies to improve continence.

Our findings demonstrate that even though UI is framed as part and parcel of life (up to a point); it profoundly affects a person's quality of life. Our findings demonstrate the complexity of: deciding whether or not I am ill enough to seek help; deciding whether to tell someone or to keep quiet; deciding to use strategies that conceal UI or strategies (although nebulous) that might make me continent again. These decisions pivot upon the success (or not) of keeping UI *'under control'*. Our model demonstrates that it is not always clear whether or not I am ill, and whether or not I should seek help. Similarly, in a meta-ethnography of chronic pelvic pain, Toye, Seers and Barker found that women with chronic pelvic pain struggled to 'know if my pain is abnormal or whether this is normal for women' [14].

Our findings also indicate that the challenge of accessing healthcare is exacerbated by a *culture of secrecy* around certain conditions, such as UI and chronic pelvic

**Table 4** GRADE-CERQUAL summary of findings

| Review finding | Studies contributing | Methodological limitations | Relevance | Coherence number of studies | Adequacy number of themes | Overall confidence |
|---|---|---|---|---|---|---|
| Am i ill or is this normal? | [116–121, 123, 125, 129–131, 133–135, 137–142, 144–146, 150, 151, 153, 154, 156] | 3 key paper, 38 satisfactory | 34 direct, 3 indirect, 3 partial | 28/41 | 80 | High 20 to 31 studies contributed 69 to 93 concepts that supported these themes. We also found rich use of narrative to support the themes |
| It effects who i am and how i feel | [126, 127, 129–131, 133–137, 139, 141–145, 148, 149, 151, 153] | 2 key paper, 39 satisfactory | 37 direct, 3 indirect 1 partial | 20/41 | 69 | |
| I feel stigmatised, ashamed and guilty | [116–119, 121–125, 127–131, 134–137, 140–145, 149, 152, 155, 156] | 4 key paper, 37 satisfactory | 38 direct, 2 indirect 1 partial | 28/41 | 80 | |
| Talking can be difficult (but it can help) | [116–120, 122–125, 128–134, 137, 138, 140, 142, 144–149, 151, 153–156] | 3 key paper, 38 satisfactory | 33 direct, 5 indirect, 3 part al | 31/41 | 93 | |
| I must keep incontinence under control | [116–123, 125, 127, 128, 131, 133–143, 150–153, 155, 156] | 4 key paper, 37 satisfactory | 34 direct, 4 indirect, 3 part al | 29/41 | 76 | |
| Have i got to the point that i need help? | [118, 125, 134, 135, 145, 146, 150, 154, 155] | 1 key paper, 40 satisfactory | 40 direct, 1 indirect | 9/41 | 17 | Moderate downgraded due to fewer studies contributing although narrative rich |

**Table 5** translation of ideas across QES

| Original Finding | Essence Of Original Finding Translated Into First Person | Am i ill or is this normal | It effects who i am and how i feel | I feel stigmatised, ashamed & guilty | Talking can be difficult (but it can help) | I must keep it under control | Have i got to the point that i need help? |
|---|---|---|---|---|---|---|---|
| Mendes & Colleague s[26]: Cultural and religious backgrounds and personal reluctance contribute to delays in seeking UI treatment | I don't want to ask for professional help. There is no opportunity to share my problems with a HCP, I want to deal with it without professional help, I don't have a clear physical symptom; I don't want to find out that I have something serious; God will cure me; he won't let me suffer. It's not serious; other things are more important | YES | | | | | YES |
| Mendes & Colleague s[26]: The inevitable and regrettable problem of UI endured silently and alone affects women's daily activities and their social roles | I regret having UI; but other people have it too. My daily life is affected. I avoid thing that I used to do; I don't go to RE and social gatherings as much now I silently endure the loneliness. I can't go out because I need the loo all the time. I worry about what others will think and keep it a secret. | | YES | YES | YES | YES | |
| Mendes & Colleague s[26]: Poor knowledge and the vague nature of the symptoms mask the fact that UI is a disease | UI is a vague condition that we don't know much about. The symptoms are vague. It is not recognised as a disease. We don't talk about it so people don't know about it. | YES | | | | | |
| Mendes & Colleagues [26]: The experiences provoked by UI and the sense of shame regarding the condition have impaired women's lives | UI makes me anxious, distressed. It carries a stigma. It is so embarrassing and humiliating when I leak in public. I feel depressed and hopeless and have low self-esteem because I can't do the things that I used to do and I can't do much to help myself. It is an emotional experience. I am ashamed | YES | | YES | | | |
| Mendes & Colleague s[26]: UI has provoked negative effects on women's intimacy and sexual satisfaction and provoked changes in the way they experience their sexuality and sexual function | I feel fear, shame, blame and guilt. It has affected intimacy and my sexual satisfaction. | YES | | YES | | | |
| Mendes & Colleague s[26]: UI is considered a consequence of pregnancy and childbirth, inherent to aging or a religious punishment | UI is a natural result of pregnancy and childbirth. It is part of ageing. It is a punishment and I must just accept it. | YES | | | | | |
| Mendes & Colleague s[26]: The women affected by UI adopt several strategies to improve their health status | I try and learn things so that I can control the consequences of UI. I seek professional help. I try and keep it under control; I manage using various strategies | | | | | YES | YES |
| Mendes & Colleague s[26]: Women have personal preferences towards care providers and treatments; they confront difficulties through UI treatment and some care needs are not met' | My health needs are not being met. Doctors lack interest. I am not being taken seriously. There are language barriers; there is no medical diagnosis or plan. It is difficult to understand / adhere to treatments prescribed. I prefer a female Hcp; I prefer my own family to translate or at least someone of my own ethnicity | | | | YES | | |

**Table 5** translation of ideas across QES *(Continued)*

| Original Finding | Essence Of Original Finding Translated Into First Person | Am i ill or is this normal | It effects who i am and how i feel | I feel stigmatised, ashamed & guilty | Talking can be difficult (but it can help) | I must keep it under control | Have i got to the point that i need help? |
|---|---|---|---|---|---|---|---|
| Siddiqui and Colleagues [25]: UI management | I need to adhere to strict routines and strategies to manage UI. I need to make plans for being in public, including knowing where toilets are. It is only a minor, it is normal so I don't seek treatment. It is difficult to communicate with the dr. they don't take it seriously. They need to talk more clearly. I would prefer to see a woman | YES | | | YES | YES | |
| Siddiqui and Colleagues [25]: UI experience | I feel fear, stigmatization, and shame. I worry what people think. I feel disgusting. | | YES | YES | | | |

pain [14]: Incontinence is experienced as taboo. Talking about UI can be a *blessing and a curse* [132], and needs to be carefully managed. Although there are clear benefits to be gained from discussing UI, the risk of exposure can be a weighty burden to bear. We see that people with UI feel stigmatised, ashamed and guilty. Healthcare encounters can contribute to this sense of guilt: for example, at times patients are made to feel that UI 'is my fault because I haven't done my exercises'. It can be difficult to reconcile the idea that incontinence is a normal and expected part of life with these associated feelings of shame: 'I feel vile'.

There are anthropological concepts that help to explain the profound sense of defilement associated with UI. For example, in the seminal text, 'Purity and Danger', Douglas explores the concept of pollution and taboo [170]. Douglas describes how feelings of abhorrence, defilement and 'dirt' stem from a cultural reaction to ambiguity and anomaly: 'Dirt offends against order' (page 2). Our findings demonstrate that UI is indeed experienced as anomalous, as it defies social categorisation: I am ill and also not ill; urination is normal and also not normal; I am an adult and also not like an adult. This sense of anomaly is intensified because the boundary between inside and outside the body is unconventionally and unexpectedly breached. Thus, people living with UI exist in a liminal social space that is 'betwixt and between' states [171]:

> 'These [liminal] persons elude or slip through the network of classifications that normally locate states and positions in cultural space. Liminal entities are neither here nor there; they are betwixt and between the positions assigned and arrayed by law, custom, convention, and ceremonial' (page 144).

The anomaly of UI can make it very difficult talk about, and this may help to explain why only the tip of the iceberg seek care or see a pelvic floor specialist [4]. Although Talcott-Parson's *Sick Role* [172] indicates that we are obliged to go to the doctor in order to access the privileges of the Sick Role, people with ambiguous or stigmatised conditions are torn between the incentive to access these privileges, and the cultural incentive to keep quiet.

Our conceptual model also highlights potential differences between patients and healthcare professionals' understanding of what it means to keep UI under control. We see that people with UI focus on *concealing* UI, rather than improving continence, and go to great lengths to avoid risky situations. In contrast to this, the NICE guidelines for incontinence recommend PFMT as the first line treatment for UI, and stipulate that concealment strategies such as, 'absorbent products, hand held urinals and toileting aids should not be considered as a treatment for UI', but only used as 'a coping strategy pending definitive treatment an adjunct to ongoing therapy' [173]. Although a Cochrane review of trials found that PFMT can 'cure and improve' UI [3], our finding show that people find exercises somewhat nebulous. This is likely to be a significant barrier to adherence for PFMT. Hay-Smith and colleagues also found that women with UI could find it difficult to understand and perform PFMT [23].

Toye and colleagues suggest that it would be 'useful to find ways in which we can be more discerning about what to include' in QES [35]. QES reviewers spend a lot of time searching for studies and this time might be more valuable spent on analysis. Toye and colleagues suggest that it is important for reviewers (and funders) to consider whether or not an exhaustive search of the literature is necessary for QES [8]. We limited our search to Medline for several reasons: firstly, previous QES have shown that Medline retrieves a large proportion of the studies included in a QES [7, 13, 14, 35]; secondly, our scoping review indicated that we were likely to find a large number of studies; thirdly, although Campbell and colleague suggest that 38 studies is sufficient for meta-ethnography [33], there is limited agreement about the optimum amount of studies required to have confidence in QES findings. Intuitively, a certain weight and spread of data appears more convincing. However, the *richness* of data contributing to a finding may make a weightier contribution to idea development. Our findings raise some concerns about the comprehensiveness of search strategies for QES. Firstly, our search of a single database using search terms developed for QES identified more studies than other QES using more than one database. Secondly, other QES exploring particular aspects of UI indicate that there are other relevant studies that were not found; for example [62, 174–177]. Finally, through serendipity we identified other relevant studies beyond our purposive search; for example [178, 179]. The question remains, how long is a piece of string? It may be that continuing to search for studies beyond the point of theoretical saturation is not time well spent. The two studies identified when we re ran our search did not highlight any additional concepts, suggesting saturation of conceptual categories [168, 169]. Our findings resonate with those in two descriptive QES of UI [25, 26]. Siddiqui and colleagues discuss the shame and secrecy of UI (experiences), the struggle to decide whether it is normal and if anything will help (understanding), the secrecy and difficulty communicating with health professionals (behaviours). Vetthanayagam and colleagues also explore 'being brushed aside' by health professionals, the feeling that I must 'put up with it' because it is normal and because I am embarrassed and also the point at which 'something has to be done'.

A growing number of researchers are appraising studies for QES; the percentage of qualitative syntheses including quality appraisal increased from 40% (1988–2004) to 72% (2005–2008) [18]. This number may increase further in the current research climate. However, Campbell and colleagues [33] argue that 'inclusion of poorer quality qualitative research. .. is unlikely to be as damaging' and do not exclude studies on the basis of poorly reported methods [33]. In contrast, Dixon Woods and colleagues exclude studies which they judge to be 'fatally flawed' [17]. We made the cost-benefit decision to appraise studies, as suggested by Dixon-Woods, as: 'key' (conceptually rich); 'satisfactory'; 'irrelevant'; or 'fatally flawed' [37]. For the purposes of meta-ethnography, we suggest that it is important to determine whether or not a study is good enough or *satisfactory* [38]. However, high quality studies that include robust ideas will influence the analytical output and weaker studies will not: thus we agree that low quality studies will do no harm. Similarly, no harm is done by including themes from studies that draw data from the same cohort. This is a key difference between meta-analysis and meta-ethnography. This is because QES relies on abstracting the essence of ideas from studies, and it is very common for different themes from the same cohort to appear in different publications. This does no harm because QES does not hinge on numerical analysis.

We aimed to use QES to further understand the experience of living with UI and the potential barriers to seeking help and therefore receiving appropriate treatment. Most of the studies explored women's experience of UI and further studies might usefully explore, and compare, what it is like for men. We did not include the experience of pregnant women or the experience within the first year peri-partum. However, we did include two studies by Mason and colleagues [137, 138] as these included the experience of 15 women who were symptomatic 1 year after childbirth. However, the first experience of involuntary leakage for many women is during pregnancy or after a birth, and childbirth is a strong predictor of UI. Further research would usefully explore the differences is experience during childbirth and peri-partum. The majority of studies explored experience of women in high income countries; only four studies explored the experience of women from in upper middle income countries (Brazil, China and Iran) and one study explored the experience in a lower income country (Ethiopia) (Table 2). It is likely that the experience of incontinence would differ between countries and further research might highlight these differences. However, we demonstrate that there are important themes that cut across age, gender and type of UI. Further primary studies would usefully explore differences in specific samples related to gender, age, pathophysiology or other factors.

## Conclusions

There are some important clinical considerations and implications that can be drawn. Firstly, the culture of secrecy and profound sense of shame felt by those with UI makes it very difficult for people to talk about it and to seek help. Proactively asking patients about UI would help to reduce the taboo and ensure that help is made available. This finding may be usefully extended to other anomalous and embarrassing health conditions. Secondly, differences in the concept of what it is to keep UI under control have direct implications for clinical care. Research indicates that PFMT can improve continence and yet this is not the focus of many people's control strategies. A cultural environment which reduces the shame and stigma of UI may help people to switch the focus to strategies that will improve continence (i.e. PFMT). At the same time, it would be useful for healthcare professionals to recognise a person's need to conceal UI, and to collaborate in a treatment approach that not only facilitates this need, but that also aims to improve continence. Finally, future research should address the issue of nebulosity of PFMT, as this is likely to have a direct effect on adherence when balanced against a person's competing needs.

### Abbreviations

GRADE-CERQual: Grading of Recommendations Assessment, Development and Evaluation-Confidence in the Evidence from Reviews of Qualitative research; NHS: National Health Service (UK); PFMT: Pelvic floor muscle training; QES: Qualitative Evidence Synthesis; STARLITE: Sampling strategy, type of study, approaches, range of years, limits, inclusion and exclusions, terms used, electronic sources; UI: Urinary Incontinence

### Acknowledgements

Not applicable.

### Authors' contributions

FT and KB made a substantial contribution to the design, acquisition, analysis and interpretation of data. FT drafted the first, subsequent and final versions. KB revised all versions for important intellectual content and approved the final version. Both authors agree to be accountable for the accuracy and integrity of the work. Both authors have read and approved the manuscript.

### Competing interests

The authors declare that they have no competing interests.

## References


1. Hay-Smith E, Herderschee R, Dumoulin C, Herbison G. Comparisons of approaches to pelvic floor muscle training for urinary incontinence in women (Review). Cochrane Database Syst Rev. 2011;12(CD009508):1–110.
2. Buckley BS, Lapitan MCM. Prevalence of urinary incontinence in men, women, and children—current evidence: findings of the fourth international consultation on incontinence. Urology. 2010;76(2):265–70.
3. Dumoulin C, Cacciari LP, Hay-Smith EJC. Pelvic floor muscle training versus no treatment, or inactive control treatments, for urinary incontinence in women. Cochrane Database Syst Rev. 2018;10:CD005654 https://doi.org/10.1002/14651858.CD005654.pub4.
4. Minassian V, Yan X, Lichtenfeld M, Sun H, Stewart W. The iceberg of health care utilization in women with urinary incontinence. Int Urogynecol J. 2012;23(1):1087–93.
5. Noyes J, Popay J, Pearson A, Hannes K, Booth A. Qualitative research and cochrane reviews. In: Higgins J, Green S, editors. Cochrane Handbook for Systematic Reviews. Chichester: Wiley; 2008.
6. Noblit G, Hare R. Meta-ethnography: Synthesising qualitative studies. California: Sage Publications; 1988.
7. Toye F, Seers K, Allcock N, Briggs M, Carr E, Andrews J, Barker K. A meta-ethnography of patients' experiences of chronic non-malignant musculoskeletal pain. Health Serv Deliv Res. 2013;1(12):1–189.
8. Toye F, Seers K, Allcock N, Briggs M, Carr E, Barker K. Meta-ethnography 25 years on: challenges and insights for synthesising a large number of qualitative studies. BMC Med Res Methodol. 2014;14:80.
9. France EF, Cunningham M, Ring N, Uny I, Duncan EA, Jepson RG, Maxwell M, Roberts RJ, Turley RL, Booth A, et al. Improving reporting of meta-ethnography: The eMERGe reporting guidance. J Adv Nurs. 0(0) p. 1-13.
10. Toye F, Seers K, Allcock N, Briggs M, Carr E, Barker K. A synthesis of qualitative research exploring the barriers to staying in work with chronic musculoskeletal pain. Disabil Rehabil. 2016;38(6):566–72.
11. Daker-White G, Donovan J, Campbell R. Redefined by illness: meta-ethnography of qualitative studies on the experience of rheumatoid arthritis. Disabil Rehabil. 2014;36(13):1061–71.
12. Mengshoel A, Marit A, Sim J, Birgitte A, Madden S. Diagnostic experience of patients with fibromyalgia - A meta-ethnography. Chronic Illn. 2017;0(0) http://journals.sagepub.com/doi/pdf/10.1177/1742395317718035.
13. Barker K, Toye F, Lowe C. A qualitative systematic review of patients' experience of osteoporosis using meta-ethnography. Arch Osteoporos. 2016;11(1):1–13.
14. Toye F, Seers K, Barker K. A meta-ethnography of patients' experiences of chronic pelvic pain: struggling to construct chronic pelvic pain as 'real'. J Adv Nurs. 2014;70(12):2713–27.
15. Sandelowski M, Barrosso J. Handbook for synthesising qualitative research. New York: Springer Publishing Company; 2007.
16. Dixon-Woods M, Booth A, Sutton A. Synthesizing qualitative research: a review of published reports. Qual Res. 2007;7:375–422.
17. Dixon-Woods M, Agarwal S, Jones D, Young B, Sutton A. Synthesising qualitative and quantitative research evidence: a review of possible methods. J Health Serv Res Policy. 2005;10(1):45–53.
18. Hannes K, Macaitis K. A move to more systematic and transparent approaches in qualitative evidence synthesis: update on a review of published papers. Qual Res. 2012;12(4):402–42.
19. Barnett-Page E, Thomas J. Methods for synthesis of qualitative research: a critical review. In: Economic and Social Research Council Research Methods, National Centre for Research Methods Working Paper Series (01/09); 2009.
20. Toye F, Seers K, Hannink E, Barker K. A mega-ethnography of eleven qualitative evidence syntheses exploring the experience of living with chronic non-malignant pain. BMC Med Res Methodol. 2017;17(1):116.
21. Toye F, Seers K, Barker K: Living life precariously with rheumatoid arthritis - A mega-ethnography of nine qualitative evidence syntheses. BMC Rheumatol 2019, accepted for publication.
22. French B, Thomas LH, Harrison J, Coupe J, Roe B, Booth J, Cheater FM, Leathley MJ, Watkins CL, Hay-Smith J. Client and clinical staff perceptions of barriers to and enablers of the uptake and delivery of behavioural interventions for urinary incontinence: qualitative evidence synthesis. J Adv Nurs. 2017;73(1):21–38.
23. Hay-Smith J, Dean S, Burgio K, McClurg D, Frawley H, Dumoulin C. Pelvic-floor-muscle-training adherence 'modifiers': a review of primary qualitative studies—2011 ICS state-of-the-science seminar research paper III of IV. Neurourol Urodyn. 2015;34(7):622–31.
24. Avery JC, Braunack-Mayer AJ, Stocks NP, Taylor AW, Duggan P. Psychological perspectives in urinary incontinence: a metasynthesis. OA Women's Health. 2013;1(1):1–10.
25. Siddiqui N, Levin P, Ammarell N, Phadtare A, Pietrobon R. Perceptions about female urinary incontinence in different racial and ethnic groups: a systematic review. Neurourol Urodyn. 2012;31(6):1000–1.
26. Mendes A, Hoga L, Goncalves B, Silva P, Pereira P. Adult women's experiences of urinary incontinence: a systematic review of qualitative evidence. JBI Database System Rev Implement Rep. 2017;15(5):1350–408.
27. Wong SSWN, Haynes RB. Developing optimal search strategies for detecting clinically relevant qualitative studies in MEDLINE. Medinfo. 2004;11(1):311–6.
28. Wilczynski NLMS, Haynes RB. Search strategies for identifying qualitative studies in CINAHL. Qual Health Res. 2007;17(5):705–10.
29. McKibbon KAWN, Haynes RB. Developing optimal search strategies for retrieving qualitative studies in PsycINFO. Eval Health Prof. 2006;29(4):440–54.
30. WN WLA, Haynes RB. Hedges team. Developing optimal search strategies for retrieving clinically relevant qualitative studies in EMBASE. Qual Health Res. 2006;16(1):162–8.
31. Toye F, Seers K, Barker K. A meta-ethnography of health-care professionals' experience of treating adults with chronic non-malignant pain to improve the experience and quality of health care. In: Health Services and Delivery Research. Edn. NIHR Journals Library: Southampton; 2018.
32. Barker K, Toye F, MinnsLowe C. A qualitative systematic review of patients' experience of osteoporosis using meta-ethnography. Arch Osteoporos. 2016;11(33) https://doi.org/10.1007/s11657-11016-10286-z.
33. Campbell R, Pound P, Morgan M, Daker-White G, Britten N, Pill R, Yardley L, Pope C, Donovan J. Evaluating meta-ethnography: systematic analysis and synthesis of qualitative research. Health Technol Assess. 2011;15(43):1–157.
34. Charmaz K. Constructing grounded theory. California: Sage Publications; 2006.
35. Toye F, Seers K, Tierney S, Barker K. A qualitative evidence synthesis to explore healthcare professionals' experience of prescribing opioids to adults with chronic non-malignant pain. BMC Fam Pract. 2017;18:94 https://www.ncbi.nlm.nih.gov/pmc/articles/PMC5702226/pdf/5712875_5702017_Article_5702663.pdf.
36. Booth A. 'Brimful of STARLITE': toward standards for reporting literature searches. J Med Libr Assoc. 2006;94(4):421–e205.
37. Dixon-Woods M, Sutton A, Shaw R, Miller T, Smith J, Young B, Bonas S, Booth A, Jones D. Appraising qualitative research for inclusion in systematic reviews: a quantitative and qualitative comparison of three methods. J Health ServRes Policy. 2007;12(1):42–7.
38. Toye F, Seers K, Allcock N, Briggs M, Carr E, Andrews J, Barker K. 'Trying to pin down jelly' - exploring intuitive processes in quality assessment for meta-ethnography. BMC Med Res Methodol. 2013;13:46.
39. Nvivo. Nvivo qualitatitve data analysis and software, QSR International Pty Ltd. In: Software for qualitative data analysis. 9th ed; 2010.
40. Tavory I, Timmermans S. Abductive analysis - theorizing qualitative research. Chicago: University of Chicago Press; 2014.
41. Pope C, Mays N, Popay J. Synthesizing qualitative and quantitative health research: a guide to methods. Berkshire: Open University Press; 2007.
42. Lewin S, Glenton C, Munthe-Kaas H, Carlsen B, Colvin CJ, Gülmezoglu M, Noyes J, Booth A, Garside R, Rashidian A. Using Qualitative Evidence in Decision Making for Health and Social Interventions: An Approach to Assess Confidence in Findings from Qualitative Evidence Syntheses (GRADE-CERQual). PLOS Med. 2016;12(10):e1001895 https://doi.org/10.1371/journal.pmed.1001895.
43. Noyes J, Booth A, Lewin S, Carlsen B, Glenton C, Colvin CJ, Garside R, Bohren MA, Rashidian A, Wainwright M, et al. Applying GRADE-CERQual to qualitative evidence synthesis findings–paper 6: how to assess relevance of the data. Implement Sci. 2018;13(suppl 1):4.
44. Munthe-Kaas H, Bohren M, Glenton C, Lewin S, Noyes J, Tunçalp Ö, Booth A, Garside R, Colvin C, Wainwright M, et al. Applying GRADE-CERQual to qualitative evidence synthesis findings—paper 3: how to assess methodological limitations. Implement Sci. 2018;13(suppl 1):9.

45. Lewin S, Booth A, Glenton C, Munthe-Kaas H, Rashidian A, Wainwright M, Bohren M, Tunçalp Ö, Colvin C, Garside R, et al. Applying GRADE-CERQual to qualitative evidence synthesis findings: introduction to the series. Implement Sci. 2018;13(Suppl 1):2.
46. Lewin S, Bohren M, Rashidian A, Munthe-Kaas H, Glenton C, Colvin C, Garside R, Noyes J, Booth A, Tunçalp Ö, et al. Applying GRADE-CERQual to qualitative evidence synthesis findings—paper 2: how to make an overall CERQual assessment of confidence and create a Summary of Qualitative Findings table. Implement Sci. 2018;13(supp1):10.
47. Glenton C, Carlsen B, Lewin S, Munthe-Kaas H, Colvin CJ, Tunçalp Ö, Bohren MA, Noyes J, Booth A, Garside R, et al. Applying GRADE-CERQual to qualitative evidence synthesis findings—paper 5: how to assess adequacy of data. Implement Sci. 2018;13(supp 1):14.
48. Colvin C, Garside R, Wainwright M, Munthe-Kaas H, Glenton C, Bohren M, Carlsen B, Tunçalp Ö, Noyes J, Booth A, et al. Applying GRADE-CERQual to qualitative evidence synthesis findings—paper 4: how to assess coherence. Implement Sci. 2018;13(suppl 1):13.
49. Booth A, Lewin S, Glenton C, Munthe-Kaas H, Toews I, Noyes J, Rashidian A, Berg RC, Nyakang'o B, Meerpoh JJ, et al. Applying GRADE-CERQual to qualitative evidence synthesis findings–paper 7: understanding the potential impacts of dissemination bias. Implement Sci. 2018;13(suppl 1):1–70.
50. Kemp K, Griffiths J, Lovell K. Understanding the health and social care needs of people living with IBD: a meta-synthesis of the evidence. World J Gastroenterol. 2012;18(43):6240–9.
51. Koch LH. Help-seeking behaviors of women with urinary incontinence: an integrative literature review. J Midwifery Women's Health. 2006;51(6):e39.
52. Mendes A, Hoga L, Gonçalves B, Silva P, Pereira P. Adult women's experiences of urinary incontinence: a systematic review of qualitative evidence protocol. JBI Database System Rev Implement Rep. 2015;13(3): 103–10.
53. Ostaszkiewicz J, O'Connell B, Dunning T. Residents' perspectives on urinary incontinence: a review of literature. Scand J Caring Sci. 2012;26(4):761–72.
54. Strickland R. Reasons for not seeking care for urinary incontinence in older community-dwelling women: a contemporary review. Urol Nurs. 2014;34(2): 63.
55. Terzoni S, Montanari E, Mora C, Destrebecq A. Urinary incontinence in adults: nurses' beliefs, education and role in continence promotion. A narrative review. Arch Ital Urol Androl. 2011;83(4):213–6.
56. Dingwall L, McLafferty E. Do nurses promote urinary continence in hospitalized older people?: an exploratory study. J Clin Nurs. 2006;15(10): 1276–86.
57. Ehlman K, Wilson A, Dugger R, Eggleston B, Coudret N, Mathis S. Nursing home staff members' attitudes and knowledge about urinary incontinence: the impact of technology and training. Urol Nurs. 2012;32(4):205–13.
58. Lyons SS. How do people make continence care happen? An analysis of organizational culture in two nursing homes. Gerontologist. 2010;50(3):327–39.
59. MacDonald CD, Butler L. Silent no more: elderly women's stories of living with urinary incontinence in long-term care. J Gerontol Nurs. 2007;33(1):14–20.
60. Mason M, Tully S. Urinary incontinence in the older acute care population: effects of knowledge, attitudes and beliefs of nurses on continence management. Perspectives. 2002;26(3):4–9.
61. Mather KF, Bakas T. Nursing assistants' perceptions of their ability to provide continence care. Geriatr Nurs (New York, NY). 2002;23(2):76–81.
62. O'Dell KK, Jacelon C, Morse AN. 'I'd rather just go on as I am'--pelvic floor care preferences of frail, elderly women in residential care. Urol Nurs. 2008; 28(1):36–47.
63. Resnick B, Keilman LJ, Calabrese B, Parmelee P, Lawhorne L, Pailet J, Ouslander J. Nursing staff beliefs and expectations about continence care in nursing homes. J Wound Ostomy Continence Nurs. 2006;33(6):610–8.
64. Robinson JP. Managing urinary incontinence in the nursing home: residents' perspectives. J Adv Nurs. 2000;31(1):68–77.
65. Sylvia CJ, Jones V. The lived experience of the wound, ostomy, and continence nurse in wound care. J Wound Ostomy Continence Nurs. 2010; 37(3):265–71.
66. Taunton RL, Swagerty DL, Lasseter JA, Lee RH. Continent or incontinent? That is the question. J Gerontol Nurs. 2005;31(9):36–44.
67. Chelvanayagam S, Stern J. Using therapeutic groups to support women with faecal incontinence. Br J Nurs. 2007;16(4):214–8 (Mark Allen Publishing).
68. Collings S, Norton C. Women's experiences of faecal incontinence: a study. Br J Community Nurs. 2004;9(12):520–3.
69. Frohlich DO. Support often outweighs stigma for people with inflammatory bowel disease. Gastroenterol Nurs. 2014;37(2):126–36.
70. Olsson F, Berterö C. Living with faecal incontinence: trying to control the daily life that is out of control. J Clin Nurs. 2015;24(1–2):141–50.
71. Peden-McAlpine C, Bliss D, Becker B, Sherman S. The experience of community-living men managing fecal incontinence. Rehabil Nurs. 2012; 37(6):298–306.
72. Peden-McAlpine C, Bliss D, Hill J. The experience of community-living women managing fecal incontinence. West J Nurs Res. 2008;30(7):817–35.
73. Rasmussen JL, Ringsberg KC. Being involved in an everlasting fight--a life with postnatal faecal incontinence. A qualitative study. Scand J Caring Sci. 2010;24(1):108–15.
74. Rimmer CJ, Gill KA, Greenfield S, Dowswell G. The design and initial patient evaluation of an integrated care pathway for faecal incontinence: a qualitative study. BMC Health Serv Res. 2015;15:444.
75. Tucker J, Clifton V, Wilson A. Teetering near the edge; women's experiences of anal incontinence following obstetric anal sphincter injury: an interpretive phenomenological research study. Aust N Z J Obstet Gynaecol. 2014;54(4):377–81.
76. Wilson M. The impact of faecal incontinence on the quality of life. Br J Nurs. 2007;16(4):204–7 (Mark Allen Publishing).
77. Wilson M. Living with faecal incontinence: follow-up to a research project. Br J Nurs. 2013;22(3):147 (Mark Allen Publishing).
78. Wilson M. Living with faecal incontinence: a 10-year follow-up study. Br J Nurs. 2015;24(5):268 (Mark Allen Publishing).
79. Brittain KR, Shaw C. The social consequences of living with and dealing with incontinence--a carers perspective. Soc Sci Med (1982). 2007;65(6): 1274–83.
80. Cassells C, Watt E. The impact of incontinence on older spousal caregivers. J Adv Nurs. 2003;42(6):607–16.
81. Coyne KS, Matza LS, Brewster-Jordan J. 'We have to stop again?!': The impact of overactive bladder on family members. Neurourol Urodyn. 2009; 28(8):969–75.
82. Hayder D, Schnepp W. Urinary incontinence - the family caregivers' perspective. Z Gerontol Geriatr. 2008;41(4):261–6.
83. Santini S, Andersson G, Lamura G. Impact of incontinence on the quality of life of caregivers of older persons with incontinence: a qualitative study in four European countries. Arch Gerontol Geriatr. 2016;63:92–101.
84. Lobchuk MM, Rosenberg F. A qualitative analysis of individual and family caregiver responses to the impact of urinary incontinence on quality of life. J Wound Ostomy Continence Nurs. 2014;41(6):589–96.
85. Butterfield YC, O'Connell B, Phillips D. Peripartum urinary incontinence: a study of midwives' knowledge and practices. Women Birth. 2007;20(2):65–9.
86. Grealish M, O'Dowd TC. General practitioners and women with urinary incontinence. Br J General Pract. 1998;48(427):975–7.
87. Hägglund D. District continence nurses' experiences of their continence service in primary health care. J Nurs Manag. 2010;18(2):225–33.
88. Hutchings J, Sutherland L. Student nurse understanding of the psychosocial impact of urinary incontinence. Urol Nurs. 2014;34(6):318–25.
89. Newman DK. Talking to patients about bladder control problems. Nurse Pract. 2009;34(12):33–45.
90. Peters S. Don't ask, don't tell. Breaking the silence surrounding female urinary incontinence. Adv Nurse Pract. 1997;5(5):41–4.
91. Rolnick S, Bliss DZ, Jackson JM, Arntson C, Mullins J, Hepburn K. Healthcare providers' perspectives on communicating incontinence and skin damage information with patients with dementia and their family caregivers: a descriptive study. Ostomy Wound Manage. 2013;59(4):62–7.
92. Shaw C, Atwell C, Wood F, Brittain K, Williams K. A qualitative study of the assessment and treatment of incontinence in primary care. Fam Pract. 2007; 24(5):461–7.
93. Siu JY-M. Communicating with mismatch and tension: treatment provision experiences of primary care doctors treating patients with overactive bladder in Hong Kong. BMC Fam Pract. 2015;16:160.
94. Tannenbaum C, Labrecque D, Lepage C. Understanding barriers to continence care in institutions. Can J Aging. 2005;24(2):151–9.
95. Teunissen D, van den Bosch W, van Weel C, Lagro-Janssen T. Urinary incontinence in the elderly: attitudes and experiences of general practitioners. A focus group study. Scand J Prim Health Care. 2006; 24(1):56–61.

96. Basu M, Duckett JRA. Barriers to seeking treatment for women with persistent or recurrent symptoms in urogynaecology. BJOG. 2009;116(5): 726–30.
97. Sevilla C, Wieslander CK, Alas AN, Dunivan GC, Khan AA, Maliski SL, Rogers RG, Anger JT. Communication between physicians and Spanish-speaking Latin American women with pelvic floor disorders: a cycle of misunderstanding? Female Pelvic Med Reconstr Surg. 2013;19(2):90–7.
98. Srikrishna S, Robinson D, Cardozo L. Qualifying a quantitative approach to women's expectations of continence surgery. Int Urogynecol J Pelvic Floor Dysfunct. 2009;20(7):859–65.
99. Buurman MBR, Lagro-Janssen ALM. Women's perception of postpartum pelvic floor dysfunction and their help-seeking behaviour: a qualitative interview study. Scand J Caring Sci. 2013;27(2):406–13.
100. Roe B, May C. Incontinence and sexuality: findings from a qualitative perspective. J Adv Nurs. 1999;30(3):573–9.
101. Lindeman K, Li Y, Palmer MH. Help-seeking for incontinence by individuals with heart failure. J Am Geriatr Soc. 2012;60(10):1994–5.
102. Bush TA, Castellucci DT, Phillips C. Exploring women's beliefs regarding urinary incontinence. Urol Nurs. 2001;21(3):211–8.
103. Bradway C, Dahlberg B, Barg FK. How women conceptualize urinary incontinence: a cultural model. J Women's Health (2002). 2010;19(8):1533–41.
104. Hart KJ, Palmer MH, Fitzgerald S. Perceived causes of urinary incontinence and reporting: a study with working women. Clin Nurs Res. 1999;8(1):84–92.
105. Chaliha C, Stanton SL. The ethnic cultural and social aspects of incontinence--a pilot study. Int Urogynecol J Pelvic Floor Dysfunct. 1999; 10(3):166–70.
106. Kang Y, Crogan NL. Social and cultural construction of urinary incontinence among Korean American elderly women. Geriatr Nurs (New York, NY). 2008; 29(2):105–11.
107. Anger JT, Le TX, Nissim HA, Rogo-Gupta L, Rashid R, Behniwal A, Smith AL, Litwin MS, Rodriguez LV, Wein AJ, et al. How dry is 'OAB-dry'? Perspectives from patients and physician experts. J Urol. 2012;188(5):1811–5.
108. Coyne KS, Sexton CC, Thompson C, Bavendam T, Brubaker L. Development and psychometric evaluation of the urgency questionnaire for evaluating severity and health-related quality of life impact of urinary urgency in overactive bladder. Int Urogynecol J. 2015;26(3):373–82.
109. Bradway C, Strumpf N. Seeking care: women's narratives concerning long-term urinary incontinence. Urol Nurs. 2008;28(2):123–9.
110. Bradway CW, Barg F. Developing a cultural model for long-term female urinary incontinence. Soc Sci Med (1982). 2006;63(12):3150–61.
111. Bradway C. Women's narratives of long-term urinary incontinence. Urol Nurs. 2005;25(5):337–44.
112. Diokno AC, Sand PK, Macdiarmid S, Shah R, Armstrong RB. Perceptions and behaviours of women with bladder control problems. Fam Pract. 2006;23(5): 568–77.
113. Filipetto FA, Fulda KG, Holthusen AE, McKeithen TM, McFadden P. The patient perspective on overactive bladder: a mixed-methods needs assessment. BMC Fam Pract. 2014;15:96.
114. Palmer MH, Newman DK. Bladder control educational needs of older adults. J Gerontol Nurs. 2006;32(1):28–32.
115. Teunissen D, van Weel C, Lagro-Janssen T. Urinary incontinence in older people living in the community: examining help-seeking behaviour. Br J General Pract. 2005;55(519):776–82.
116. Andersson G, Johansson J-E, Nilsson K, Sahlberg-Blom E. Accepting and adjusting: older women's experiences of living with urinary incontinence. Urol Nurs. 2008;28(2):115–21.
117. Andersson G, Johansson JE, Nilsson K, Sahlberg-Blom E. Perceptions of urinary incontinence among Syrian Christian women living in Sweden. J Transcult Nurs. 2009;20(3):296–303.
118. Ashworth PD, Hagan MT. The meaning of incontinence: a qualitative study of non-geriatric urinary incontinence sufferers. J Adv Nurs. 1993;18(9):1415–23.
119. Cochran A. Response to urinary incontinence by older persons living in the community. J Wound Ostomy Continence Nurs. 1998;25(6):296–303.
120. Doshani A, Pitchforth E, Mayne CJ, Tincello DG. Culturally sensitive continence care: a qualitative study among south Asian Indian women in Leicester. Fam Pract. 2007;24(6):585–93.
121. Dowd TT. Discovering older women's experience of urinary incontinence. Res Nurs Health. 1991;14(3):179–86.
122. Getliffe K, Fader M, Cottenden A, Jamieson K, Green N. Absorbent products for incontinence: 'treatment effects' and impact on quality of life. J Clin Nurs. 2007;16(10):1936–45.
123. Gjerde JL, Rortveit G, Muleta M, Blystad A. Silently waiting to heal: experiences among women living with urinary incontinence in Northwest Ethiopia. Int Urogynecol J. 2013;24(6):953–8.
124. Griffiths F, Pepper J, Jørstad-Stein EC, Smith JF, Hill L, Lamb SSE. Group versus individual sessions delivered by a physiotherapist for female urinary incontinence: an interview study with women attending group sessions nested within a randomised controlled trial. BMC Womens Health. 2009;9:25.
125. Hägglund D, Wadensten B. Fear of humiliation inhibits women's care-seeking behaviour for long-term urinary incontinence. Scand J Caring Sci. 2007;21(3):305–12.
126. Hägglund D, Ahlström G. The meaning of women's experience of living with long-term urinary incontinence is powerlessness. J Clin Nurs. 2007; 16(10):1946–54.
127. Hamid TA, Pakgohar M, Ibrahim R, Dastjerdi MV. 'Stain in life': the meaning of urinary incontinence in the context of Muslim postmenopausal women through hermeneutic phenomenology. Arch Gerontol Geriatr. 2015;60(3): 514–21.
128. Hayder D, Schnepp W. Experiencing and managing urinary incontinence: a qualitative study. West J Nurs Res. 2010;32(4):480–96.
129. Hayder D. The effects of urinary incontinence on sexuality: seeking an intimate partnership. J Wound Ostomy Continence Nurs. 2012;39(5):539–44.
130. Higa R, Chvatal VLS, de Moraes Lopes MHB, Turato ER. The meanings of silence in Brazilian women with urinary incontinence. J Wound Ostomy Continence Nurs. 2011;38(5):565–8.
131. Horrocks S, Somerset M, Stoddart H, Peters TJ. What prevents older people from seeking treatment for urinary incontinence? A qualitative exploration of barriers to the use of community continence services. Fam Pract. 2004; 21(6):689–96.
132. Jackson CB, Botelho EM, Welch LC, Joseph J, Tennstedt SL. Talking with others about stigmatized health conditions: implications for managing symptoms. Qual Health Res. 2012;22(11):1468–75.
133. Kao H-T, Hayter M, Hinchliff S, Tsai C-H, Hsu M-T. Experience of pelvic floor muscle exercises among women in Taiwan: a qualitative study of improvement in urinary incontinence and sexuality. J Clin Nurs. 2015;24(13–14):1985–94.
134. Komorowski L, Chen B. Female urinary incontinence in China: experiences and perspectives. Health Care Women Int. 2006;27(2):169–81.
135. Li FLW, Low LPL, Lee DTF. Chinese women's experiences in coping with urinary incontinence. J Clin Nurs. 2007;16(3):610–2.
136. MacInnes CL. Why women leave therapy for stress incontinence. Nurs Times. 2008;104(41):50–3.
137. Mason L, Glenn S, Walton I, Appleton C. The experience of stress incontinence after childbirth. Birth (Berkeley, Calif). 1999;26(3):164–71.
138. Mason L, Glenn S, Walton I, Hughes C. Women's reluctance to seek help for stress incontinence during pregnancy and following childbirth. Midwifery. 2001;17(3):212–21.
139. Milne JL, Moore KN. Factors impacting self-care for urinary incontinence. Urol Nurs. 2006;26(1):41–51.
140. Nicolson P, Kopp Z, Chapple CR, Kelleher C. It's just the worry about not being able to control it! A qualitative study of living with overactive bladder. Br J Health Psychol. 2008;13:343–59.
141. Peake S, Manderson L. The constraints of a normal life: the management of urinary incontinence by middle aged women. Women Health. 2003;37(3): 37–51.
142. Peake S, Manderson L, Potts H. 'Part and parcel of being a woman': female urinary incontinence and constructions of control. Med Anthropol Q. 1999; 13(3):267–85.
143. Roos A-M, Thakar R, Sultan AH, Burger CW, Paulus ATG. Pelvic floor dysfunction: women's sexual concerns unraveled. J Sex Med. 2014;11(3): 743–52.
144. Sange C, Thomas L, Lyons C, Hill S. Urinary incontinence in Muslim women. Nurs Times. 2008;104(25):49–52.
145. Shaw C, Tansey R, Jackson C, Hyde C, Allan R. Barriers to help seeking in people with urinary symptoms. Fam Pract. 2001;18(1):48–52.
146. Shaw C, Brittain K, Tansey R, Williams K. How people decide to seek health care: a qualitative study. Int J Nurs Stud. 2008;45(10):1516–24.
147. Shaw C, Williams KS, Assassa RP. Patients' views of a new nurse-led continence service. J Clin Nurs. 2000;9(4):574–82.
148. Siu JY-M. 'Seeing a doctor is just like having a date': a qualitative study on doctor shopping among overactive bladder patients in Hong Kong. BMC Fam Pract. 2014;15:27.

149. Siu JY-M. Communicating under medical patriarchy: gendered doctor-patient communication between female patients with overactive bladder and male urologists in Hong Kong. BMC Womens Health. 2015;15:44.
150. Skoner MM, Haylor MJ. Managing incontinence: women's normalizing strategies. Health Care Women Int. 1993;14(6):549–60.
151. St John W, James H, McKenzie S. 'Oh, that's a bit of a nuisance': community-dwelling clients ' perspectives of urinary continence health service provision. J Wound Ostomy Continence Nurs. 2002;29(6):312–9.
152. van den Muijsenbergh ME, Lagro-Janssen TA. Urinary incontinence in Moroccan and Turkish women: a qualitative study on impact and preferences for treatment. Br J General Pract. 2006;56(533):945–9.
153. Welch LC, Botelho EM, Joseph JJ, Tennstedt SL. A qualitative inquiry of patient-reported outcomes: the case of lower urinary tract symptoms. Nurs Res. 2012;61(4):283–90.
154. Welch LC, Taubenberger S, Tennstedt SL. Patients' experiences of seeking health care for lower urinary tract symptoms. Res Nurs Health. 2011;34(6): 496–507.
155. Wilkinson K. Pakistani women's perceptions and experiences of incontinence. Nurs Standard (Royal College of Nursing (Great Britain) : 1987). 2001;16(5):33–9.
156. Zeznock DE, Gilje FL, Bradway C. Living with urinary incontinence: experiences of women from 'The last frontier'. Urol Nurs. 2009;29(3):157.
157. Hatchett L, Hebert-Beirne J, Tenfelde S, Lavender MD, Brubaker L. Knowledge and perceptions of pelvic floor disorders among african american and Latina women. Female Pelvic Med Reconstr Surg. 2011;17(4): 190–4.
158. Welch LC, Botelho EM, Tennstedt SL. Race and ethnic differences in health beliefs about lower urinary tract symptoms. Nurs Res. 2011;60(3):165–72.
159. Wells M, Wagg A. Integrated continence services and the female Bangladeshi population. Br J Nurs. 2007;16(9):516–9.
160. Akyuz A, Kok G, Kilic A, Guvenc G. In her own words: living with urinary incontinence in sexual life. Sex Disabil. 2014;32(1):23–33.
161. Coyne KS, Margolis MK, Jumadilova Z, Bavendam T, Mueller E, Rogers R. Overactive bladder and women's sexual health: what is the impact? J Sex Med. 2007;4(3):656–66.
162. Delarmelindo RCA, CMGdL P, RAP R, SCM B. Between suffering and hope: rehabilitation from urinary incontinence as an intervening component. Ciênc Saúde Colet. 2013;18(7):1981–91.
163. Siu L-SK, Lopez V. Chinese women's experiences of stress incontinence: a descriptive qualitative study. Int J Urol Nurs. 2012;6(3):125–36.
164. Elstad EA, Taubenberger SP, Botelho EM, Tennstedt SL. Beyond incontinence: the stigma of other urinary symptoms. J Adv Nurs. 2010; 66(11):2460–70.
165. Brown JS, Subak LL, Gras J, Brown BA, Kuppermann M, Posner SF. Urge incontinence: The patient's perspective. J Womens Health. 1998;7(10):1263–9.
166. Klemm LW, Creason NS. Self-care practices of women with urinary incontinence--a preliminary study. Health Care Women Int. 1991;12(2):199–209.
167. Higa R, CRSFd R, Campos LK, MHdM L, Turato ER. Vivências de mulheres brasileiras com incontinência urinária. Texto Contexto Enfermagem. 2010;19: 627–35.
168. Siddiqui NY, Ammarell N, Wu JM, Sandoval JS, Bosworth HB. Urinary incontinence and health-seeking behavior among White, black, and Latina women. Female Pelvic Med Reconstr Surg. 2016;22(5):340–5.
169. Vethanayagam N, Orrell A, Dahlberg L, McKee KJ, Orme S, Parker SG, Gilhooly M. Understanding help-seeking in older people with urinary incontinence: an interview study. Health Soc Care Community. 2017;25(3): 1061–9.
170. Douglas M. Purity and danger: an analysis of the concepts of pollution and taboo. London: Routledge; 1966.
171. Turner V. The ritual process structure and anti-structure. Ithaca: Cornell University Press; 1966.
172. Talcott-Parsons. The social system. New York: New York Free Press; 1951.
173. National-Institute-for-Health-and-Care-Excellence: Urinary incontinence in women: management - Clinical Guideline. 2013. https://www.niceorguk/guidance/cg171/resources/urinary-incontinence-in-women-management-pdf-35109747194821.
174. Hay-Smith EJC, Ryan K, Dean S. The silent, private exercise: experiences of pelvic floor muscle training in a sample of women with stress urinary incontinence. Physiotherapy. 2007;93(1):53–61.
175. Hemachandra NN, Rajapaksa LC, Manderson L. A 'usual occurrence:' stress incontinence among reproductive aged women in Sri Lanka. Soc Sci Med. 2009;69(9):1395–401.
176. Kincade JE, Johnson TM, Ashford-Works C, Clarke MK, Busby-Whitehead J. A pilot study to determine reasons for patient withdrawal from a pelvic muscle rehabilitation program for urinary incontinence. J Appl Gerontol. 1999;18(3):379–96.
177. Teunissen D, Van Den Bosch W, Van Weel C, Lagro-Janssen T. 'It can always happen': the impact of urinary incontinence on elderly men and women. Scand J Prim Health Care. 2006;24(3):166–73.
178. Hamid T-A, Ibrahim R, Vahid-Dastjerdi M. Portrait representation of postmenopausal Women's experiences of living with urinary incontinence AU - Pakgohar. Minoo. J Women Aging. 2015;27(1):81–95.
179. Roin A, Nord C. Urine incontinence in women aged sixty to sixty-five: negotiating meaning and responsibility. Scand J Caring Sci. 2015; 29(4):625–32.

# 6

# Multiple inferior vena cava aneurysms mimic a retroperitoneal tumor

Yuzhi Zuo, Zhenyu Zhang, Bingbing Shi, Zhigang Ji and Zhongming Huang*

**Abstract**

**Background:** Inferior vena cava (IVC) aneurysms are extremely rare with variable clinical manifestations. Patients are usually asymptomatic or present with complications of thrombosis and rupture. To date, there have been only a few reports of the condition in the literature, and diagnosis of IVC aneurysms may be difficult.

**Case presentation:** A 33-year-old male patient presented to hospital because of a retroperitoneal mass found by computerized tomography during a health examination. He was asymptomatic, and post medical history and physical examination were unremarkable. Laboratory tests including tests for paraganglioma were all negative. Contrast-enhanced computed tomography scan revealed a stenosis of IVC in the suprarenal segment and two retroperitoneal mass on the right side of IVC. The larger one is about 3 cm in diameter and the smaller one is about 1 cm in diameter, which was considered as a retroperitoneal tumor with an enlarged lymph node. However, two IVC diverticular aneurysms were confirmed during the retroperitoneal laparoscopic exploration. The larger aneurysm was resected from the IVC successfully. Since the smaller aneurysm was about 1 cm in diameter without thrombosis, we did not resect it during surgery. The patient recovered well from surgery and discharged from our department successfully.

**Conclusions:** This is the first report of multiple IVC aneurysms. Because of the extremely low prevalence of IVC diverticular aneurysm, it may be misdiagnosed as other disease. Due to the high rate of thrombosis, surgical treatment especially retroperitoneal laparoscopy is recommended for small diverticular aneurysms.

**Keywords:** Inferior vena cava, Diverticular aneurysm, Retroperitoneal laparoscopy, Case report

## Background

Aneurysms are local vascular dilatations that develop when part of the vascular wall weakens, which mostly occur in arterial system. Although venous aneurysms can also occur throughout the body [1], they are relatively uncommon, and inferior vena cava (IVC) aneurysms are extremely rare. The first case of an IVC aneurysm was reported in 1972 by Conn [2]. To date, there have been only a few reports of the condition in the literature, and diagnosis of IVC aneurysms may be difficult. Here, we describe a case involving multiple IVC malformations, including aneurysms that mimicked a retroperitoneal tumor with an enlarged lymph node.

## Case presentation

A 33-year-old Chinese male patient presented to Urology Department because of a retroperitoneal mass that was incidentally found by computerized tomography (CT) during a health examination. He was asymptomatic and had no abdominal or back pain, episodic hypertension, palpitation, or lower limb edema. Post medical history and physical examination were unremarkable.

* Correspondence: zhmhuang@hotmail.com
Department of Urology, Peking Union Medical College Hospital, Peking Union Medical College and Chinese Academy of Medical Sciences, No.1 Shuaifuyuan, Beijing 100730, P.R. China

Laboratory tests including complete blood count, liver and renal function and D-Dimer were normal. Tests for paraganglioma such as 24-h urinary catecholamine and somatostatin receptor imaging were negative. Contrast-enhanced CT scan revealed a stenosis of IVC in the suprarenal segment (Fig. 1a), a 34 mm × 30 mm × 33 mm retroperitoneal mass on the right side of the infrarenal IVC (Fig. 1a and b) and a small mass about 10 mm in diameter in the retroperitoneal area that was considered an enlarged lymph node (Fig. 1c). No thrombosis was found in the IVC. Therefore, a diagnosis of retroperitoneal tumor with possible lymph node metastasis was considered.

To further confirm our diagnosis, a retroperitoneal laparoscopic exploration was performed. During the surgery, we found that both mass were diverticular aneurysms of IVC (Fig. 2a). There was a very narrow neck between the larger aneurysm and IVC (Fig. 2b). A hem-o-lok clamp was applied on the neck of aneurysm (Fig. 2c), and the aneurysm was resected from the IVC successfully. Since the smaller aneurysm was about 1 cm in diameter without thrombosis, we did not resect it during surgery. However, the stenosis of IVC may cause venous hypertension which can be a risk factor for aneurysms progression. Therefore, we referred the patient to Vascular Surgery Department for pressure gradient test across the suprarenal IVC to determine the following therapy. They suggested to monitor the size of aneurysm annually to determine further treatment. The patient recovered well from surgery and discharged from our department successfully. The pathology shows vascular wall tissue with a lot fibrous tissue, which is consistent with the diagnosis of IVC aneurysm. However, there is no intact vascular wall identified.

## Discussion and conclusions

Our patient had multiple IVC malformations, including two IVC aneurysms. IVC aneurysms are extremely rare with variable clinical manifestations. They may be discovered incidentally in asymptomatic patients, as it was in our case, or may present with complications, such as leg swelling, pulmonary embolism and retroperitoneal mass related effects, like abdominal/low back pain, hydronephrosis and bowel obstruction [3–5]. Because the symptoms are non-specific, imaging tests like ultrasonography, contrast-enhanced CT, magnetic resonance imaging and cavography play a vital role in the diagnosis of IVC aneurysms [6]. However, some IVC aneurysms could be confused with retroperitoneal tumors, such as renal carcinoma, sarcomas, enlarged lymph nodes, neurogenic tumors and primary IVC tumors [7–9], especially when the lumen of the aneurysm is completely thrombosed [8]. Therefore, comprehensive consideration of various imaging tests results can increase the accuracy

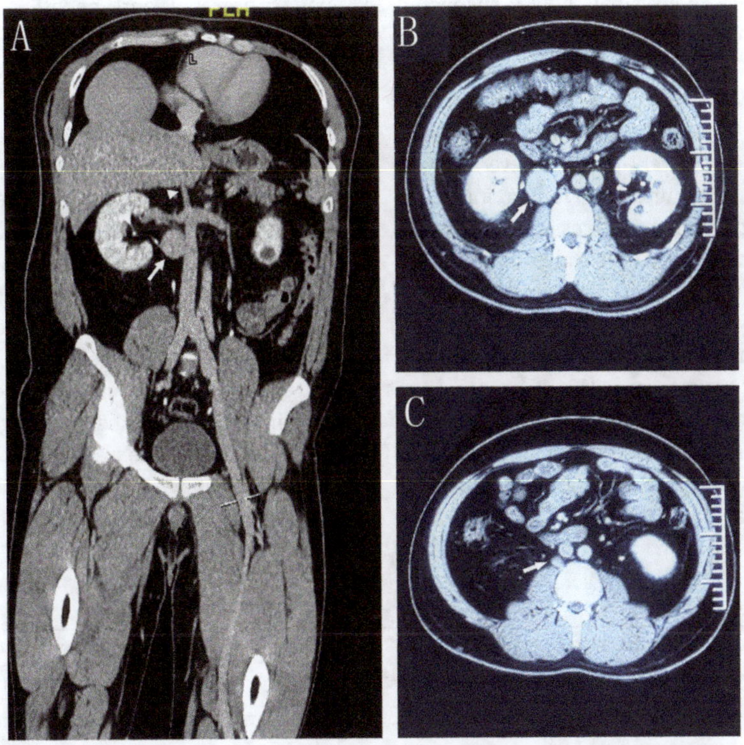


**Fig. 1** Contrast-enhanced CT imaging. **a** Coronal view showing the stenosis of IVC (arrowhead) and a retroperitoneal mass on the right side of the infrarenal IVC (long arrow). **b** and **c** Axial view showing the two retroperitoneal mass (long arrow)

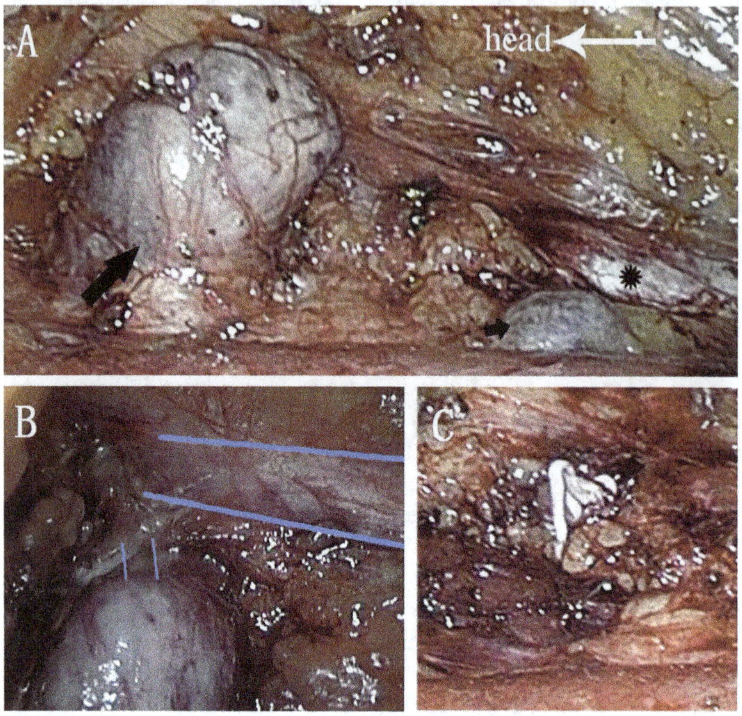


**Fig. 2** Intra-operative photographs. **a** IVC (black star) and two aneurysms (black long arrow and short arrow). **b** A narrow neck between the larger aneurysm and IVC (blue thick lines showing edges of IVC and thin lines showing the neck of the aneurysm). **c** Hem-o-lok in the neck of aneurysm after resection

of diagnosis. Cavography or surgical exploration is recommended when an IVC aneurysm is highly suspected. Biopsy should be more carefully chosen when the nature of the mass is unclear.

Pathological studies have revealed that IVC aneurysms are composed of all three layers of the normal venous wall with thinning elastic and muscular layers [10]. However, the etiology of IVC aneurysms is still unclear. Trauma, injury, inflammation, longstanding venous hypertension secondary to heart failure, cardiomyopathy, tricuspid valve lesions, constrictive pericarditis and stenosis of IVC are all risk factors of IVC aneurysms. As many cases are diagnosed in childhood, congenital defects like embryological venous malformations are considered the most common cause [11–15].

Embryological development of IVC is complex. Through complex sequential processes of development, anastomosis and regression of three parallel veins (the postcardinal, subcardinal and supracardinal veins), the mature IVC forms [16, 17]. The normal IVC is composed of four segments, including the infrarenal, renal, suprarenal and hepatic IVC, which are derived from supracardinal veins, subcardinal-supracardinal vein anastomoses, subcardinal veins and subcardinal-hepatic vein anastomoses, respectively [18, 19]. Our patient presented with no risk factors, and multiple IVC malformations were observed, indicating that an embryological development anomaly may be the cause of his condition.

In the literature, there are two classification systems for IVC aneurysms (Table 1). The Thompson and Lindenauer classification includes three types based on the etiology of aneurysm [20]. However, application of this classification is limited, since the etiology of aneurysm is unclear in most cases. Gradman and Steinberg classified IVC aneurysms into four types depending on the relation to the hepatic vein and the resultant obstruction [21]. Type I IVC aneurysms were most common, followed by type III. Type IV IVC aneurysms were rare [12]. This classification has more utility in clinic and is used in our article.

**Table 1** IVC aneurysm classification system

| | Gradman and Steinberg classification | Thompson and Lindenauer classification |
|---|---|---|
| Type I | Aneurysms of the suprahepatic IVC without venous obstruction | Congenital aneurysm |
| Type II | Aneurysms associated with interruption of the IVC above or below the hepatic vein | Acquired aneurysm |
| Type III | Aneurysms confined to the infrarenal IVC without associated venous anomaly | Aneurysm secondary to arteriovenous fistula |
| Type IV | Miscellaneous | |

**Table 2** Reported diverticular IVC aneurysms

| Author | Year | Age (year) | Gender | Presentation | Location | Thrombosis | Treatment | Outcome |
|---|---|---|---|---|---|---|---|---|
| Hasan, et al. [16] | 1992 | 59 | Male | Abdominal pain | Infrarenal | No | Open surgical resection | Good |
| Levesque, et al. [27] | 1993 | 70 | Male | Asymptomatic | Infrarenal | Yes | Monitoring | No changes in thrombosis or aneurysm size |
| Gradman, et al. [21] | 1993 | 45 | Male | Back and chest pain, swelling of left lower extremity | Infrarenal | Yes | Open surgical resection | Good |
| Davidovic, et al. [3] | 2008 | 27 | Male | Abdominal pain and swelling of bilateral lower extremities | Infrarenal | Yes | Open surgical resection | Good |
| Deshpande, et al. [28] | 2010 | 40 | Male | Bilateral lower extremity swelling and pain | Infrarenal | Yes | Open surgical resection and anticoagulation | Good |
| Weber, et al. [29] | 2011 | 13 | Male | Left lower extremity swelling and pain | Infrarenal | Yes | Open surgical resection and anticoagulation | Good |
| Tadayon, et al. [22] | 2019 | 22 | Male | Abdominal pain | Infrarenal | No | Open surgical resection | Good |
| Ladurner, et al. [30] | 2019 | 23 | Male | NM | Infrarenal | Yes | Anticoagulation | NM |

*NM* Not mentioned

However, both of the classification systems have limited guidance for treatment and prognosis.

Due to potential life-threatening morbidities, such as thromboembolic events and rupture, treatment of IVC aneurysms is recommended [3, 12, 22]. However, there is no consensus on patient management. In some literature reviews, surgical treatment such as resection and reconstruction is recommended for types II–IV or symptomatic patients [3, 11, 12]. Endovascular techniques were also recently reported in the treatment of IVC aneurysm. Michel et al. [23] successfully embolized a congenital large saccular aneurysm of the infrarenal IVC in a 2.5-year-old male with coils and an Amplatzer vascular plug device. Falkowski et al. [24] implanted a custom-made stent-graft in an infrarenal IVC aneurysm to exclude it from the circulation completely. Walsh et al. [25] performed balloon angioplasty to improve the congenital stenosis of IVC in a type II aneurysm, and aneurysm size was decreased during the follow-up. Asymptomatic type I IVC aneurysm can be managed conservatively by regularly monitoring aneurysm size and the development of any complications [26]. Medical management can include anticoagulation and IVC filter placement in patients with thrombosis.

In our case, it was difficult to classify the IVC aneurysms accurately. There were two infrarenal IVC aneurysm and stenosis of suprarenal IVC. It was unclear whether the aneurysm was associated with the stenosis of IVC. In our opinion, there was no obvious dilation of the distal IVC, and the aneurysms were relatively far from the stenosis. Therefore, the infrarenal IVC aneurysms were probably not associated with the stenosis, and thus, are type III IVC aneurysms. IVC aneurysms can be saccular, fusiform or diverticular. The diverticular type is rare, and to date there have been only eight cases reported in the literature [3, 16, 21, 22, 27–30] (Table 2). All reported patients were male, and all aneurysms were located at the infrarenal IVC segment, which is different from the IVC aneurysm entity. Therefore, diverticular IVC aneurysms may be a special type of IVC aneurysm, and it is probably caused by the incomplete regression of supracardinal vein branches. Due to the high rate of thrombosis associated with diverticular IVC aneurysms, surgical treatment is recommended. Compared to open surgical operation, retroperitoneal laparoscopy is less invasive with a shorter in-hospital duration and less blood loss, and it is especially suitable for treating small aneurysm. Endovascular treatment is an alternative method for patients without thrombosis.

Table 2. Reported diverticular IVC aneurysms (in the end of the file).

IVC aneurysms are extremely rare, and this is the first report of multiple IVC diverticular aneurysms. It should be a differential diagnosis in the evaluation of retroperitoneal tumors. In addition, IVC diverticular aneurysms may be a special type. Due to the high rate of thrombosis, surgical treatment is recommended and retroperitoneal laparoscopy is suitable for small aneurysms.

**Abbreviations**

IVC: Inferior vena cava; CT: Computerized tomography

**Acknowledgements**

We thank the nurses for taking good care of our patient, which enhanced his discharge successfully.

**Authors' contributions**

ZH, ZZ and BS performed the surgery and collected the patient clinical data. YZ wrote the manuscript and ZJ was a major contributor in manuscript revision. All authors read and approved the final manuscript.

**Competing interests**

The authors declare that they have no competing interests.

**References**

1. French JR, Moncrieff NJ, Englund R, Hanel KC. Thrombotic complications of venous aneurysms. ANZ J Surg. 2003;73(6):384–6.
2. Conn HO, Ramsby GR. Aneurysm of the inferior vena cava after portacaval anastomosis. Surgery. 1972;71(6):828–33.
3. Davidovic L, Dragas M, Bozic V, Takac D. Aneurysm of the inferior vena cava: case report and review of the literature. Phlebology. 2008;23(4):184–8.
4. Jegananthan R, Reid JA, Hannon RJ. Aneurysm of the inferior vena cava. Surgeon. 2003;1(3):164–5.
5. Debing E, Vanhulle A, van Tussenbroek F, von Kemp K, Van den Brande P. Idiopathic aneurysm of the inferior vena cava as a cause of massive penile bleeding. Eur J Vasc Endovasc Surg. 1998;15(4):365–8.
6. Momeni M, Momeni F. Ruptured inferior vena cava aneurysm in the setting of mural vascular malformation: a case report. J Clin Ultrasound. 2019;47(7): 423–5.
7. Rodríguez-González M, Castellano-Martinez A. Inferior vena cava aneurysm in children: a case report. Ann Vasc Surg. 2017;38:315.e9–315.e13.
8. Unzueta-Roch JL, García-Abós M, Sirvent-Cerdá S, de Prada I, Martínez de Azagra A, Ollero JM, et al. Inferior vena cava aneurysm in an infant presenting with a renal mass. J Pediatr Hematol Oncol. 2014;36(7):583–5.
9. de Bree E, Klaase JM, Schultze Kool LJ, van Coevorden. Aneurysm of the inferior vena cava complicated by thrombosis mimicking a retroperitoneal neoplasm. Eur J Vasc Endovasc Surg. 2000;20(3):305–7.
10. Calligaro KD, Ahmad S, Dandora R, Dougherty MJ, Savarese RP, Doerr KJ, et al. Venous aneurysms: surgical indications and review of the literature. Surgery. 1995;117(1):1–6.
11. Gusani R, Shukla R, Kothari S, Bhatt R, Patel J. Inferior vena cava aneurysm presenting as deep vein thrombosis - a case report. Int J Surg Case Rep. 2016;29:123–5.
12. Montero-Baker MF, Branco BC, Leon LL Jr, Labropoulos N, Echeverria A, Mills JL Sr. Management of inferior vena cava aneurysm. J Cardiovasc Surg. 2015; 56(5):769–74.
13. Makaloski V, Schmidli J. Giant symptomatic aneurysm of the inferior vena cava. Eur J Vasc Endovasc Surg. 2015;49(3):247.
14. Inoue M, Sudo T, Yamaguchi M, Seo S, Miyamoto T, Misumi T, et al. Aneurysm of the inferior vena cava with thrombosis. Clin Case Rep. 2018; 6(2):402–6.
15. Wells IT, Bhatnagar R. Presumed rupture of a massive inferior vena cava aneurysm associated with right heart failure; a unique case. Clin Radiol. 2008;63(10):1181–3.
16. Hasan F, Gleeson F, Lock MR, Williams R, Grant D. Diverticulum of the inferior vena cava: a case report. J Vasc Surg. 1992;15(3):578–80.
17. Sürücü HS, Erbil KM, Tastan C, Yener N. Anomalous veins of the retroperitoneum: clinical considerations. Surg Radiol Anat. 2001;23(6):443–5.
18. Mookadam F, Rowley VB, Emani UR, Al-Harthi MS, Baxter CM, Wilansky S, et al. Aneurysmal dilatation of the inferior vena cava. Echocardiography. 2011;28(8):833–42.
19. Woo K, Cook P, Saeed M, Dilley R. Inferior vena cava aneurysm. Vascular. 2009;17(5):284–9.
20. Thompson NW, Lindenauer SM. Central venous aneurysms and arteriovenous fistulas. Ann Surg. 1969;170(5):852–6.
21. Gradman WS, Steinberg F. Aneurysm of the inferior vena cava: case report and review of the literature. Ann Vasc Surg. 1993;7(4):347–53.
22. Tadayon N, Kalantar-Motamedi SM, Zarrintan S, Tayyebi A. Isolated inferior vena cava aneurysm: a case report. J Cardiovasc Thorac Res. 2019;11(1):72–4.
23. Michel LL, Alomari AI. Embolization of a large inferior vena cava aneurysm in a child. J Vasc Interv Radiol. 2008;19(10):1509–12.
24. Falkowski A, Wiernicki I. Stent-graft implantation to treat an inferior vena cava aneurysm. J Endovasc Ther. 2013;20(5):714–7.
25. Walsh K, O'Connor D, Wilderman M, Ratnathicam A, Simonian G, Napolitano MM. Balloon angioplasty for symptomatic inferior vena cava aneurysm. J Vasc Surg Venous Lymphat Disord. 2018;6(5):661 3.
26. Le Moigne F, Jarry J, Michel P, Vitry T, Rode A. Aneurysm of the retrohepatic inferior vena cava. J Mal Vasc. 2013;38(1):58–9.
27. Levesque H, Cailleux N, Courtois H, Clavier E, Milon P, Benozio M. Idiopathic saccular aneurysm of the inferior vena cava: a new case. J Vasc Surg. 1993; 18(3):544–5.
28. Deshpande A, Sahoo S, Chaudhari P, Abhijit R. Aneurysm of the inferior vena cava: accurate preoperative diagnosis and surgical excision. ANZ J Surg. 2010;80(7–8):552–3.
29. Weber C, Jones K, Milner R. Resection and primary repair of an inferior vena cava aneurysm in a 13-year-old male. Vascular. 2011;19(4):218–22.
30. Ladurner R, Strohaeker J, Bongers M. The rare occurrence of an aneursym of the inferior vena cava. Dtsch Arztebl Int. 2019;116:841.

7

# Rationale, design and methods of electroencephalography-based investigation of the effects of oral desmopressin on improving slow-wave sleep time in nocturnal polyuria patients (the DISTINCT study): Protocol for a single-arm, open-label, single-assignment trial

Kazumasa Torimoto*, Makito Miyake, Yasushi Nakai, Katsuya Aoki, Nobumichi Tanaka and Kiyohide Fujimoto

**Abstract**

**Background:** Nocturia is one of the most bothersome lower urinary tract symptoms and often impairs sleep quality in the elderly. Although previous studies on nocturia have indicated that the successful treatment of nocturia improves sleep quality, most used questionnaires and activity devices to analyze sleep/wake patterns. Therefore, there is little information about the treatment effects of desmopressin on objective sleep quality. The aim of the DISTINCT study is to investigate the change in subjective and objective sleep quality using electroencephalography (EEG) and the Pittsburgh Sleep Quality Index (PSQI) after the administration of desmopressin in patients with nocturia due to nocturnal polyuria.

**Methods:** A total of 20 male patients, ≥65 years old, with nocturnal polyuria, defined as a nocturnal polyuria index (NPi) (nocturnal urine volume / 24 h urine volume) value ≥0.33, will participate in this study. The participants must have a nocturnal frequency of ≥2 and the first uninterrupted sleep period (FUSP) must occur within < 2.5 h. Desmopressin 50 μg per day will be orally administered before going to bed for 4 weeks. Urinary frequency volume charts (FVC) and EEG will be recorded prior to treatment and at 1 week and 4 weeks after the initiation of treatment. The PSQI will be completed before and 4 weeks after treatment. The primary endpoint is the change from baseline in the mean time of slow-wave sleep (sleep stages N3 and N4) at 4 weeks. The secondary endpoints include the change in the mean value of each sleep variable, the mean delta power during the FUSP, the correlation between nocturnal urinary frequency and slow-wave sleep time, and the change in PSQI score before and after treatment.

(Continued on next page)

* Correspondence: torimoto@naramed-u.ac.jp
Department of Urology, Nara Medical University, 840 Shijocho, Kashihara, Nara 634-8522, Japan

(Continued from previous page)
**Discussion:** The DISTINCT study will provide valuable evidence to indicate that oral desmopressin treatment for nocturnal polyuria prolongs the FUSP, resulting in the extension of slow-wave sleep time associated with sleep quality.

**Keywords:** Nocturia, Nocturnal polyuria, Desmopressin, Sleep quality, Slow-wave sleep, Delta power

## Background

Nocturia is a common disease in the elderly. One consequence of nocturia is the complaint of poor sleep quality due to polyuria and nocturnal voids [1]. Nocturia is defined by the International Continence Society as "The number of times urine is passed during the main sleep period. Having woken to pass urine for the first time, each urination must be followed by sleep or the intention to sleep" [2]. The prevalence of nocturnal urinary frequency ≥ 2 is 47% in Japanese residents ≥65 years old [3], 36% in European residents from 60 to 80 years old [4], and 14.2% in the United States (mean age of patients is 46 years) [5]. Nocturia correlates with age, race/ethnicity, medical problems (such as hypertension, diabetes, and stroke), psychological aspects, tasting habits, quality of life, and even mortality [6].

Nocturia causes poor sleep quality by prompting nocturnal voids during the first uninterrupted sleep period (FUSP) [7, 8]. Nocturia increases the number of nocturnal voids, and nocturnal voiding has been shown to be an independent predictor of both self-reported insomnia (75% increased risk) and reduced sleep quality (71% increased risk), along with female gender and other medical psychiatric conditions [7]. Nocturia decreases the FUSP, and the FUSP is a potentially valuable metric that correlates with changes in perceived sleep duration, depth, quality of sleep for the entire night, efficiency, and latency, as evaluated by Pittsburgh Sleep Quality Index (PSQI) [8]. The FUSP has a close relationship with slow-wave, or non-REM, sleep. Sleep stages are divided from 1 to 4, and slow-wave sleep occurs during stages N3 and N4. Stages N3 and N4 commonly occur during the first two sleep cycles (about 180 min after falling asleep) and are considered important for high-quality sleep [9].

We hypothesize that desmopressin treatment for nocturia will improve subjective and objective sleep quality. Desmopressin 25 and 50 μg orally disintegrating tablets are now available worldwide for nocturia and have been shown to decrease the number of nocturnal voids [10]. It is reported that subjective sleep quality, estimated by a quality of life questionnaire, was improved by desmopressin treatment [11]. Desmopressin prolonged the FUSP, suggesting that the slow-wave sleep time might also have been prolonged, although this has not been investigated.

The aim of the DISTINCT study is to use electroencephalography (EEG) and PSQI to investigate the change in subjective and objective sleep quality after the administration of desmopressin to patients with nocturia due to nocturnal polyuria.

## Methods/design

This is a single-arm, open-label, single-assignment study. It is an exploratory study to compare subjective and objective sleep qualities after 1 week and 4 weeks of desmopressin treatment for nocturnal polyuria (Fig. 1). Qualifying patients will be males, ≥65 years old, and suffering from insomnia due to nocturnal polyuria, defined as a nocturnal polyuria index (NPi) value (nocturnal urine volume / 24 h urine volume) of ≥0.33 [2].

This study will be conducted at Nara Medical University Hospital in compliance with both the articles of the Declaration of Helsinki (revised in October 2013) and the Ethical Guidelines for Medical and Health Research Involving Human Subjects established by the Ministry of Health, Labor, and Welfare in Japan.

### Planned outcomes

#### *Primary endpoint*

The primary endpoint is the change in mean time of slow-wave sleep (stages N3 and N4) as evaluated by EEG at 28 days from baseline (Table 1).

#### *Secondary endpoints*

The secondary endpoints are listed in Table 1.

**Safety endpoints** Data on the clinical trial results, vital sign measurements, and adverse events (AEs), especially signs of hyponatremia, will be collected at each visit. The severity, causal relationship to desmopressin, and outcomes of all AEs will be assessed.

### Study population

A total of 20 male patients, ≥65 years old, with nocturnal polyuria, will participate in this study. The participants must have nocturnal frequency ≥ 2 and NPi ≥0.33, which will be recorded by 2-days FVC. Patients will be considered eligible for the study if they fulfill all of the inclusion criteria and none of the exclusion criteria, as defined in Table 2. The investigator will provide a suffi-

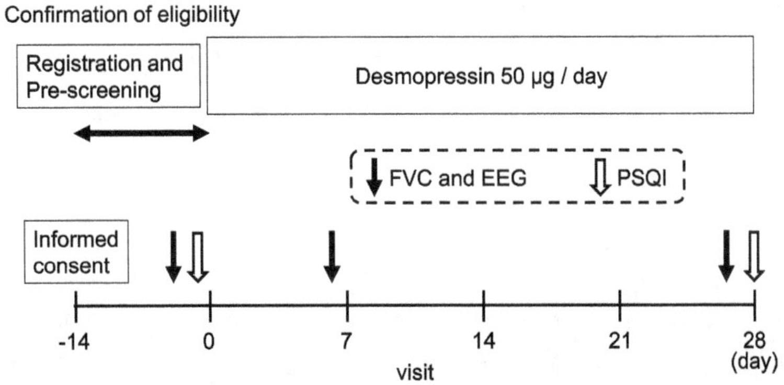


**Fig. 1** Study design. A total of 20 patients with nocturnal polyuria will participate in this study. After the conformation of eligibility, the enrolled patients will be treated with oral desmopressin 50 µg per day. In the pre-screening period, 2-day frequency volume chart (FVC) and sleep encephalography (EEG) will be recorded and the Pittsburgh Sleep Questionnaire Index (PSQI) will be completed. Before visit Day 0, 2-day FVC and EEG will be recorded. Before visit Day 7 and Day 28, 2-day FVC and EEG will be recorded. On visit Day 28, the PSQI will be completed

cient explanation of the study to each patient and obtain written informed consent prior to the initiation of any study procedures.

### Treatment

Patients will be provided with desmopressin 50 µg (as MINIRINMELT® OD Tablets 25 µg / 50 µg; Ferring Pharmaceuticals Co., Ltd., Tokyo, Japan) to be orally administered once daily prior to going to bed. The drug has been approved only for male patients with nocturnal polyuria in Japan.

### Measurements

The schedule of data collection is detailed in Table 3. A window of ±2 days is acceptable.

#### *Informed consent and registration*

The principal investigator or co-investigator will explain the study to each eligible participant, using the informed consent documents. Participants who give written informed consent will be registered in this study. Registration will be closed when the planned total number of participants (20 participants) is reached.

#### *Data collection*

Patient characteristics will include age, height, weight, and medical history. Blood tests performed at pre-screening will evaluate the following clinical chemistry analytes: serum creatinine, estimated glomerular filtration rate, sodium (Na), potassium, chlorine (Cl), brain natriuretic peptide, fasting blood glucose, white blood cell count, red blood cell count, hemoglobin content, hematocrit, platelet count, total protein, albumin, blood urea nitrogen, aspartate aminotransferase, alanine aminotransferase, alkaline phosphatase, and gamma-glutamyl transferase. Blood tests performed during the treatment period will evaluate Na and Cl.

A mobile EEG device, Sleep Graph® (Proassist, Ltd., Osaka, Japan), will be used for EEG recordings. The device is small, easy to carry, and well-validated by standard methods (polysomnography) [12]. The device records brain-waves during sleep, which indicate sleep stages.

The FVC will be recorded by the patients independently to assess the nocturnal frequency and nocturnal urine volume. The results of the visual analog scale (VAS) will be used as additional indicators of subjective sleep quality on days when FVC and EEG

**Table 1** Primary and secondary endpoints of the DISTINCT Study

| Primary endpoint | Secondary endpoints |
|---|---|
| Change in mean time of slow-wave sleep (N3 + N4) as evaluated by EEG at 28 days from baseline | 1. Change is PSQI before and after desmopressin administration |
| | 2. Change in nocturnal urinary frequency, the first nocturnal urinary volume, and the FUSP before and after desmopressin administration |
| | 3. Change in sleep time, sleep effiency, and sleep quality as estimated by VAS before and after desmopressin administration |
| | 4. Correlation between slow-wave sleep time (N3 + N4) and PSQI, VAS, FUSP, nocturnal urinay frequency at 28 days from baseline |
| | 5. Change is delta power during the FUSP before and after desmopressin administration |

*N1–4* non-rapid eye movement sleep stage 1–4, *EEG* eletroecephalography, *PSQI* Pittsburgh sleep quality index, *FUSP* the first uninterrupted sleep period, *VAS* visual analogue scale

**Table 2** Inclusion and exclusion criteria of the DISTINCT Study

| Inclusion criteria | Exclusion criteria |
|---|---|
| 1. Nocturnal urinary frequency is 2 or more. | 1. Concentration of serum sodium is less than 135 mEq/L |
| 2. Nocturnal polyuria index is 0.33 or more. | 2. Habitual or psychogenic polydipsia |
| 3. FUSP is 2.5 h or less. | 3. Heart failure, the history of heart failure, or suspected heart failure |
| 4. Concentration of serum sodium is 135 mEq/L or more. | 4. Fluid retention that requires diuretic treatment, whether currently or in the patient's medical history |
| 5. Creatinine clearance or eGFR is 50 mL/min/1.73m$^2$ or more. | 5. Antidiuretic hormone incompatible secretion syndrome |
| 6. Patients with BPH or OAB are acceptable if the storage symptoms (urgency and daytime frequency) are well managed and stable for 3 months or more by any treatments or 6 months or more by 5-alpha reductase inhibitors. | 6. Moderate or severe renal failure (Creatinine clearance or eGFR < 50 mL/min/1.73m$^2$) |
| | 7. Hypersensitivity to desmopressin or the history, whether currently or in the patient's medical history |
| | 8. Concomitant or scheduled administration of thiazides, thiazide-like diuretics, or loop diuretics |
| | 9. Concomitant or scheduled administration of corticosteroids |
| | 10. Cardiac pacemaker implantation |
| | 11. Judged to be inappropriate by the principal investigator or subinvestigators |

*FUSP* the first uninterrupted sleep period, *BPH* benign prostatic hyperplasia, *OAB* overactive bladder, *eGFR* estimate glomerular filtration rate

are recorded. The VAS is a measurement instrument that asks patients to rate their sleep from "I could sleep well" (left end of the scale) to "I could not sleep at all" (right end of the scale). Subjective sleep quality will be assessed by the length between the left end and the point at which a patient records their sleep rating.

### Sample size calculation

This study is designed to demonstrate a statistically significant difference in the change from baseline in slow-wave sleep time in patients treated with desmopressin 50 μg with overall power of 80% and an overall Type 1 error rate of 5% (two-sided). The R program was used for sample size calculation. Bliwise et al. reported that in

**Table 3** Schedule of enrollment, interventions, and assessments

| | Study period | | | | | | | | |
|---|---|---|---|---|---|---|---|---|---|
| | Pre-screening | | Treatment | | | | | | |
| **Timepoint:** | Visit 1 | Visit 2 | Visit 3 | | | Visit 4 | | | Visit 5 |
| | Day −28 to −14 | Day −14 to − 1 | Day 0 | Day 5 | Day 6 | Day 7 | Day 26 | Day 27 | Day 28 |
| **Enrollment:** | | | | | | | | | |
| Eligibility screen | X | | | | | | | | |
| Informed concent | X | | | | | | | | |
| Registration | | X | | | | | | | |
| **Intervention:** | | | | | | | | | |
| Desmopressin | | | | | | | | | |
| **Assessment:** | | | | | | | | | |
| Patient characteristcs | X | | | | | | | | |
| Blood test | X | X | | | | X | | | X |
| PSQI | | X | | | | | | | X |
| EEG | | X | | X | X | | X | X | |
| VAS | | | X | | | X | | | X |
| FVC | | X | | X | X | | X | X | |
| Checking for AEs | | | | | | X | | | X |

*AEs* adverse events

15 patients studied, 8 patients had one or two voids, and 7 patients had three or four voids, showing a trend for higher amounts of N3 sleep at 81.4 ± 28.8 min vs 48.2 ± 40.7 min, respectively, assuming a total sleep time of 6 h [13]. Based on these data, we assumed 33.2 min as the difference between both groups and 35.7 min as the standard deviation, and determined that data from 13 subjects will be needed to detect a significant difference from baseline. Considering subject withdrawal, missing data, and feasibility, we assume 20 subjects will be sufficient.

### Statistical analysis

#### *Primary endpoint*

A Wilcoxon matched-pairs signed rank test would be used to compare the mean time of slow-wave sleep (N3 + N4) at Day 26 or 27 with that at baseline.

#### *Secondary endpoints*

A Wilcoxon matched-pairs signed rank test will be used to compare the mean score of the PSQI at Day 28 with that at baseline, and the mean time of slow-wave sleep (N3 + N4) at Day 5 or 6 with that at baseline. Friedman's test and Dunn's multiple comparisons test will be used to compare the change in mean total sleep time, mean sleep efficiency, mean sleep latency, mean VAS, mean time of sleep stages, and delta power during the FUSP from baseline to Day 26 or 27. The dependency between the mean time of slow-wave sleep (N3 + N4), the score of the PSQI, VAS, FUSP, number of voids, delta power during the FUSP, and other baseline characteristics will be analyzed using a linear regression model at Day 28. The significance level for statistical tests will be 0.05 on two sides.

## Discussion

The aim of the DISTINCT study is to investigate the change in subjective (measured by PSQI) and objective (measured by EEG) sleep quality after the administration of desmopressin to patients with nocturia due to nocturnal polyuria. One of the treatment goals for nocturia is to prolong the FUSP because slow-wave sleep, which is important for brain rest, appears early in sleep. Desmopressin, which has world-wide marketing authorization, has been demonstrated as safe and efficacious in prolonging the FUSP. However, the prolongation of slow-wave sleep time following desmopressin use has not been studied. The DISTINCT study addresses this gap in the research.

Additionally, this study will rely on a novel approach for measuring objective sleep quality. The standard method for analyzing sleep stages is polysomnography, which requires placing many sensors on a patient's head and body, and can be performed only in laboratories. Therefore, it is difficult for nocturia patients who go to the toilet for voiding to undergo polysomnography, which fixes patients to the bed during the sleep period. The portable EEG device used in this study does not restrain patients and was demonstrated as useful in our previous study, which demonstrated the linkage between sleep quality assessed by the PSQI and slow-wave sleep time [14].

This study has several limitations, including a small number of patients, and an open-label, single-arm modality. However, the results will provide valuable evidence by which to demonstrate the positive effects of desmopressin on objective sleep quality, which is associated with the occurrence of deeper sleep stages in patients with nocturnal polyuria.

#### Abbreviations

FUSP: First uninterrupted sleep period; PSQI: Pittsburgh Sleep Quality Index; EEG: Electroencephalography; NPi: Nocturnal polyuria index; AE: Adverse event; Na: Sodium; Cl: Chlorine; VAS: Visual analog scale; FVC: Frequency volume chart

#### Acknowledgements

We would like to thank Dr. Nagaaki Marugami, who belongs to Department of Radiology and Nuclear Medicines, Nara Medical University and has agreed to monitor this study.

#### Authors' contributions

All authors were involved in the planning and execution of the DISTINCT study. TK was a major contributor in writing the manuscript with help of NY. MM was responsible for statistical design and analysis. AK and TN interpreted the existing patient data regarding nocturnal polyuria and sleep disorder. FK critically reviewed the manuscript. All authors read and approved the final manuscript.

#### Competing interests

The funding of this protocol by the manufacturer of desmopressin is a competing interest.

#### References

1. Asplund R. Nocturia, nocturnal polyuria, and sleep quality in the elderly. J Psychosom Res. 2004;56:517–25.
2. Hashim H, Blanker MH, Drake MJ, Djurhuus JC, Meijlink J, Morris V, et al. International Continence Society (ICS) report on the terminology for nocturia and nocturnal lower urinary tract function. Neurourol Urodyn. 2019;38:179–83.
3. Hirayama A, Torimoto K, Mastusita C, Okamoto N, Morikawa M, Tanaka N, et al. Evaluation of factors influencing the natural history of nocturia in elderly subjects: results of the Fujiwara-kyo study. J Urol. 2013;189:980–6.
4. Bing MH, Moller LA, Jennum P, Mortensen S, Skovgaard LT, Lose G. Prevalence and bother of nocturia, and causes of sleep interruption in a Danish population of men and women aged 60-80 years. BJU Int. 2006;98: 599–604.
5. Coyne KS, Zhou Z, Bhattacharyya SK, Thompson CL, Dhawan R, Versi E. The prevalence of nocturia and its effect on health-related quality of life and sleep in a community sample in the USA. BJU Int. 2003;92:948–54.
6. Yoshimura K. Correlates for nocturia: a review of epidemiological studies. Int J Urol. 2012;19:317–29.
7. Bliwise DL, Foley DJ, Vitiello MV, Ansari FP, Ancoli-Israel S, Walsh JK. Nocturia and disturbed sleep in the elderly. Sleep Med. 2009;10:540–8.
8. Bliwise DL, Holm-Larsen T, Goble S. Increases in duration of first uninterrupted sleep period are associated with improvements in PSQI-measured sleep quality. Sleep Med. 2014;15:1276–8.
9. Stanley N. The underestimated impact of nocturia on quality of life. Eur Urol. 2005;Suppl 4:17 9.

10. Weiss JP, Herschorn S, Albei CD, van der Meulen EA. Efficacy and safety of low dose desmopressin orally disintegrating tablet in men with nocturia: results of a multicenter, randomized, double-blind, placebo controlled, parallel group study. J Urol. 2013;190:965–72.
11. Kerrebroeck P, Rezapour M, Cortesse A, Thüroff J, Riis A, Nørgaard JP. Desmopressin in the treatment of nocturia: a double-blind, placebo-controlled study. Eur Urol. 2007;52:221–9.
12. Nonoue S, Mashita M, Haraki S, Mikami A, Adachi H, Yatani H, et al. Inter-scorer reliability of sleep assessment using EEG and EOG recording system in comparison to polysomnography. Sleep Biol Rhythms. 2017;15:39–48.
13. Bliwise D, Dijk DJ, Juul KV. Nocturia is associated with loss of deep sleep independently from sleep apnea. Neurourol Urodyn. 2015;34:392.
14. Matsushita C, Torimoto K, Goto D, Morizawa Y, Kiba K, Shinohara M, et al. Linkage of lower urinary tract symptoms to sleep quality in elderly men with nocturia: a community based study using home measured electroencephalogram data. J Urol. 2017;197:204–9.

# 8

# Five testicles in the genital area of a thirteen-month-old baby

Telma Zahirian Moghadam[1], Hamed Mohseni Rad[2], Hamed Zandian[1] and Ali Hosseinkhani[2*]

**Abstract**

**Background:** Polyorchidism is a congenital anomaly of the urogenital system and means more than two testes. It is a rare phenomenon, where there are no more than 200 reported cases in the literature. In this case, we report a 13-month year's old case with five testicles.

**Case presentation:** We report a rare five testicles in the genital area of a 13-month-old baby. The initial diagnosis was undescended testis (UDT) based on ultrasound findings where a testis in the abdomen and a testis in the inguinal canal were detected. Surgery with general anaesthesia was performed to diagnose and treat this case. Before surgery, four HCG 1200u injections were administered. During the operation, it was determined that the case had had five testicles. Testicles were on the left in the proximal inguinal canal, and the sac hernia was ligated parallel to the inner ring. The patient was followed up several times after surgery by a urologist, and the results showed that there were no problems, and the intervention was uncomplicated.

**Conclusion:** Based on the result, it is not possible to diagnose such cases only by examination or ultrasound in infant patients, as the patient often presents with undescended testis (UDT), so the disease is diagnosed only through surgery.

**Keywords:** Testicles, Genital area, Undescended testis (UDT)

## Background

One of the congenital anomalies of the urogenital system is polyorchidism or supernumerary testis, which means more than two testes. It is a sporadic phenomenon, where there are no more reported cases in the literature. More than 50% of the all reported cases (about less than 200 cases) are detected in people between 10 to 25 years old [1, 2] and most of the discovered cases had less than four testicles [3]. In this case, we report a 13-month old case with five testicles.

## Case presentation

The case was a 13-month-old baby with 9.7 kg, which was 3.5 kg at birth, and second male child of a family habitant in a village in Ardabil, Iran. He was referred to the hospital because of undescended testis (UDT) with a testis in the abdomen and one inguinal canal that was detected by ultrasound. Because the case was infant, the family history was asked to examine the problem in more detail. Accordingly, there was UDT history in the family, where the baby's old brother also underwent orchiopexy surgery 4 years ago for UDT. During the pregnancy, the progesterone was injected to the mother for Hemorrhage every day for a week. The pregnancy was healthy and the baby is born by cesarean section.

Because of complete similar appearance to testis as the images show, we did not perform biopsy fearing of primary testicular delicate perfusion impairment. The baby referred to our centre because of bilateral UDT and non-palpable testicle on the right side. However, sonography revealed both testicles in the proximal inguinal canal. The scrotum was not grown, HCG therapy had been

* Correspondence: drhosseinkhani@yahoo.com
[2]Department of Surgery, School of Medicine and Allied Medical Sciences, Imam Reza Hospital, Ardabil University of Medical Sciences, Ardabil, Iran

started by pediatrician, and Other clinical signs were typical.

Surgical intervention was considered for the patient. Before surgery, four HCG 1200u injections were administered to the patient in four times at 1 month (one for per week) for testicular descent. However, the intervention did not completely resolve the problem, and there were no more diagnostic challenges. The patient underwent surgical procedure with general anaesthesia to diagnosis and as a final treatment stage. It was diagnosed that the testicles were on the left in the proximal inguinal canal and the sac hernia was ligated parallel to the inner ring. The left testis was a small component in the proximal without the epididymis. Two testes were closely connected in the lower part by a common epididymis, which all of them were situated in the left scrotum (Fig. 1).

Also, two testes in the proximal inguinal canal were connected by a long epididymis with the incision in the right inguinal region. We did not remove supernumerary testis, which lacks vas or epididymis, because of afraid of impairing to main testis delicate artery.

However, we do not perform genetic evaluations because of cost lacking. We played ultra-sonography before surgery. The patient was followed and examined by a urologist for placement of testis in the scrotum sac within 48 h, 10 days, one and 3 months after the surgery. We accomplished scrotal sonography after surgery and detected all five testicles with two main testicles in standard size rendering to age and also supernumerary ones in smaller sizes. Finally, the 12 months later, sonography results in the testicles showed that there were no problems, and the intervention was uncomplicated according to the baby age (Fig. 2).

## Discussion and conclusion

Blasisus in 1670 was the first one who described polyorchidism in an autopsy material, incidentally. Ahlfeld made the first histological description in 1880, and the first clinical case was reported on by Lane in 1895 [2, 4, 5]. The aetiology of polyorchidism is related to embryological period; however, this claim is not entirely clear [5, 6].

Leung classified polyorchidism into four groups based on testis embryology: 1) polyorchidism with novas differences or epididymis in the supernumerary testis, 2) testes sharing these two structures with the ipsilateral testicle, 3) testes with their epididymis and sharing the vas deferens, and 4) supernumerary testes with their annexes [7]. The patient was considered to be in group 1.

The scrotum is the most common region that Extra testicles could be seen. The other testis is usually seen

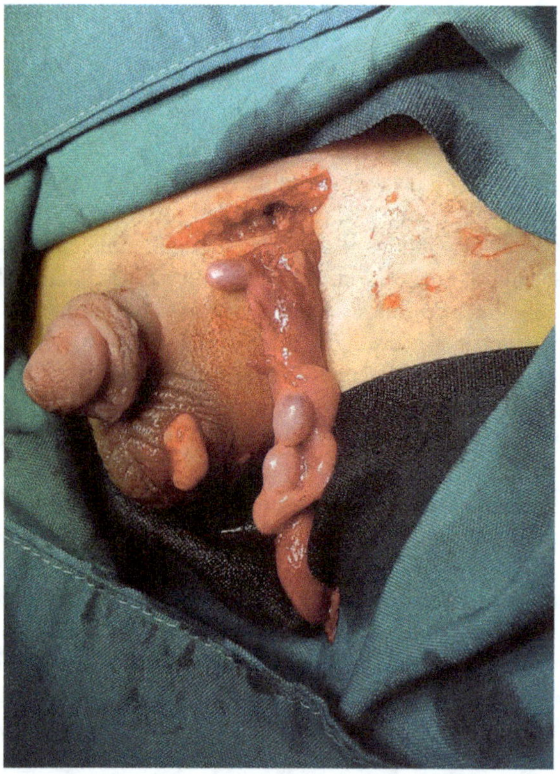

**Fig. 1** left testis, where the testicles were on the left in the proximal inguinal canal, and the sac hernia was ligated parallel to the inner ring

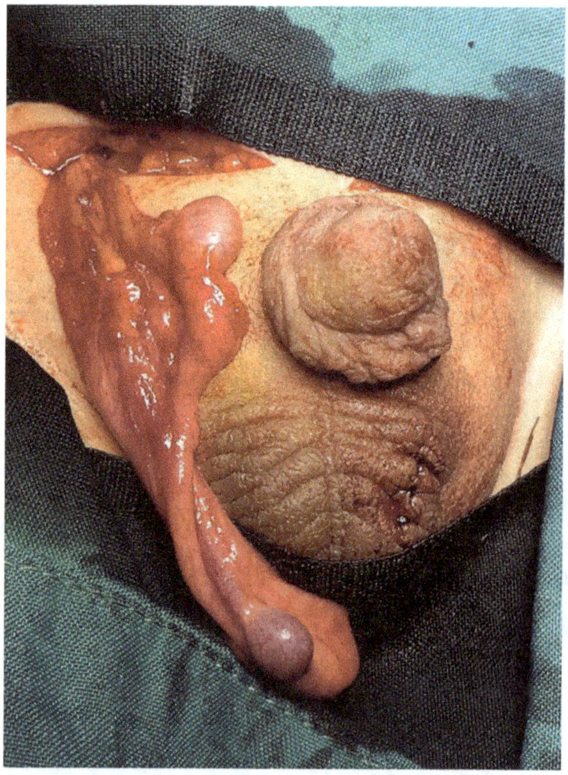

**Fig. 2** right testis, where a long epididymis connected two testes in the proximal inguinal canal with an incision in the right inguinal region

on the left side [4], similar to our study. Three and four testes are the most common form [4, 7]. Five testes have not been reported so far, and our case is the first.

The aetiology is still unclear. It is thought to be an accidental division of the genital ridge before 8th week of gestation. Although there are many embryological theories in the literature, none are sufficient to explain the pathogenesis of polyorchidism alone [7]. Our report showed that there were two right testicles with one common epididymis and one left testis without epididymis. The most common disorders of the male genital tract, which are diagnosed by clinical examination and sonography, are undescended testis, hydrocele, hypospadias, inguinal hernia, micropenis or penis enlargement and testicular defect. Treatment is often done through surgery [8, 9]. The presence of five testes, in this case, was one of the rare disorders of the genital tract in children. Aetiology and mechanism of polyorchidism are not entirely defined. However, some genetic and gestational factors may be involved, because the baby's brother also underwent orchiopexy surgery 4 years ago for UDT and his mother was injected progesterone every day for a week of pregnancy for Hemorrhage. Therefore, further studies are recommended to investigate the factors affecting these disorders.

The case with five testes is rare and undesirable in children. In both sides, testicles were in the proximal inguinal canal and nor in the abdomen. Diffusion-weighted imaging (DWI) combined with conventional magnetic resonance imaging (MRI) increase sensitivity and specificity of MRI for nonpalpable UDT detection [10]. While in our case, because of clinical finding and sonography confirmation, we did not render an abdominal MRI. Laparoscopy is standard in abdominal nonpalpable testicles, but it could be omitted if sonography confirmed their inguinal presence [11]. It has been shown that along with surgery, neo-adjuvant human chorionic gonadotropin (HCG) therapy may induce and improve testis descending [12]. In this case, surgery was performed to diagnose and treat this case. The patient needs to be monitored at different intervals. Rare cases should be handled carefully; particularly in patients with reported undescended testicles by ultrasound. During surgery, it is essential to note that more testicles may be found and we must search carefully. It is also advisable during orchiopexy, and all testes are mixed without separation to prevent damage to the epididymal system, sperm transfer, and the spermatozoa.

**Abbreviations**

UDT: Undescended testis

**Acknowledgements**

The authors thank all participants and all staffs who had provided helping to our study in ARUMS special urology hospital and deputy of research.

**Authors' contributions**

TZM, AH and HMR contributed to the conception or design of the work. TZM and HZ drafted the manuscript. All authors have read and approved the manuscript, and ensure that this is the case. All authors have agreed both to be personally accountable for the author's own contributions and to ensure that questions related to the accuracy or integrity of any part of the work.

**Competing interests**

The authors declare that there is no conflict of interests.

**Author details**

[1]Social Determinants of Health Research Center, Ardabil University of Medical Sciences, Ardabil, Iran. [2]Department of Surgery, School of Medicine and Allied Medical Sciences, Imam Reza Hospital, Ardabil University of Medical Sciences, Ardabil, Iran.

**References**

1. Myers A, Morganstern B, Fine R. A unique case of Pentaorchidism. Urology. 2017;104:196–7.
2. Artul S, Habib G. Polyorchidism: two case reports and a review of the literature. J Med Case Rep. 2014;8(1):464.
3. Savas M, Yeni E, Ciftci H, Cece H, Topal U, Utangac M. Polyorchidism: a three-case report and review of the literature. Andrologia. 2010;42(1):57–61.
4. Duymuş M, Menzilcioğlu MS, Çetinçakmak M, Avcu S. A rare case of polyorchidism: four testes. Pol J Radiol. 2016;81:39.
5. Kumar B, Sharma C, Sinha D. Supernumerary testis: a case report and review of literature. J Pediatr Surg. 2008;43(6):e9–e10.
6. Arslanoglu A, Tuncel SA, Hamarat M. Polyorchidism: color Doppler ultrasonography and magnetic resonance imaging findings. Clin Imaging. 2013;37(1):189–91.
7. Bergholz R, Wenke K. Polyorchidism: a meta-analysis. J Urol. 2009;182(5): 2422–7.
8. Saab MM, Landers M, Hegarty J. Males' awareness of benign testicular disorders: an integrative review. Am J Mens Health. 2018;12(3):556–66.
9. Délot EC, Vilain EJ. Nonsyndromic 46, XX testicular disorders of sex development. GeneReviews®[Internet]. Seattle: University of Washington; 2015.
10. Emad-Eldin S, Abo-Elnagaa N, Hanna SA, Abdel-Satar AH. The diagnostic utility of combined diffusion-weighted imaging and conventional magnetic resonance imaging for detection and localization of non palpable undescended testes. J Medical Imag Rad Oncol. 2016;60(3):344–51.
11. Jamalalail YA, Guerra LA, Leonard MP. Selective use of laparoscopy in nonpalpable undescended testes. Urology Ann. 2016;8(1):81.
12. Kucharski P, Niedzielski J. Neoadjuvant human chorionic gonadotropin (hCG) therapy may improve the position of undescended testis: a preliminary report. Central Eur J Urol. 2013;66(2):224.

# 9

# Ambient sulfur dioxide could have an impact on testicular volume from a observational study on a population of infertile male

Yu-An Chen[1,2], Yi-Kai Chang[1], Yann-Rong Su[3] and Hong-Chiang Chang[1*]

**Abstract**

**Background:** The effect of ambient pollutants on the male reproductive system is controversial. This retrospective study investigated the effect of environmental pollutants on male reproductive health.

**Methods:** Male patients with primary infertility ($n = 282$) were identified from a single center between January 2016 and December 2017. Patients were physically examined for the presence of varicocele and for the volume of both testicles. Semen quality was measured in terms of the total sperm count, sperm concentration, and the percentage of sperm cells with motility and normal morphology. Data were acquired on the concentration of ambient pollutants, namely particulate matters of diameter < 2.5 μm, sulfur dioxide ($SO_2$), nitrogen oxides ($NO_x$), and ozone ($O_3$), measured on daily and hourly basis, from the Environmental Protection Administration Executive Yuan, Taiwan. Individual exposure to pollutants was estimated based on the reported residential address of each participant. Statistical analysis indicated the effect of each pollutant on the testicular volume, sex hormone profile, and semen parameters.

**Results:** The mean ± standard deviation of age was 36.7 ± 7.3 years. The average sperm count and concentration were 41.9 million/mL and 34.1 million/mL, respectively. The mean levels of serum testosterone, follicle-stimulating hormone, and luteinizing hormone were 3.57 ± 1.68 ng/mL, 7.59 ± 6.3 IU/L, and 4.68 ± 3.49 IU/L, respectively. According to the multivariate linear regression model, $NO_x$ exposure was a risk factor for decreased sperm concentration and motility ($p = 0.043$ and 0.032). Furthermore, $SO_2$ exposure was negatively associated and testicular volume ($p < 0.01$).

(Continued on next page)

* Correspondence: changhong@ntu.edu.tw



[1]Department of Urology, National Taiwan University Hospital and National Taiwan University College of Medicine, No.1, Changde St., Zhongzheng Dist, Taipei City 10048, Taiwan

(Continued from previous page)

**Conclusions:** $NO_2$ and $SO_2$ exposure were negatively associated with the seminal parameter and decreased testicular volume, respectively, in a population of men with infertility. However, additional prospective studies are needed to ascertain the cause–effect relation of current results.

**Keywords:** Infertility, Air pollution, Sperm quality, Testicular volume

## Background

Following industrialization, increasing attention has been focused on the effects of environmental toxicants on the human reproductive system. Occupational exposure to heavy metals, including arsenic, lead, and mercury, disrupts male reproductive functions through altered sex hormone levels and decreased testicular volume. Furthermore, environmental and occupational exposure to synthetic organic compounds, such as organochlorides and organophosphate, reduce sperm quality. Methyl parathion, a known pesticide, is a type of organophosphate [1–3]. Ambient pollutants resulting from the increasing number of automobiles and factories include particulate matters with aerodynamic diameter < 2.5 μm ($PM_{2.5}$), nitrogen oxides ($NO_x$), and sulfur oxides. These ambient pollutants have been shown to not only impair human fertility but also interfere with male reproductive functions [4–10].

Several mechanisms have been proposed to explain how inhaled ambient particles disrupt reproductive function. First, ambient particles could induce oxidative stress (OS) in the gonad along with increased proinflammatory cytokine gene expression [8]. Second, ambient pollutants could interrupt germ cell maturation through altering the expression of the gene regulating differentiation or apoptosis in mice germ cells [11, 12].

Previous studies on the disruption of male reproductive function due to air pollution have almost always only focused on semen quality. The outcomes of other parameters of reproductive function, particularly testicular volume and the presence of varicocele, were not evaluated [3, 13, 14]. Furthermore, the effect of a particular gaseous molecule, for example, sulfur oxides or ozone ($O_3$), is still inconclusive, and the results of several studies have been conflicting each another [6, 12, 15–17]. This fueled our interest in conducting a study to evaluate the relationship between ambient pollutants and male reproductive functions based on semen parameters, sex hormone profile, and physical examination, namely examining testicular size and the presence of varicocele.

## Methods

### Ethic approval

The present study followed all standards for ethics regarding the experimentation and research. The institutional review board of the National Taiwan University approved our study and waived the informed consent requirement because of the retrospective design of the present study (approval number: 20190311 RIND).

### Study design

We retrospectively analyzed data from a medical chart database. Patient data were recorded, including age at the time of diagnosis, body mass index (BMI), and lifestyle factors, such as smoking and the presence of diabetes. Furthermore, blood test for fasting blood sugar and sex hormone profile were recorded. At least one semen sample was obtained from each participant. If a patient had more than one semen sample, the first sample was used for the analysis. Air pollution data were acquired from the Environmental Protection Administration Executive Yuan, Taiwan. Outcomes were seminal parameter, sex hormone profile, and change in testicular volume.

### Participants

We analyzed data of men diagnosed with primary infertility obtained from a single center (National Taiwan University Hospital, Taipei, Taiwan) from January 2016 to December 2017. Primary infertility was defined as the inability to conceive under an unprotected sexual encounter in ≥12 months as defined by the World Health Organization (WHO) [18].

Participants with aberrant chromosomes, previous chemotherapy/radiotherapy due to malignancy, or bone marrow transplantation were excluded. Furthermore, patients who were previously diagnosed with obstructive azoospermia, such as the absence of vas deferens or had received vasectomies or orchiectomy, were excluded.

### Physical examination

Physical examination consisted of determining the presence and grading of varicocele and recording the volume of both testicles. The testicular volume was estimated using the Prader orchidometer (Bayer, Müllerstraße 178, Berlin, Germany). Genital malformation, if any, was recorded. Body weight, height, and smoking habits, if any, were recorded.

### Blood and hormonal analysis

Venous blood samples were collected at 9:00–11:00 in the morning. Hormonal assays were conducted in accordance with the instructions of our institute. The testosterone level was recorded in ng/mL, and luteinizing hormone (LH) and follicle-stimulating hormone (FSH) levels were recorded in IU/L.

### Semen analysis

Patients were asked to practice abstinence for 3–5 days before semen collection. Each man was provided a wide-mouth plastic container. The semen sample was collected through masturbation and was sent to the laboratory at our institute. Each sample was smeared, stained, and preserved. The following semen variables were used as outcomes: total sperm count (million), sperm concentration (million/mL), percentage of motile sperm cells, and the percentage of sperm cells with normal morphology.

### Ambient pollutant data and analysis

Data were acquired from the Environmental Protection Administration Executive Yuan, Taiwan (https://airtw.epa.gov.tw). The concentrations of air pollutants, namely sulfur dioxide ($SO_2$), $O_3$, $NO_x$ [nitrogen monoxide (NO) and nitrogen dioxide ($NO_2$)], and $PM_{2.5}$, were automatically recorded at 78 monitoring stations throughout Taiwan. The data collected from these stations were recorded automatically, and the measures were previously validated manually by using linear regression to check concentrations. The concentration of each pollutant was continuously measured on daily and hourly bases. The monthly average of each pollutant was calculated if ≥20 daily average records were available for a month. In this study, individual exposure to air pollution was estimated on the basis of current residential address reported by the study participants and the mean concentrations of air pollutants in the study period (January 2016 to December 2017).

### Statistical analysis

Values are expressed as the mean ± standard deviation. Linear regression with a regression coefficient β and a 95% confidence interval was applied to indicate the effect of each unit of pollutant on the testicular volume and semen parameter. Smoking and medical comorbidities, including obesity and the varicocele status, were adjusted in the multivariate regression model. Furthermore, we examined the effect of ambient pollutants on sex hormone by using the multivariate linear regression model. Because serum sex hormone is associated with testicular size, an individual linear regression was performed for testicular volume after adjusting for sex hormone. We set the significance level at $p < 0.05$. All data analyses were performed using SPSS version 12 (SPSS Inc., Chicago, IL, USA).

## Results

The demographic characteristics of the included participants are summarized in Table 1a and 1b. In the study, 282 participants residing in Taiwan were included. The mean (±standard deviation) age, BMI, and the sizes of the right and left testes of all the participants were 36.7 ± 7.3 years, 24.6 ± 4.2 kg/m$^2$, and 14.18 ± 2.7 and 14.30 ± 2.4 mL, respectively. In total, 64 participants (22%) had varicocele, and 212 participants (77%) were nonsmokers. The majority of the participants ($n = 265$, 93%) resided in northern Taiwan; 3, 3, and 1% of the patients were from central, southern, and other parts of Taiwan, respectively.

### Sperm parameters

The average sperm count was 41.9 ± 56.6 million, and the average sperm concentration was 34.1 ± 38.8 million/mL. The percentages of sperms with total motility and normal morphology were 30.5 ± 16% and 23.6 ± 9.2%, respectively (Table 2). The mean values of the total sperm count, concentration, and normal morphology were higher in these participants than the cut-off values according to WHO standards [19]. However, the percentage of the progressively motile spermatozoa was low.

### Sex hormone profile

The sex hormone profile of the study population is summarized in Table 2. The mean levels of serum testosterone, FSH, and LH were 3.57 ± 1.68 ng/mL, 7.59 ± 6.3 IU/L, and 4.68 ± 3.49 IU/L, respectively. The mean

**Table 1** a and b. Demographic characteristics of the study participants

| Characteristics | Mean ± standard deviation | | Range |
|---|---|---|---|
| Age | 36.7 ± 7.3 years | | 19–69 |
| BMI | 24.6 ± 4.2 kg/m$^2$ | | 17.3–36 |
| Right testis | 14.18 ± 2.7 ml | | 6–20 |
| Left testis | 14.30 ± 2.4 ml | | 5–20 |
| Characteristics | N, total = 282 | % | |
| Cigarette | | | |
| Smoker | 65 | 23 | |
| Nonsmoker | 217 | 77 | |
| Varicocele | | | |
| Present | 64 | 22 | |
| Absent | 218 | 78 | |
| Residency | | | |
| Northern Taiwan | 265 | 93 | |
| Central Taiwan | 7 | 3 | |
| Southern Taiwan | 7 | 3 | |
| Other | 3 | 1 | |

**Table 2** Distribution of sperm parameters and sex hormone profile

| | Mean ± standard deviation | Range |
|---|---|---|
| Sperm quality parameters | | |
| Sperm count | 41.9 ± 56.6 mln | 0.25–280 |
| Sperm concentration | 34.1 ± 38.8 mln/ml | 0.1–420 |
| Sperm motility | 30.5% ± 16% | 0–75 |
| Normal form | 23.6% ± 9.2% | 0–80 |
| Sex hormone profile | | |
| FSH | 7.59 ± 6.3 IU/L | 1.2–56.28 |
| LH | 4.68 ± 3.49 IU/L | 0.32–33.5 |
| Testosterone | 3.57 ± 1.68 ng/mL | 0.98–12.8 |

*Abbreviations*: *FSH* Follicle Stimulating Hormone, *LH* Luteinizing hormone

testosterone level was higher than the cutoff value of hypogonadism as defined by the American urological association [20].

### Air pollution levels

The average levels of $PM_{2.5}$, $O_3$, $SO_2$, and $NO_x$ were 18.0 μg/m$^3$ (range = 10.9–27.2 μg/m$^3$), 27.3 ppb (parts per billion) (range = 21.0–40.6 ppb), 2.9 ppb (range = 1.7–5.6 ppb), and 29.0 (range = 3.7–91.9 ppb), respectively. According to WHO air quality guidelines, the recommended annual mean for $PM_{2.5}$, $O_3$, $SO_2$, and $NO_2$ were 10 μg/m$^3$, 100 ppb, 20 ppb, and 40 ppb, respectively [21]. Except for $PM_{2.5}$, the mean concentrations of particulate matter in Taiwan were within reference values suggested by the WHO air quality guidelines. The eastern part of Taiwan, which consists of mostly rural regions, had low $SO_2$, $NO_x$, and $PM_{2.5}$ levels. The distribution of $O_3$ did not considerably vary between the different parts of Taiwan, but a high $O_3$ level was observed in Kinmen, an island located on the east coast of China. All ambient pollutants were at the highest concentration in the southern part of Taiwan, including Tainan, Kaohsiung, and Kinmen, in all seasons. The $PM_{2.5}$ level was high in winter and low in summer, and the regional concentration difference of $PM_{2.5}$ was particularly obvious in January and February (Figs. 1, 2, 3, 4, 5).

Tables 3, 4, 5 summarize multiple regression analysis results for the semen parameter, sex hormone profile, and testicular volume after adjusting for blood sugar, BMI, varicocele, and smoking. The exposed mean concentrations of $NO_x$ in the study period were negatively associated with the sperm concentration and total motility ($p < 0.05$). No statistically significant relationship was observed between exposure to $PM_{2.5}$, $SO_2$ or $O_3$ and sperm parameters. In this study, linear regression did not show an effect of ambient pollutant on the sex hormone profile. Only age was found to be an independent predicting factor for increased follicle stimulating hormone (Table 4).

The testicular volume was negatively associated with the exposed mean concentration of $SO_2$ ($p < 0.01$). The effect of $SO_2$ on testicular volume was statistically significant even after adjusting for sex hormone (Table 6).

## Discussion

The current study investigated the effects of air pollutants on the reproductive health of men with infertility. As air pollutants are known to be hazardous to humans, it is unethical to conduct an interventional study on humans. Most studies on the effects of ambient pollutants on humans have been retrospective or observational, and the majority of them focused solely on the effects of pollutants on semen quality [6, 10, 13, 15–17, 22, 23].

Observational studies analyzing the effect of $SO_2$ and $NO_2$ on sperm quality have reported an unfavorable effect of these ambient particles on the sperm concentration and total count [9, 10, 15]. Our study suggested that $NO_2$ exposure was negatively associated with the sperm concentration and sperm motility, which is consistent with the finding of Broggia [9]. Nevertheless, Zhang reported that $SO_2$, $NO_2$, and PMs were not associated with poor semen quality [16].

The reported effect of $O_3$ on the reproductive function of men was deleterious. Data obtained from country-wide air quality monitoring showed high $O_3$ exposure to be an independent factor predicting low semen quality, including total sperm count, sperm concentration, and percentage of normal form [16, 22, 24]. However, our results did not show a significant association between $O_3$ and seminal parameters. The inconsistency with the previous literature could be due to the small sample size and retrospective study design, which failed to detect statistically significant effects of $O_3$ on male reproductive function.

The detailed mechanism through which ambient pollutants interfere with the male reproductive system is not well elucidated. One of the most frequently proposed mechanisms is the induction of OS in the reproductive system.

A rat model biopsy showed that $PM_{2.5}$ increased OS in the testes. First, expression of superoxide dismutase (SOD) decreased, which is one of the crucial enzymes that protect cells from reactive oxygen species (ROS). Second, an increase in heme oxygenase (HO) was observed. HO participates in ROS metabolism. An increased HO level signified increased OS [25].

Similarly, a testicular biopsy of $SO_2$-exposed mice showed decreased expression of antioxidation enzymes, including SOD and glutathione peroxidase (GPx). GPx catalyzed the reduction of peroxide radicals to alcohols and oxygen and thereby reduced OS [7].

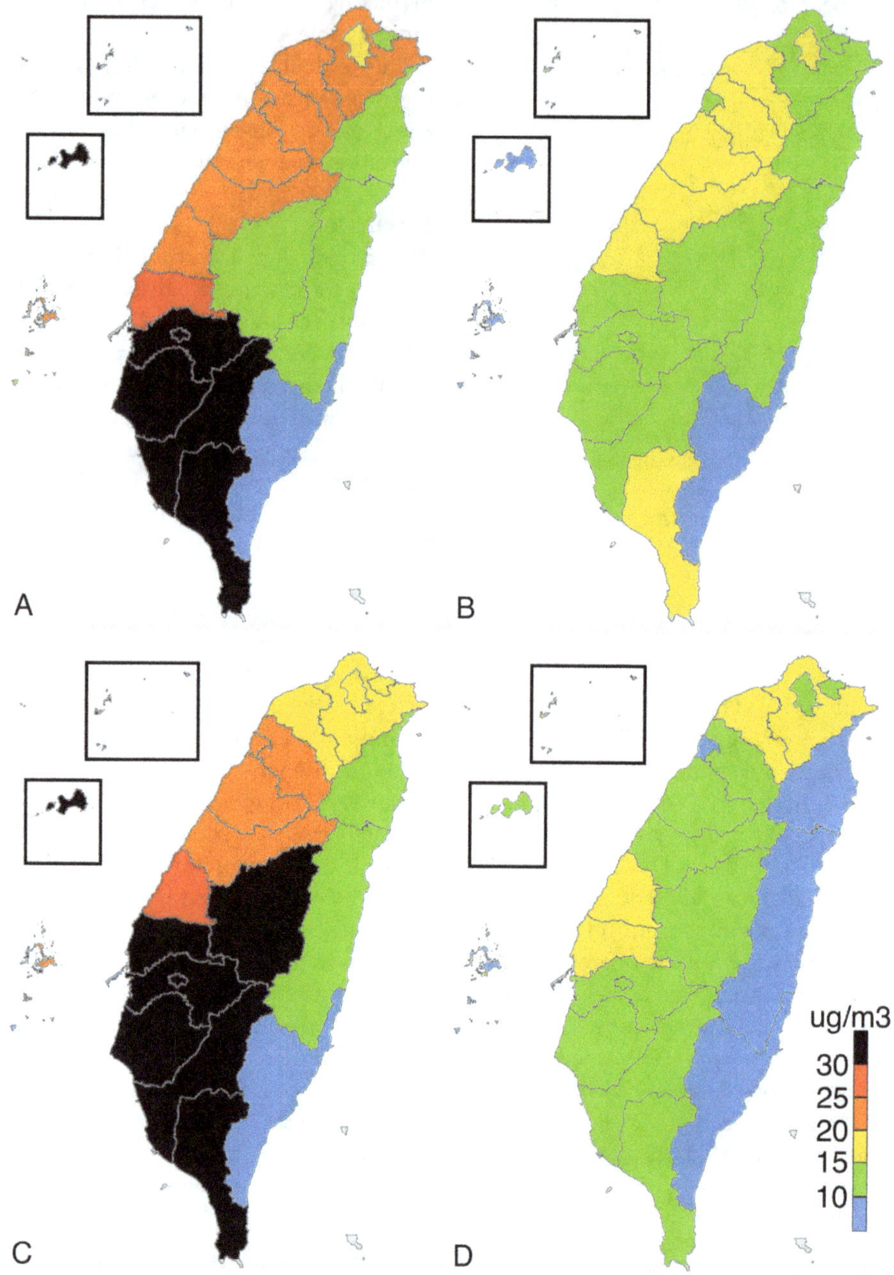


**Fig. 1** Distribution of 2.5-μm particulate matter in **a** January 2016; **b** July 2016; **c** January 2017; and **d** July 2017. (This work is adapted from the datasets of the National Land Surveying and Mapping Center MOI 2019–20, which is available to the public under the Open Government Data Licenses and is licensed under the Creative Commons Attribution-Share Alike 4.0 International license)

$NO_2$ and $O_3$ led to an increased expression of oxidative-stress-related gene, heme oxygenase (decycling) 1 ($HMOX_1$), which encodes HO in human bronchial epithelial cells. As aforementioned, an increased level of HO indicates increased OS. With exposure to $NO_2$ and $O_3$, the expression of $HMOX_1$ and proinflammatory-related genes, including interleukin-6 and interleukin-8, increased [26]. More importantly, these molecules not only are deposited in the respiratory system but also travel to diverse organ systems through circulation [26–28].

OS and ROS could compromise male reproductive fucntion through altering the reproductive hormone profile and impairing spermatogenesis. ROS has been reported to be responsible for reduction in testosterone production, and a low testosterone level had a negative effect on spermatogenesis and male fertility [29–31]. Testosterone can protect the testicular microenvironment from

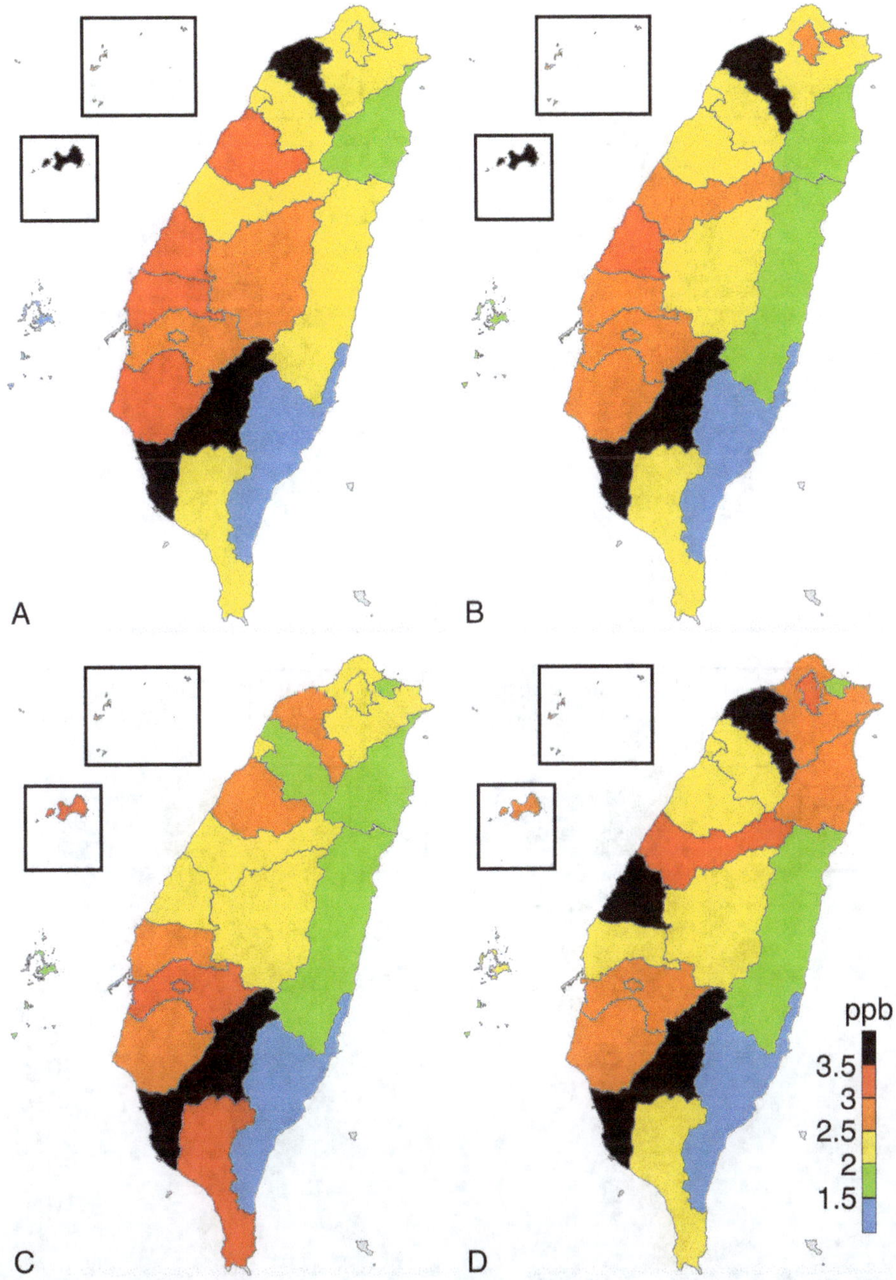


**Fig. 2** Distribution of sulfur dioxide in **a** January 2016; **b** July 2016; **c** January 2017; and **d** July 2017. (This work is adapted from the datasets of the National Land Surveying and Mapping Center MOI 2019–20, which is available to the public under the Open Government Data Licenses and is licensed under the Creative Commons Attribution-Share Alike 4.0 International license)

damage by ROS [32, 33]. Activating hypothalamus-pituitary-gonadal (HPG) axis with leptin in rat could induce high FSH and LH levels. High levels of FSH and LH were associated with high OS and DNA fragementation [34]. Similar results were reported by Beattie et al. after administering exogenous LH to rat Leydig cells [35]. ROS, on the other hand, downregulates the HPG axis through hormonal cross-link through activation of the hypothalamus-pituitary-adrenal axis. Cortisone secretion increased in response to increased stress, a high level of which suppresses FSH and LH secretion, finally leading to decreased testosterone production [31].

Exposing an animal model to air pollution reduced its testosterone level [36]. However, in the present study, the toxic ambient pollutants did not show a statistically significant effect on the sex hormone profile in our study population. Calogero el al reported similar results. Compared with the control group, Tollgate workers exposed

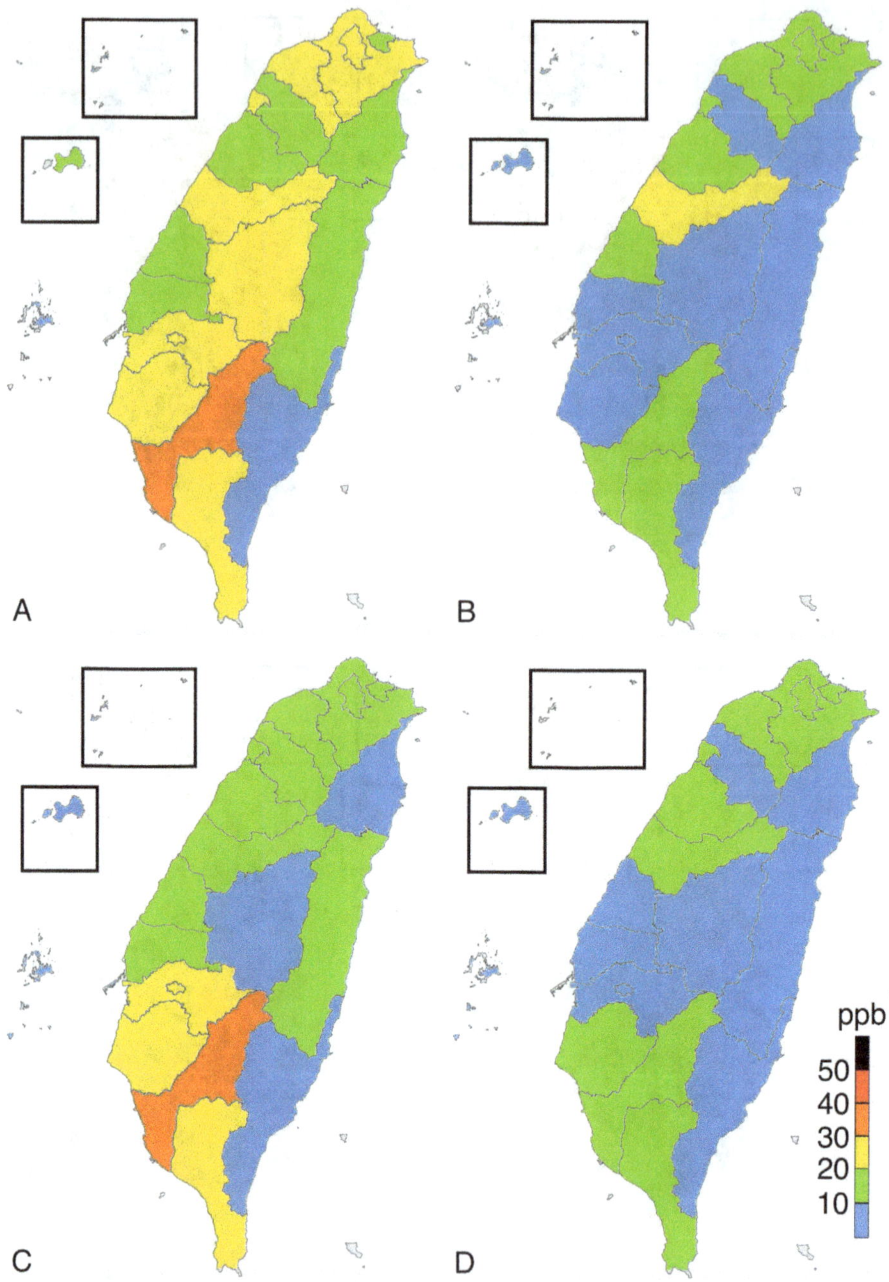


**Fig. 3** Distribution of nitrogen oxides in **a** January 2016; **b** July 2016; **c** January 2017; and **d** July 2017. (This work is adapted from the datasets of the National Land Surveying and Mapping Center MOI 2019–20, which is available to the public under the Open Government Data Licenses and is licensed under the Creative Commons Attribution-Share Alike 4.0 International license)

to a high level of car exhaust did not have significantly different serum levels of LH, FSH, and testosterone [37]. However, additional studies are required to evaluate OS by using markers, such as SOD and GPx, after exposure to ambient pollutants to further establish the link between ambient pollutants, OS, and male sexual endocrinological function.

Spermatozoon is a cell type that generates ROS independently, which is crucial in the acrosome reaction [38]. However, excessive ROS attacks the fluidity of the sperm plasma membrane and induces DNA damage in the sperm nucleus [27, 28]. Moreover, spermatozoa are more vulnerable to OS than oocytes because they lack downstream enzymes that participate in base excision repair [7, 11, 39, 40]. Human testicular development mainly occurs during puberty, and different cell types, including Sertoli cells, spermatogonia, and spermatocytes, play a role. In childhood, the elongation of

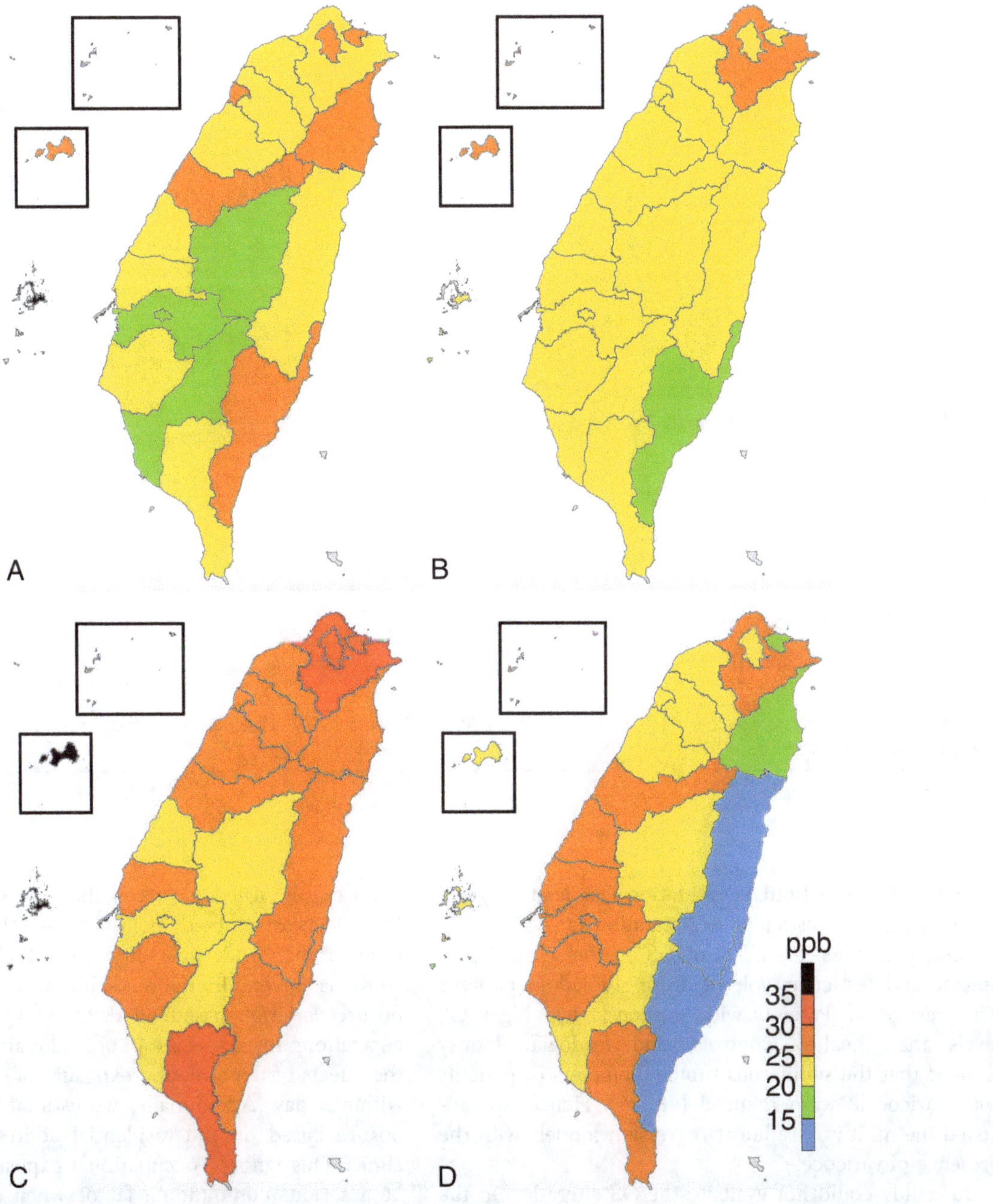


**Fig. 4** Distribution of ozone in **a** January 2016; **b** July 2016; **c** January 2017; and **d** July 2017. (This work is adapted from the datasets of the National Land Surveying and Mapping Center MOI 2019–20, which is available to the public under the Open Government Data Licenses and is licensed under the Creative Commons Attribution-Share Alike 4.0 International license)

seminiferous tubules contributes to testicular growth. In puberty, the testicles enlarge due to increase in the diameter of the seminiferous tubules [41, 42]. Later, the exponential growth of germ cells during spermatogenesis increases the testicular volume [21, 43].

The effect of OS on testicular development was studied in mice models. Mice exposed to excessive OS caused by crotonaldehyde, a food preservative, had significantly low levels of GPx and SOD with an increased malondialdehyde (MDA) level, which was a direct indicator of lipid peroxidation-induced injury caused by ROS. Following increased ROS and OS, lower testicular and epididymal weights were observed in the experimental group [44]. Furthermore, mice exposed to doxorubicin-induced OS had similar outcomes. After a week's treatment, testicular volume, epididymal sperm count, and seminiferous tubule diameter decreased compared with the control group.

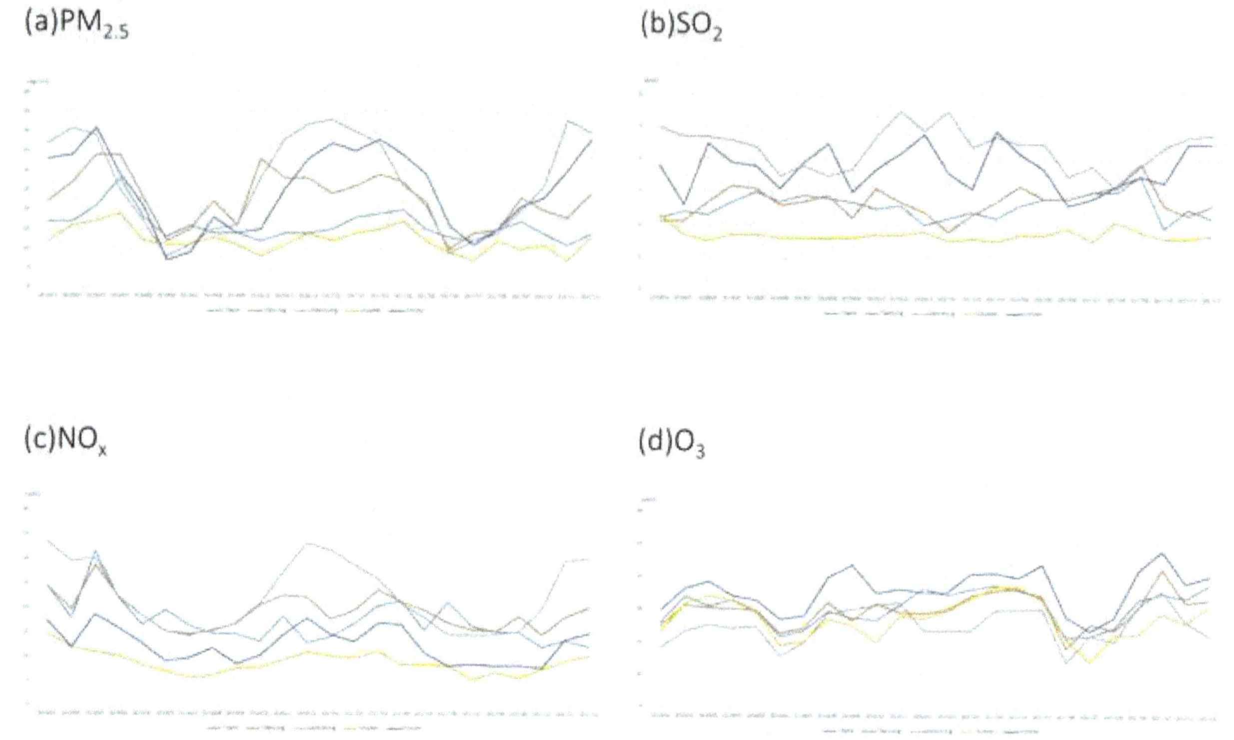


**Fig. 5** Ambient pollutants concentration in Taiwan from January 2016 to December 2017: **a** particulate matter of 2.5 μm; **b** sulfur dioxide; **c** nitrogen oxides; and **d** ozone

Excessive OS and lipid peroxidation can lead to germ cell damage and testicular degeneration [45–47].

Among humans, the effect of OS on the seminal parameter and testicular volume were studied in patients with varicocele. Patients with varicocele had higer OS levels than healthy controls, and testicular biopsy showed that the semiferous tubule diameters of patients with varicocele were reduced [48, 49]. Hence, we adjusted the multivariate linear regression models with the presence of varicocele.

Our study could not evaluate the OS alteration in the male reproductive system that results from ambient pollutant exposure. A future study with OS markers from the semen testicular tissue after exposure to ambient pollution should be conducted. If semen quality and testicular volume change, the sperm structure should be observed in relation to increased OS to further establish the link between OS and the male reproductive system. In participants exposed to ambient pollutants, the enzymes that partake in redox could be analyzed, including SOD, GPx, MDA, and HO. Furthermore, DNA fragmentation could be analyzed, as it has been reported to result from OS and could lead to sperm apoptosis [27, 28, 38, 50].

To our knowledge, this is the first study to evaluate the effects of ambient pollutants on the testicular volume of men with infertility. Nevertheless, the current study has several limitations. First, we considered the exposure variation based on daily average exposure concentrations for a specific period (2 years) while ignoring the effects of the peak and exposure of certain pollutants within a day. Additionally, we estimated individual exposure based on the residential address record at the clinic. This ignored occupational exposure, which could be a serious confounding factor when occupational exposure to air pollution is profound; for example, if a participant is a factory worker. Moreover, if the patient spends only a little time at home, estimating the exposure based on residential address could be misleading. Second, our study was retrospective and observatory in design because intentionally exposing participants to air pollutants is unethical. Moreover, the present study lacked serum or seminal marker for OS, which we believe participates in the alteration of seminal parameter and testicular volume. We aim to conduct further studies by using surrogate markers to determine OS in the semen and testicular tissue of patients with infertility who needed testicle biopsy. Third, our study population

**Table 3** Multivariable linear regression by using a sperm parameter for exposure to ambient pollutants

| Sperm parameters | Regression coefficients (95% confidence interval) | $p$ value |
|---|---|---|
| Sperm count | | |
| PM2.5 | 0.896 (−16.113 to 40.225) | 0.382 |
| $SO_2$ | −0.891 (− 169.427 to 68.260) | 0.384 |
| NOx | −1.136 (− 12.614 to 3.738) | 0.270 |
| $O_3$ | −0.196 (−18.947 to 15.698) | 0.846 |
| Sperm concentration | | |
| PM2.5 | 0.109 (−13.821 to 15.340) | 0.914 |
| $SO_2$ | −1.302 (−99.796 to 23.235) | 0.208 |
| NOx | −2.174 (−8.627 to −0.164) | 0.043* |
| $O_3$ | −1.749 (−16.458 to 1.475) | 0.096 |
| Sperm motility | | |
| PM2.5 | −0.303 (−7.508 to 5.608) | 0.765 |
| $SO_2$ | 0.049 (−27.026 to 28.308) | 0.962 |
| NOx | −2.321 (−4.014 to −0.207) | 0.032* |
| $O_3$ | −1.248 (−6.437 to 1.624) | 0.227 |
| Sperm normal form | | |
| PM2.5 | 1.248 (−3.566 to 13.322) | 0.234 |
| $SO_2$ | −0.617 (−46.216 to 25.681) | 0.548 |
| NOx | 1.400 (−1.147 to 5.369) | 0.185 |
| $O_3$ | 0.992 (−4.546 to 12.267) | 0.339 |

*$p < 0.05$

**Table 4** Multivariable linear regression by using sex hormone for exposure to ambient pollutants

| Sex hormone | Regression coefficients (95% confidence interval) | $p$ value |
|---|---|---|
| FSH | | |
| PM2.5 | 0.073 (−0.651 to 0.931) | 0.704 |
| $SO_2$ | 0.262 (−2.613 to 7.24) | 0.324 |
| NOx | −0.431 (−0.218 to 0.004) | 0.057 |
| $O_3$ | 0.122 (−0.503 to 0.852) | 0.582 |
| Age | 1.053 (0.290 to 0.639) | < 0.01** |
| LH | | |
| PM2.5 | 0.014 (−0.357 to 0.371) | 0.966 |
| $SO_2$ | 0.170 (−1.857 to 2.680) | 0.697 |
| NOx | 0.276 (−0.032 to 0.070) | 0.436 |
| $O_3$ | 0.559 (−0.093 to 0.531) | 0.150 |
| Testosterone | | |
| PM2.5 | 0.052 (−0.50 to 0.576) | 0.880 |
| $SO_2$ | −0.376 (−4.572 to 2.042) | 0.421 |
| NOx | 0.156 (−0.061 to 0.090) | 0.678 |
| $O_3$ | −0.044 (− 0.469 to 0.424) | 0.914 |

*Abbreviations: FSH* Follicle Stimulating Hormone, *LH* Luteinizing hormone, **$p < 0.01$

**Table 5** Multivariable linear regression by using the testicular volume for exposure of ambient pollutant

| | Regression coefficients (95% confidence interval) | $p$ value |
|---|---|---|
| Right testicle | | |
| PM2.5 | −0.472 (− 0.956 to 0.607) | 0.643 |
| $SO_2$ | −3.101 (−8.279 to −1.575) | 0.006** |
| NOx | −0.967 (− 0.376 to 0.140) | 0.347 |
| $O_3$ | −1.337 (− 1.007 to 0.226) | 0.199 |
| Left testicle | | |
| PM2.5 | 0.472 (−0.956 to 0.607) | 0.643 |
| $SO_2$ | −3.101 (−8.279 to −1.575) | 0.006** |
| NOx | −0.967 (− 0.376 to 0.140) | 0.347 |
| $O_3$ | −1.337 (− 1.007 to 0.226) | 0.199 |

**$p < 0.01$

was relatively small, and some data were missing. Therefore, the statistical power to detect the effects of pollutants on the reproductive system and sex hormone profile may be weakened. Selection bias was inevitable, as most of our patients were from northern Taiwan. Moreover, as data were obtained from men with infertility, a future study with a healthy population is needed to extrapolate the result to the general population. Recruiting patients from other parts of Taiwan and data from healthy individuals, such as from volunteers undergoing health examination during college entrance, are recommended to strengthen the statistical power.

## Conclusions

The result of the present study suggests that ambient $NO_x$ are a risk factor for poor sperm motility and decreased sperm concentration. Moreover, exposure to

**Table 6** Multivariable linear regression by using the testicular volume for exposure of ambient pollutant after adjusting for sex hormone

| | Regression coefficients (95% confidence interval) | $p$ value |
|---|---|---|
| Right testicle | | |
| PM2.5 | 0.147 (−0.492 to 1.031) | 0.476 |
| $SO_2$ | −0.520 (−4.696 to − 0.0474) | 0.018* |
| NOx | 0.170 (−0.067 to 0.155) | 0.424 |
| $O_3$ | −0.188 (− 0.834 to 0.317) | 0.366 |
| Left testicle | | |
| PM2.5 | 0.141 (−0.465 to 0.929) | 0.502 |
| $SO_2$ | −0.506 (−4.193 to − 0.328) | 0.023* |
| NOx | 0.199 (−0.055 to 0.147) | 0.362 |
| $O_3$ | −0.009 (− 0.538 to 0.516) | 0.967 |

*$p < 0.01$

$SO_2$ was negatively associated with testicular volume. However, the strength of the result is limited by the retrospective nature and small sample size of the study. Future prospective studies with healthy control and oxidative markers should be conducted to further establish the cause–effect relation between ambient pollutants and the male reproductive system and determine the mechanism behind it.

### Abbreviations

WHO: World Health Organization; Ppb: Parts per billion; $PM_{2.5}$: Particulate matters 2.5; $O_3$: Ozone; $SO_2$: Sulfur dioxide; NO: Nitrogen monoxide; $NO_2$: Nitrogen dioxide; FSH: Follicle stimulating hormone; LH: Luteinizing hormone; BMI: Body mass index; SOD: Superoxide dismutase; HO: Heme oxygenase; ROS: Reactive oxygen species; $HMOX_1$: Heme oxygenase (decycling) 1; GPx: Glutathione peroxidase; MDA: Malondialdehyde; NOx: Nitrogen oxides; OS: Oxidative stress; HPG: Hypothalamus-pituitary-gonadal

### Acknowledgements

This manuscript was edited for language by Wallace Academic Editing.

### Authors' contributions

HC Chang and YK Chang conceived the study design and contributed to data collection. YA Chen analyzed and interpreted the patient data regarding the sperm and physical examination and was a major contributor in writing the manuscript. HC Chang and YK Chang revised the article. All authors read and approved the final manuscript.

### Competing interests

The authors declare that they have no competing interests.

### Author details

[1]Department of Urology, National Taiwan University Hospital and National Taiwan University College of Medicine, No.1, Changde St., Zhongzheng Dist, Taipei City 10048, Taiwan. [2]Department of Urology, Cardinal Tien Hospital, School of Medicine Fu-Jen Catholic University, No.362, Zhongzheng Rd., Xindian Dist, New Taipei City 231, Taiwan. [3]Department of Urology, National Taiwan University Hospital Hsin-Chu Branch, NO.25, Lane 442, Sec.1, Jingguo Rd, Hsinchu City 300, Taiwan.

### References

1. Sengupta P. Environmental and occupational exposure of metals and their role in male reproductive functions. Drug Chem Toxicol. 2013;36(3):353–68.
2. Sengupta P, Banerjee R. Environmental toxins: alarming impacts of pesticides on male fertility. Hum Exp Toxicol. 2013;33(10):1017–39.
3. Ruth De Celis MS, Feria-Velasco A, Marco Gonza' lez-Unzaga MS, Torres-Calleja J, Pedro' n-Nuevo N. Semen quality of workers occupationally exposed to hydrocarbons. Fertil Steril. 2000;73(2):221–8.
4. Nieuwenhuijsen MJ, Basagaña X, Dadvand P, Martinez D, Cirach M, Beelen R, et al. Air pollution and human fertility rates. Environ Int. 2014;70:9–14.
5. Frutos V, González-Comadrán M, Solà I, Jacquemin B, Carreras R, Checa Vizcaíno MA. Impact of air pollution on fertility: a systematic review. Gynecol Endocrinol. 2015;31(1):7–13.
6. Farhat J, Farhat SCL, Braga ALF, Cocuzza M, Borba EF, Bonfá E, et al. Ozone decreases sperm quality in systemic lupus erythematosus patients. Rev Bras Reumatol Engl Ed. 2016;56(3):212–9.
7. Meng Z, Bai W. Oxidation damage of sulfur dioxide on testicles of mice. Environ Res. 2004;96(3):298–304.
8. Pires A, de Melo EN, Mauad T, Nascimento Saldiva PH, de Siqueira Bueno HM. Pre- and postnatal exposure to ambient levels of urban particulate matter (PM2.5) affects mice spermatogenesis. Inhal Toxicol. 2011;23(4):237–45.
9. Boggia B, Carbone U, Farinaro E, et al. Effects of working posture and exposure to traffic pollutants on sperm quality. J Endocrinol Investig. 2009; 32(5):430–4.
10. Zhou N, Cui Z, Yang S, Han X, Chen G, Zhou Z, et al. Air pollution and decreased semen quality: A comparative study of Chongqing urban and rural areas. Environ Pollut. 2014;187:145–52.
11. Wei Y, Cao X-N, Tang X-L, Shen L-J, Lin T, He D-W, et al. Urban fine particulate matter (PM2.5) exposure destroys blood–testis barrier (BTB) integrity through excessive ROS-mediated autophagy. Toxicol Mech Methods. 2017;28(4):302–19.
12. Zhang J, Zheng F, Liang C, Zhu Y, Shi Y, Han Y, et al. Sulfur dioxide inhalation lowers sperm quality and alters testicular histology via increasing expression of CREM and ACT proteins in rat testes. Environ Toxicol Pharmacol. 2016;47:47–52.
13. Hansen C, Luben TJ, Sacks JD, Olshan A, Jeffay S, Strader L, et al. The effect of ambient air pollution on sperm quality. Environ Health Perspect. 2010; 118(2):203–9.
14. Selevan SG, Borkovec L, Slott VL, Zudová Z, Rubes J, Evenson DP, et al. Semen quality and reproductive health of young Czech men exposed to seasonal air pollution. Environ Health Perspect. 2000;108(9):887–94.
15. Liu Y, Zhou Y, Ma J, Bao W, Li J, Zhou T, et al. Inverse association between ambient sulfur dioxide exposure and semen quality in Wuhan, China. Environ Sci Technol. 2017;51(21):12806–14.
16. Zhang HT, Zhang Z, Cao J, Tang WH, Zhang HL, Hong K, et al. Ambient ozone pollution is associated with decreased semen quality: longitudinal analysis of 8945 semen samples from 2015 to 2018 and during pollution-control period in Beijing, China. Asian J Androl. 2019;21(5):501–7.
17. Nobles CJ, Schisterman EF, Ha S, Kim K, Mumford SL, Buck Louis GM, et al. Ambient air pollution and semen quality. Environ Res. 2018;163:228–36.
18. Cooper TG, Noonan E, von Eckardstein S, Auger J, Baker HWG, Behre HM, et al. World Health Organization reference values for human semen characteristics*‡. Hum Reprod Update. 2009;16(3):231–45.
19. Menkveld R. Clinical significance of the low normal sperm morphology value as proposed in the fifth edition of the WHO Laboratory manual for the examination and processing of human semen. Asian J Androl. 2010; 12(1):47–58.
20. Mulhall JP, Trost LW, Brannigan RE, Kurtz EG, Redmon JB, Chiles KA, et al. Evaluation and Management of Testosterone Deficiency: AUA guideline. J Urol. 2018;200(2):423–32.
21. Krzyzanowski M, Cohen A. Update of WHO air quality guidelines. Air Qual Atmos Health. 2008;1(1):7–13.
22. Wdowiak A, Wdowiak E, Bien A, Bojar I, Iwanowicz-Palus G, Raczkiewicz D. Air pollution and semen parameters in men seeking fertility treatment for the first time. Int J Occup Med Environ Health. 2019;32(3):387–99.
23. Fathi Najafi T, Latifnejad Roudsari R, Namvar F, Ghavami Ghanbarabadi V, Hadizadeh Talasaz Z, Esmaeli M. Air Pollution and Quality of Sperm: A Meta-Analysis. Iran Red Crescent Med J. 2015;17(4):e26930.
24. Sokol RZ, Kraft P, Fowler IM, Mamet R, Kim E, Berhane KT. Exposure to environmental ozone alters semen quality. Environ Health Perspect. 2006; 114(3):360–5.
25. Wei Y, Cao X-N, Tang X-L, Shen L-J, Lin T, He D-W, et al. Urban fine particulate matter (PM2.5) exposure destroys blood–testis barrier (BTB) integrity through excessive ROS-mediated autophagy. Toxicol Mech Methods. 2018;28(4):302–19.
26. Mirowsky JE, Dailey LA, Devlin RB. Differential expression of pro-inflammatory and oxidative stress mediators induced by nitrogen dioxide and ozone in primary human bronchial epithelial cells. Inhal Toxicol. 2016; 28(8):374–82.
27. Aitken J, Fisher H. Reactive oxygen species generation and human spermatozoa: the balance of benefit and risk. BioEssays. 1994;16(4):259–67.
28. Agarwal A, Saleh RA, Bedaiwy MA. Role of reactive oxygen species in the pathophysiology of human reproduction. Fertil Steril. 2003;79(4):829–43.
29. Kahn BE, Brannigan RE. Obesity and male infertility. Curr Opin Urol. 2017; 27(5):441–5.
30. Syriou V, Papanikolaou D, Kozyraki A, Goulis DG. Cytokines and male infertility. Eur Cytokine Netw. 2018;29(3):73–82.
31. Darbandi M, Darbandi S, Agarwal A, Sengupta P, Durairajanayagam D, Henkel R, et al. Reactive oxygen species and male reproductive hormones. Reprod Biol Endocrinol. 2018;16(1):87.
32. Chainy GB, Samantaray S, Samanta L. Testosterone-induced changes in testicular antioxidant system. Andrologia. 1997;29(6):343–9.

33. Shang X, Huang Y, Ye Z, Yu X, Gu W. Protection of melatonin against damage of sperm mitochondrial function induced by reactive oxygen species. Zhonghua Nan Ke Xue. 2004;10(8):604–7.
34. Abbasihormozi S, Shahverdi A, Kouhkan A, Cheraghi J, Akhlaghi AA, Kheimeh A. Relationship of leptin administration with production of reactive oxygen species, sperm DNA fragmentation, sperm parameters and hormone profile in the adult rat. Arch Gynecol Obstet. 2013;287(6):1241–9.
35. Beattie MC, Chen H, Fan J, Papadopoulos V, Miller P, Zirkin BR. Aging and luteinizing hormone effects on reactive oxygen species production and DNA damage in rat Leydig cells. Biol Reprod. 2013;88(4):100.
36. Sobolewski M, Anderson T, Conrad K, Marvin E, Klocke C, Morris-Schaffer K, et al. Developmental exposures to ultrafine particle air pollution reduces early testosterone levels and adult male social novelty preference: risk for children's sex-biased neurobehavioral disorders. NeuroToxicology. 2018;68:203–11.
37. Calogero AE, La Vignera S, Condorelli RA, Perdichizzi A, Valenti D, Asero P, et al. Environmental car exhaust pollution damages human sperm chromatin and DNA. J Endocrinol Investig. 2011;34(6):e139–43.
38. Dutta S, Henkel R, Sengupta P, Agarwal A. Physiological Role of ROS in Sperm Function. Male Infertility. 2020:337–45.
39. Aitken RJ, Smith TB, Jobling MS, Baker MA, De Iuliis GN. Oxidative stress and male reproductive health. Asian J Androl. 2014;16(1):31–8.
40. Cao XN, Shen LJ, Wu SD, Yan C, Zhou Y, Xiong G, et al. Urban fine particulate matter exposure causes male reproductive injury through destroying blood-testis barrier (BTB) integrity. Toxicol Lett. 2017;266:1–12.
41. Koskenniemi JJ, Virtanen HE, Toppari J. Testicular growth and development in puberty. Curr Opin Endocrinol Diabetes Obes. 2017;24(3):215–24.
42. Cortes D, Müller J, Skakkebaek NE. Proliferation of Sertoli cells during development of the human testis assessed by stereological methods. Int J Androl. 1987;10(4):589–96.
43. Rodolfo A, Rey SMC, Bedecarras P, Nagle CA, Hetor E. CHEMES is infancy a quiescent period of testicular development? Histological, morphometric, and functional study of the seminiferous tubules of the Cebus monkey from birth to the end of puberty. J Clin Endocrmol Metab. 1993;76(5):1325–31.
44. Li SSZB, Zhang ZH. Study on oxidative stress damage of reproductive organs in male rats induced by long-term exposure to crotonaldehyde. Chin J Ind Hygiene Occup Dis. 2019;37(4):241–6.
45. Farsani BE, Karimi S, Mansouri E. Pravastatin attenuates testicular damage induced by doxorubicin - a stereological and histopatological study. J Basic Clin Physiol Pharmacol. 2018;30(1):103-9.
46. Mirzaei Khorramabadi K, Reza Talebi A, Abbasi Sarcheshmeh A, Mirjalili A. Protective effect of vitamin E on oxidative stress and sperm apoptosis in diabetic mice. Int J Reprod Biomed (Yazd). 2019;17(2):127–34.
47. Koksal IT, Usta M, Orhan I, Abbasoglu S, Kadioglu A. Potential role of reactive oxygen species on testicular pathology associated with infertility. Asian J Androl. 2003;5(2):95–9.
48. Agarwal A, Makker K, Sharma R. Clinical relevance of oxidative stress in male factor infertility: an update. Am J Reprod Immunol. 2008;59(1):2–11.
49. Boujbiha MA, Hamden K, Guermazi F, Bouslama A, Omezzine A, Kammoun A, et al. Testicular toxicity in mercuric chloride treated rats: association with oxidative stress. Reprod Toxicol. 2009;28(1):81–9.
50. Muratori M, Tamburrino L, Marchiani S, Cambi M, Olivito B, Azzari C, et al. Investigation on the origin of sperm DNA fragmentation: role of apoptosis, Immaturity and Oxidative Stress. Mol Med. 2015;21(1):109–22.

# 10

# Urinary tract infection is associated with hypokalemia

Ai-Ling Shen[1], Hsiu-Li Lin[1,2], Hsiu-Chen Lin[3,4], Yuan-Fu Tseng[1], Chien-Yeh Hsu[2,5] and Che-Yi Chou[6,7,8*]

**Abstract**

**Background:** Hypokalemia is a common clinical problem. The association between urinary tract infection (UTI) and hypokalemia is not clear. Hypokalemia is common in patients with UTI in clinical observation. The aim of the study is to determine if UTI is associated with hypokalemia.

**Methods:** Patients hospitalized with UTI and the control group were retrieved from the Longitudinal Health Insurance Database 2005. The control group was patients hospitalized with other reasons and were matched for the confoundings of UTI and hypokalemia. We analyze the risk of hypokalemia using logistic regression and calculate the odds ratio (OR) and 95% confidence interval (CI) of OR.

**Results:** We analyzed 43,719 UTI patients and control patients. Hypokalemia was found in 4540 (10.4%) patients with UTI and 1842 (4.2%) control patients. The percentage of patients with hypokalemia was higher in UTI patients (chi-square, $p < 0.001$). UTI was associated with hypokalemia and the odds ratio (OR) was 2.27 [95% confidence interval (CI): 2.17–2.41]. Cerebrovascular accident, chronic obstructive pulmonary disease, hypertension, congestive heart failure, diarrhea, medications including thiazides, sulfonamides, xanthines, and laxatives were independently associated with hypokalemia. Recurrent UTI was associated with hypokalemia in UTI patients (OR: 1.13, 95% CI: 1.05–1.23, $p < 0.001$).

**Conclusions:** Urinary tract infection is associated with hypokalemia among inpatients. The association is independent of patients' comorbidities and medications. Recurrent UTI is associated with increased hypokalemia in UTI patients.

**Keywords:** UTI, Hypokalemia, Recurrent UTI, Comorbidities, Diarrhea, Thiazides, Sulfonamides

## Background

Hypokalemia is a common electrolyte abnormality in hospitalized patients. Unrecognized hypokalemia may trigger arrhythmias [1] and is associated with increased mortality in patients with chronic diseases such as heart failure, diabetes, or chronic kidney disease [2, 3]. Urinary tract infection (UTI) is a common bacterial infection in women and the elderly [4–6]. Clinical manifestations of UTI include dysuria, frequency, urgency, fever, nausea, vomit, and gross hematuria. It may not be surprised that hypokalemia may be occurred because of increased potassium loss after vomit and fever. However, the association between UTI and hypokalemia is not clear [7–11]. We observed that hypokalemia is common among UTI patients in clinical settings. This study was conducted to determine the association between UTI and hypokalemia. Inpatients were selected because serum potassium is rarely measured in outpatient settings as UTI has not been considered as a risk factor for hypokalemia.

* Correspondence: cychou.chou@gmail.com
[6]Division of Nephrology, Asia University Hospital, NO 222, Fuxin Rd, Wufeng Dist, Taichung 413, Taiwan
[7]Department of Post-baccalaureate Veterinary Medicine, Asia University, NO 222, Fuxin Rd, Wufeng Dist, Taichung 413, Taiwan

## Methods

We extracted data from the Longitudinal Health Insurance Database 2005 (LHID2005) as prescribed in the previous study [12]. The dataset used in this study is a de-identified secondary data and is released to the public for research purposes. A review of the institutional review board is not required. All inpatients with UTI between 1 January 2000 and 31 December 2008 were extracted. The first hospitalization for UTI was selected in the patients with more than one episode of UTI. The control patients were patients who are hospitalized for other reasons with matching for confoundings at a 1:1 ratio. The confoundings include cerebrovascular accident (CVA), chronic obstructive pulmonary disease (COPD), diabetes mellitus (DM), hypertension (HTN), acute kidney injury (AKI), chronic kidney disease (CKD), Cushing syndrome, hyperthyroidism, leukorrhea, medications, and urethral catheterization. These confoundings were used because they are associated with UTI or hypokalemia in the literature.

The patients hospitalized with UTI were identified with ICD-9-CM code 599 on discharge. Patients on dialysis were excluded in this study because pyuria is common in auric dialysis patients. The development of hypokalemia was identified using ICD-9-CM code (276.8) in the same hospitalization. The comorbidities diagnosed before the episode of UTI in at least 3 visits were retrieved. The comorbidities include CVA (ICD-9-CM code 430–436 and 438), COPD (490–496), DM (250), HTN (401–405), CHF (428), AKI (584.9), CKD (585), Cushing's syndrome (255.0), hyperthyroidism (242), hypothyroidism (244), alkalosis (276.3), diarrhea (787.91), malnutrition (269.9, 262, 263), poor intake (783.0), magnesium disorder (275.2), and leukorrhea (616 and 623.5). Urethral catheterization in 1 week before hospitalization was identify using procedure code 47013–47014. Recurrent UTI was defined as individuals who had more than two episodes of UTI in 6 months or three episodes in 1 year [13]. Medications used for more than 14 days in 1 month before the UTI diagnosed were extracted. Medications include potassium-sparing diuretics (ATC code C03D, C03E), thiazides (C03A, C03B), sulfonamides (C03CA01, C03CA02), beta-2-adrenoreceptor agonists (R03CC), xanthines (R03DA, R03DB), antibiotics (J01CA, J01CR, J01GB, A01AB04), meropenem (J01DH02), insulin (A10), steroids (H02AB), potassium binders (V03AE01), and laxatives (A06AG07).

### Statistical analysis

Data are expressed as number (percentage), or mean (standard deviation) where appropriate. Chi-square tests and *t*-test was used to test the differences of variables between two groups. The association of hypokalemia and UTI was estimated using univariable logistic regression. Variables with a $p < 0.05$ in univariable logistic regression were further analyzed by multivariable logistic regression. The odds ratios (ORs) and 95% confidence interval (CIs) of ORs were calculated. All statistical analyses were carried out using SAS statistical package, version 9.3 (SAS, Inc., NC, USA). All comparison tests were two-sided and a *P*-value of less than 0.05 was considered as statistically significant.

## Results

A total of 43,719 inpatients with UTI and matched control patients were analyzed (Table 1). 4540 (10.4%) UTI patients and 1842 (4.2%) control patients had hypokalemia ($p < 0.001$, chi-square test). The duration of hospitalization was longer in UTI patients 12.7 ± 24.8 days vs 7.4 ± 14.5 days in the control patients ($p < 0.001$). The average age of UTI patients was 63.5 ± 17.7 years old and 63.6 ± 18.2 years old in the control patients ($p =$ 0.492). 39.3% of UTI patients and 39.2% of control patients were male. The percentage of patients with different comorbidities were similar in UTI patients and control patients after matching. The percentage of CVA was 28.8% in UTI patients and 28.4% in control patients. COPD 30.9 and 30.7%, DM 33.8 and 33.4%, HTN 59.2 and 58.9%, CHF 14.1 and 14.0%, AKI 0.3 and 0.3%, CKD 7.2 and 7.2%. Diarrhea, poor intake, and malnutrition were identified in 0.1% of the patients. The percentage of patients on potassium-sparing diuretics was 0.1% in UTI patients and 0.2% in control patients. Thiazides 0.6 and 0.6%, sulfonamides 0.4 and 0.5%, beta-2-adrenoreceptor agonists 0.7 and 0.7%, xanthiums 4.1 and 4.1%, antibiotics 0.7 and 0.7%, insulin 1.7 and 1.7%, steroids 1.5 and 1.5%, potassium binders 0.2 and 0.2%, laxatives 10.2 and 10.1%. The percentage of patients with urethral catheterization was 6.7% in both groups.

UTI was associated with hypokalemia in univariable and multivariable logistic regression (Table 2). The ORs were 2.48 (95% CI: 2.33–2.64, $p < 0.001$) in univariable logistic regression and 2.27 (95% CI: 2.13–2.41, $p < 0.001$) in multivariable logistic regression. Factors associated with hypokalemia in univariable logistic regression include age, CVA, COPD, DM, HTN, CHF, CKD, diarrhea, potassium-sparing diuretics, thiazides, sulfonamides, beta-2-adrenoreceptor agonists, xanthines, steroids, and laxatives. DM, CKD, beta-2-adrenoreceptor agonists, and steroids were not significantly associated with hypokalemia in multivariable logistic regression. The ORs of age was 1.01 (95% CI: 1.01–1.01) for every one additional year, CVA 1.29 (95% CI: 1.20–1.39), COPD 1.47 (95% CI: 1.37–1.57), HTN 1.56 (95% CI: 1.44–1.68), CHF 1.40 (95% CI: 1.28–1.53), diarrhea 2.25 (95% CI: 1.24–3.82), thiazides 1.57 (95% CI: 1.21–2.00), sulfonamides 1.44 (95% CI: 1.03–1.97), xanthines 1.44 (95% CI: 1.22–1.69), and laxatives 1.32 (95% CI: 1.16–1.52).

**Table 1** Clinical characteristics of patients with and without urinary tract infection (UTI)

| Factor | UTI *N* = 43,719 | Control *N* = 43,719 | *P* |
|---|---|---|---|
| Hypokalemia n (%) | 4540 (10.4) | 1842 (4.2) | < 0.001 |
| Duration of hospitalization (day) | 12.7 ± 24.8 | 7.4 ± 14.5 | < 0.001 |
| Age | 63.6 ± 18.2 | 63.5 ± 17.7 | 0.492 |
| Male n (%) | 17,177 (39.3) | 17,152 (39.2) | 0.87 |
| Comorbidity n (%) | | | |
| CVA | 12,574 (28.8) | 12,412 (28.4) | 0.23 |
| COPD | 13,519 (30.9) | 13,428 (30.7) | 0.51 |
| DM | 14,776 (33.8) | 14,615 (33.4) | 0.25 |
| HTN | 25,860 (59.2) | 25,752 (58.9) | 0.46 |
| CHF | 6154 (14.1) | 6128 (14.0) | 0.81 |
| AKI | 119 (0.3) | 117 (0.3) | 0.95 |
| CKD | 3162 (7.2) | 3125 (7.1) | 0.64 |
| Cushing syndrome | 283 (0.6) | 279 (0.6) | 0.90 |
| Hyperthyroidism | 660 (1.5) | 654 (1.5) | 0.89 |
| Leukorrhea | 350 (0.8) | 332 (0.8) | 0.51 |
| Diarrhea | 59 (0.1) | 62 (0.1) | 0.85 |
| Poor intake | 40 (0.1) | 46 (0.1) | 0.59 |
| Malnutrition | 22 (0.05) | 25 (0.06) | 0.77 |
| Medications n (%) | | | |
| Potassium-sparing diuretics | 63 (0.1) | 75 (0.2) | 0.35 |
| Thiazides | 261 (0.6) | 283 (0.6) | 0.37 |
| Sulfonamides | 175 (0.4) | 208 (0.5) | 0.10 |
| Beta-2-adrenoreceptor agonists | 176 (0.4) | 204 (0.5) | 0.17 |
| Xanthiums | 1777 (4.1) | 1782 (4.1) | 0.94 |
| Antibiotics | 298 (0.7) | 296 (0.7) | 0.97 |
| Insulin | 752 (1.7) | 763 (1.7) | 0.79 |
| Steroids | 648 (1.5) | 663 (1.5) | 0.69 |
| Potassium binders | 105 (0.2) | 105 (0.2) | – |
| Laxatives | 4458 (10.2) | 4412 (10.1) | 0.61 |
| Urethral catheterization | 3034 (6.7) | 3034 (6.7) | – |

*CVA* cerebrovascular accident, *COPD* chronic obstructive pulmonary disease, *DM* diabetes mellitus, *HTN* hypertension, *AKI* acute kidney injury, *CKD* chronic kidney disease, *CHF* congestive heart failure

Recurrent UTI was significantly associated with hypokalemia in UTI patients (Table 3). The ORs were 1.31 (95% CI: 1.21–1.41) in univariable logistic regression and 1.13 (95% CI: 1.05–1.23) in multivariable logistic regression. Patient's age, CVA, COPD, HTN, CHF, thiazides, sulfonamides, xanthines, and laxatives were independently associated with hypokalemia in UTI patients in univariable logistic regression, but diarrhea was not. The OR of age in the multivariable logistic regression was 1.01 (95% CI: 1.01–1.01), CVA 1.16 (95% CI: 1.08–1.24), COPD 1.45 (95% CI: 1.35–1.55), HTN 1.42 (95% CI: 1.31–1.53), CHF 1.41 (95% CI: 1.31–1.53), xanthines 1.42 (95% CI: 1.25–1.62), and laxatives 1.29 (95% CI: 1.17–1.41).

## Discussion

In this case-control cross-sectional study, we demonstrated the association between UTI and hypokalemia among inpatients. This finding is supported by the increased OR of hypokalemia in the multivariable logistic regression. The association between hypokalemia and UTI is independent of comorbidities and mediations. Besides, recurrent UTI is also associated with hypokalemia in UTI patients. Hypokalemia in UTI may explain the cardiac arrest following infectious disease in the previous study [14]. Inpatients with UTI were selected in this study because the serum potassium was more likely to be measured in inpatient settings. The development of hypokalemia in the patients with UTI may be explained

**Table 2** Factors associated with hypokalemia in univariable and multivariable logistic regression

| Factors | Univariable | | | Multivariable | | |
|---|---|---|---|---|---|---|
| | ORs | 95% | CIs | ORs | 95% | CIs |
| UTI | 2.48 | 2.33 | 2.64 | 2.27 | 2.13 | 2.41 |
| Age | 1.03 | 1.03 | 1.03 | 1.01 | 1.01 | 1.01 |
| Comorbidity | | | | | | |
| CVA | 2.29 | 2.14 | 2.44 | 1.29 | 1.20 | 1.39 |
| COPD | 2.21 | 2.08 | 2.34 | 1.47 | 1.37 | 1.57 |
| DM | 1.56 | 1.46 | 1.66 | 1.02 | 0.95 | 1.09 |
| HTN | 2.62 | 2.46 | 2.79 | 1.56 | 1.44 | 1.68 |
| CHF | 2.49 | 2.28 | 2.71 | 1.40 | 1.28 | 1.53 |
| CKD | 1.42 | 1.21 | 1.66 | 0.98 | 0.84 | 1.15 |
| Diarrhea | 2.29 | 1.28 | 3.82 | 2.25 | 1.24 | 3.82 |
| Medications | | | | | | |
| Potassium-sparing diuretics | 1.96 | 1.12 | 3.19 | 1.24 | 0.69 | 2.08 |
| Thiazides | 1.98 | 1.53 | 2.51 | 1.57 | 1.21 | 2.00 |
| Sulfonamides | 2.26 | 1.64 | 3.06 | 1.44 | 1.03 | 1.97 |
| Beta-2-adrenoreceptor agonists | 2.04 | 1.48 | 2.76 | 0.91 | 0.64 | 1.26 |
| Steroids | 1.57 | 1.29 | 1.89 | 1.12 | 0.91 | 1.37 |
| Xanthines | 2.38 | 2.05 | 2.74 | 1.44 | 1.22 | 1.69 |
| Laxatives | 2.07 | 1.81 | 2.35 | 1.32 | 1.16 | 1.52 |

*UTI* urinary tract infection, *CVA* cerebral vascular accident, *COPD* chronic obstructive pulmonary disease, *DM* diabetes mellitus, *CHF* congestive heart failure, *CKD* chronic kidney disease

**Table 3** Risk of hypokalemia among patients with urinary tract infection

| Factors | Univariable | | | Multivariable | | |
|---|---|---|---|---|---|---|
| | ORs | 95% | CIs | ORs | 95% | CIs |
| Recurrent UTI | 1.31 | 1.21 | 1.41 | 1.13 | 1.05 | 1.23 |
| Age | 1.02 | 1.02 | 1.03 | 1.01 | 1.01 | 1.01 |
| Comorbidity | | | | | | |
| CVA | 1.71 | 1.60 | 1.82 | 1.16 | 1.08 | 1.24 |
| COPD | 2.08 | 1.95 | 2.21 | 1.45 | 1.35 | 1.55 |
| HTN | 2.20 | 2.05 | 2.36 | 1.42 | 1.31 | 1.53 |
| CHF | 2.16 | 2.01 | 2.33 | 1.41 | 1.31 | 1.53 |
| Diarrhea | 1.61 | 0.85 | 2.82 | 1.82 | 0.95 | 3.23 |
| Medications | | | | | | |
| Thiazide | 1.60 | 1.34 | 1.90 | 1.16 | 0.97 | 1.38 |
| Sulfonamides | 1.74 | 1.52 | 1.98 | 1.14 | 0.99 | 1.31 |
| Xanthines | 2.29 | 2.02 | 2.59 | 1.42 | 1.25 | 1.62 |
| Laxatives | 1.80 | 1.65 | 1.97 | 1.29 | 1.17 | 1.41 |

*UTI* urinary tract infection, *CVA* cerebral vascular accident, *COPD* chronic obstructive pulmonary disease, *DM* diabetes mellitus, *CHF* congestive heart failure

by multiple factors including renal [9, 15, 16], medications [17], gastrointestinal loss. Medications including thiazides, sulfonamides, xanthines, and laxatives were independently associated with hypokalemia. We hypothesized that hypokalemia developed because of renal potassium loss. The renal tubule potassium resorption was impaired after tubule injury in UTI and therefore the urine potassium loss is increased [18, 19]. We measured the urine potassium of several UTI patients (data not shown) and the urine potassium secretion was increased in patients with UTI. More studies are needed to verify our findings.

Because hypokalemia may be related to multiple comorbidities, we include comorbidities that may be associated with both UTI [20, 21] and hypokalemia [22] in the analysis. DM, CKD, potassium-sparing diuretics, beta-2-adrenoreceptor agonists, and steroids were associated with hypokalemia in univariable regression but not in multivariable regression. This suggests that these may be not major contributors to hypokalemia in UTI patients. A few patients (0.1%) had diarrhea, malnutrition, or poor intake in our study. We suspected these conditions were underdiagnosed because physicians rarely coded these conditions in the diagnosis. Although the numbers of patients are limited, diarrhea was associated with hypokalemia in univariable and multivariable regressions. Duration of hospitalization, alkalosis, malnutrition, poor intake, magnesium disorder, and meropenem [23] were analyzed and was not linked to hypokalemia.

### Limitations

The limitations to the study include: First, LHID only recorded the ICD-9-CM code on discharge, it is not possible to discriminate community acquired hypokalemia and hypokalemia developed in hospital. There may be many factors which may cause hypokalemia in hospital. The causal relationship can not be determined. Some of the recurrent UTI may be caused by the hypokalemia that results in the elaboration of alkaline urine, bladder dysfunction, and urinary stasis [24]. Second, the serum potassium readings and symptoms associated with hypokalemia were not available in the LHID, we were not able to report the severity of hypokalemia in this study, and symptoms associated with hypokalemia. In our clinical practice, most of the hypokalemia was asymptomatic and potassium replacement was rarely acquired. Third, we hypothesized that the renal parenchyma injury in UTI may be responsible for the development of hypokalemia. Acute pyelonephritis may be associated with more severe renal parenchyma injury than lower UTI and is more likely to develop hypokalemia. However, we did not find a significant association between acute pyelonephritis and hypokalemia. We suspected that most acute pyelonephritis may be recorded as UTI in the LHID.

## Conclusion

Urinary tract infection is associated with an increased risk of hypokalemia and measurements of serum potassium should be considered in clinical practice. UTI and hypokalemia are associated with multiple chronic diseases and medications. The association of hypokalemia and UTI is independent of comorbidities and medications.

### Abbreviations

LHID: Longitudinal Health Insurance Database; ICD-9-CM: International Classification of Disease, Ninth. Revision, Clinical Modification; UTI: Urinary tract infection; CVA: Cerebral vascular accident; COPD: Chronic obstructive pulmonary disease; DM: Diabetes mellitus; CHF: Congestive heart failure; CKD: Chronic kidney disease

### Acknowledgements

None.

### Authors' contributions

HL and HC analyzed and interpreted the data. YF and CY1 made substantial contributions to the conception. CY2 have drafted the work. AL substantively revised the work. CY1 corresponds to Chien-Yeh Hsu and CY2 corresponds to Che-Yi Chou. All authors read and approved the final manuscript.

### Competing interests

The authors declare that they have no competing interests.

### Author details

[1]Department of Neurology, Sijhih Cathay General Hospital, No.2, Ln. 59, Jiancheng Rd., Sijhih Dist, New Taipei City 221, Taiwan. [2]Graduate Institute of Biomedical Informatics, Taipei Medical University, No. 252, Wu-Xing Street, Taipei 110, Taiwan. [3]Department of Pediatrics, School of Medicine, College of Medicine, Taipei Medical University, No. 252, Wu-Xing Street, Taipei 110, Taiwan. [4]Department of Laboratory Medicine, Taipei Medical University Hospital, No. 252, Wu-Xing Street, Taipei 110, Taiwan. [5]Department of Information Management, National Taipei University of Nursing and Health Science, No. 365, Mingde Rd, Taipei 112, Taiwan. [6]Division of Nephrology, Asia University Hospital, NO 222, Fuxin Rd, Wufeng Dist, Taichung 413, Taiwan. [7]Department of Post-baccalaureate Veterinary Medicine, Asia University, NO 222, Fuxin Rd, Wufeng Dist, Taichung 413, Taiwan. [8]Division of Nephrology, China Medical University Hospital, Tacihung, Taiwan.

### References

1. Skogestad J, Aronsen JM. Hypokalemia-induced arrhythmias and heart failure: new insights and implications for therapy. Front Physiol. 2018;9:1500.
2. Jensen HK, Brabrand M, Vinholt PJ, Hallas J, Lassen AT. Hypokalemia in acute medical patients: risk factors and prognosis. Am J Med. 2015;128(1):60–7 e61.
3. Collins AJ, Pitt B, Reaven N, Funk S, McGaughey K, Wilson D, et al. Association of Serum Potassium with all-cause mortality in patients with and without heart failure, chronic kidney disease, and/or diabetes. Am J Nephrol. 2017;46(3):213–21.
4. Kolman KB. Cystitis and pyelonephritis: diagnosis, treatment, and prevention. Prim Care. 2019;46(2):191–202.
5. Foxman B. Urinary tract infection syndromes: occurrence, recurrence, bacteriology, risk factors, and disease burden. Infect Dis Clin N Am. 2014; 28(1):1–13.
6. Moskowitz D, Lee U. Patient distress in women with recurrent urinary tract infections: how can physicians better meet patients needs? Curr Urol Rep. 2018;19(12):97.
7. Wu KL, Cheng CJ, Sung CC, Tseng MH, Hsu YJ, Yang SS, et al. Identification of the causes for chronic hypokalemia: importance of urinary sodium and chloride excretion. Am J Med. 2017;130(7):846–55.
8. Melnick JZ, Preisig PA, Haynes S, Pak CY, Sakhaee K, Alpern RJ. Converting enzyme inhibition causes hypocitraturia independent of acidosis or hypokalemia. Kidney Int. 1998;54(5):1670–4.
9. Weiner ID, Wingo CS. Hypokalemia--consequences, causes, and correction. J Am Soc Nephrol. 1997;8(7):1179–88.
10. Lindeman RD. Hypokalemia: causes, consequences and correction. Am J Med Sci. 1976;272(1):5–17.
11. Kogika MM, de Morais HA. A quick reference on hypokalemia. Vet Clin North Am Small Anim Pract. 2017;47(2):229–34.
12. Shen AL, Lin HL, Lin HC, Tseng YF, Hsu CY, Chou CY. Increased risk of bullous pemphigoid after first-ever stroke: a population-based study. Neurodegener Dis. 2017;17(4–5):166–70.
13. Foxman B. Recurring urinary tract infection: incidence and risk factors. Am J Public Health. 1990;80(3):331–3.
14. Zhou X, Zhang Z, Li J, Ye Y, Tang G, Ding B. Cardiac arrest among patients with infections. Clin Microbiol Infect. 2017;23(10):782.
15. Stein JH. Hypokalemia. Common and uncommon causes. Hosp Pract (Off Ed). 1988;23(3A):55–64 66, 70.
16. Steigerwalt SP. Unraveling the causes of hypertension and hypokalemia. Hosp Pract (1995). 1995;30(7):67–71 74–65, 79.
17. Buckley MS, Leblanc JM, Cawley MJ. Electrolyte disturbances associated with commonly prescribed medications in the intensive care unit. Crit Care Med. 2010;38(6 Suppl):S253–64.
18. Melis K, Vandevivere J, Hoskens C, Vervaet A, Sand A, Van Acker KJ. Involvement of the renal parenchyma in acute urinary tract infection: the contribution of 99mTc dimercaptosuccinic acid scan. Eur J Pediatr. 1992; 151(7):536–9.
19. Ronald A. The etiology of urinary tract infection: traditional and emerging pathogens. Am J Med. 2002;113(Suppl 1A):14S–9S.
20. Medina M, Castillo-Pino E. An introduction to the epidemiology and burden of urinary tract infections. Ther Adv Urol. 2019;11:1756287219832172.
21. Mody L, Juthani-Mehta M. Urinary tract infections in older women: a clinical review. JAMA. 2014;311(8):844–54.
22. Marti G, Schwarz C, Leichtle AB, Fiedler GM, Arampatzis S, Exadaktylos AK, et al. Etiology and symptoms of severe hypokalemia in emergency department patients. Eur J Emerg Med. 2014;21(1):46–51.
23. Zaki SA, Shanbag P. Meropenem-induced hypokalemia and metabolic alkalosis. Indian J Pharm. 2012;44(2):276–7.
24. Cohen PG. The pathogenesis of recurrent urinary tract infection: the bowel, bladder hypokalemia connection. Med Hypotheses. 1983;10(1):1–4.

# 11

# Unmet needs in sexual health in bladder cancer patients

Agustina Bessa[1*], Rebecca Martin[2], Christel Häggström[1,3,4], Deborah Enting[1,5], Suzanne Amery[6], Muhammad Shamim Khan[6], Fidelma Cahill[1], Harriet Wylie[1], Samantha Broadhead[6], Kathryn Chatterton[6], Sachin Malde[6], Rajesh Nair[6], Ramesh Thurairaja[6], Pardeep Kumar[2], Anna Haire[1], Saran Green[1], Margaret Northover[6], Karen Briggs[6] and Mieke Van Hemelrijck[1]

**Abstract**

**Background:** Bladder cancer (BC) treatment can have a detrimental effect on the sexual organs of patients and yet assessment of sexual health needs has been greatly overlooked for these patients compared to those who have undergone other cancer therapies.

**Methods:** This review was conducted in accordance with the Preferred Reporting Items for Systematic Reviews and Meta-analyses (PRISMA) guidelines in July 2019. Studies were identified by conducting searches for Medline (using the PubMed interface), the Cochrane Central Register of Controlled Trials (CENTRAL) and Ovid Gateway (Embase and Ovid) using a list of defined search terms.

**Results:** 15 out of 37 studies included men only, 10 studies women only and 11 both sexes. Most participants were aged 50 to 65 years. Most studies ($n = 34$) focused on muscle invasive BC and only three on non-muscle invasive BC. Measurements of sexual dysfunction, including erection, ejaculation, firmness and desire, were the most commonly used measurements to report sexual health in men. In women, lubrification/dryness, desire, orgasm and dyspareunia were the most commonly reported. Twenty-one studies evaluated sexual dysfunction based on validated questionnaires, two with a non-validated questionnaire and through interviewing participants.

**Conclusion:** While recognition of the importance of the inclusion of psychometric measurements to assess sexual health is growing, there is a lack of consistent measures to assess sexual health in BC. With the focus on QoL arising in cancer survivorship, further studies are needed to develop, standardize and implement use of sexual health questionnaires with appropriate psychometrics and social measures to evaluate QoL in BC patients.

**Trial registration:** "PROSPERO does not currently accept registrations for scoping reviews, literature reviews or mapping reviews. PROSPERO is therefore unable to accept your application or provide a registration number. This decision should not stop you from submitting your project for publication to a journal."

**Keywords:** Bladder cancer, Sexual health, Radical cystectomy, Health-related quality of life, Mental wellbeing

* Correspondence: Agustina.m.bessa@gmail.com
[1]King's College London, School of Cancer and Pharmaceutical Studies, Translational Oncology & Urology Research (TOUR), TOUR, Guy's Hospital, 3rd Floor Bermondsey Wing, London SE1 9RT, UK

## Background

It is well known that the diagnosis and treatment of cancer causes significant physical, psychological, and social effects that interfere with a person's sexual health. Indeed, it has been estimated that between 40 and 100% of cancer patients will experience a degree of sexual dysfunction [1]. Sexual dysfunction is characterized by disturbances in sexual desire and in the psychophysiological changes associated with the sexual response cycle in men and women or pain during intercourse [2, 3]. The degree to which sexual dysfunction has been studied in different cancer types varies, with most studies performed in patients with prostate, breast or gynaecological cancers. The World Health Organization (WHO) defines sexual health as a state of physical, emotional, mental, and social wellbeing related to sexuality, and is not merely the absence of disease, dysfunction or infirmity [4]. Therefore, sexual health has to be evaluated holistically due to the complex interactions between biological, psychological, interpersonal and social/cultural factors [5], as all these factors may effect sexual function and wellbeing [6].

Bladder cancer (BC) treatments are known to have a potential detrimental effect on both the genitals and the internal sexual organs of patients and yet it has been greatly overlooked compared to other cancer therapies [7]. Research of the treatment impact on sexual health has been widely identified as an unmet need in bladder cancer patients [8, 9].

Non-muscle invasive bladder cancer (NMIBC) accounts for about 70% of all bladder cancers [10] and those are mostly treated with transurethral resection of the bladder tumor (TURBT), followed by intravesical chemotherapy (22%) or immunotherapy with bacillus CalmetteGuerin (BCG, 29%) [11]. Muscle invasive bladder cancer (MIBC) are commonly treated with cystectomy [11, 12]. The vast majority of studies currently available for bladder cancer focus on those who have undergone a radical cystectomy. Among those, many studies evaluate sexual-sparing radical cystectomy with the goal of reaching definitive oncologic control while attempting preservation of sexual function [13].

Current European Association of Urology (EAU 2019) guidelines [14] recommend that a standard radical cystectomy in men should include removal of the bladder, prostate, seminal vesical, distal ureters and regional lymph nodes, while in women removal of the bladder, entire urethra and adjacent vagina, uterus, distal ureters and regional lymph nodes is recommended. The guidelines also stated that a prostate-sparing radical cystectomy could be considered in carefully selected patients if oncologically safe. However, a sexual organ preserving operation in women is not advised, largely due to a paucity of available evidence [14]. Such treatments can induce serious complications and greatly impact the patient's body image and quality of life (QoL) [11]. Health-related QoL (HRQoL) can be formally defined as the extent to which one's usual or expected physical, emotional, and social wellbeing are affected by a medical condition or its treatment [15]. HRQoL issues of special concern to patients with BC include, among others, threats to body image and sexuality [16, 17].

With the focus on HRQoL arising in cancer survivorship, it is needed to closely address and evaluate post-treatment sexual dysfunction and offer goal-directed treatment. To date no detailed assessment of the overall burden of sexual health in bladder cancer patients has been made. This systematic literature review aimed to provide a consolidated overview of studies that address sexual health in bladder cancer patients. We specifically aimed to assess the methodology used to evaluate sexual health in terms of coverage and validation after BC treatment, which may provide a basis for future studies.

## Methods

This review was conducted in accordance with the Preferred Reporting Items for Systematic Reviews and Meta-analyses (PRISMA) guidelines in July 2019. A detailed overview of the protocol is provided in Appendix 1.

### Search strategy and inclusion criteria

Studies were identified by conducting searches for Medline (using the PubMed interface), the Cochrane Central Register of Controlled Trials (CENTRAL) and Ovid Gateway (Embase and Ovid) between May and July 2019 using a list of defined search terms (see Appendix 2). To be included in the analysis, the studies must have met the following criteria: study on the impact of bladder cancer treatment on sexual health/dysfunction and reported outcomes specifically for sexual health/dysfunction (e.g. erection, ejaculation, dryness).

### Data collection and analysis

Initially, the titles of the studies were screened to identify the relevant studies. The abstracts and subsequently full texts were then carefully read to identify those which met the inclusion criteria. Two independent reviewers (AB and RM) used the exact same search strategy and inclusion criteria and after each screening phase, a discussion was conducted with a third party (MVH) to match and decide on the included studies. Information on patient characteristics, number of study participants and type of treatment, as well as sexual health outcomes and mental wellbeing information was extracted from each study. The latter data was collected as sexual dysfunction may also have an impact on HRQoL through effects on mental wellbeing (4). The references of the included studies were also reviewed to ensure no relevant citation was missed.

## Results

### Quantity of evidence identified

The selection process for records to be included in the review was carried out according to PRISMA protocol, and this is demonstrated in a PRISMA flowchart in Fig. 1. A total of 667 records were collected from the literature search and 108 duplicates were removed. All titles were initially screened and 226 remained for abstracts screening. Of those, 71 remained for full text analysis. After the full text was read, 37 studies matched the inclusion and exclusion criteria and were included in this systematic review (Table 1, Appendix 3).

#### Characteristics of the patient profiles

Of the 37 studies included in the systematic review, 15 studies (40.5%) included men only, 10 studies (27.0%), women only and 12 studies (32.4%) included both sexes. The exact number of women and men in the studies that included both sexes is not clearly described for all studies. With respect to age, in 28 studies (75.6%) participants were

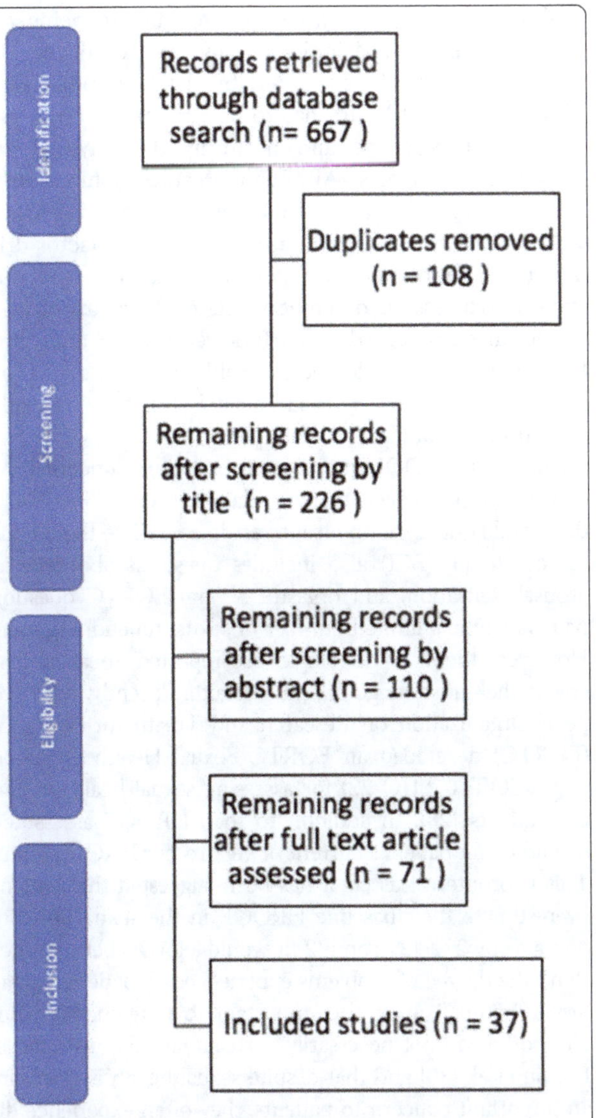


**Fig. 1** PRISMA Flow diagram for selection of studies in systematic review

**Table 1** Characteristics of the patient profile included in the studies

| Patient profile | Studies (n) |
|---|---|
| **Sex (%)** | |
| Only men | 15 (39.5%) |
| Only women | 10 (28.9%) |
| Both sex | 12 (32.4%) |
| **Age** | |
| 26–49 | 5 (13.5%) |
| 50–65 | 28 (75.6%) [a] |
| 66–80 | 4 (10.8%) |
| 81–95 | 0 |
| **Disease stage (%)** | |
| MIBC | 34 (91.9%) |
| NMIBC | 3 (8.10%) |

[a]One study does not provide the mean age but state that patients were between 56 and 75 years old

aged between 50 to 65 years, in five studies (13.5%) 26 to 49 years, in four studies (10.8%) 66 to 80 years and none included participants above 80 years old. The vast majority of studies [$n = 34$ (91.9%)] included MIBC and only three (8.10%) focused on NMIBC. Patient profiles for each study are described in Table 1.

#### Measurement of sexual health by sex

Measurements of sexual dysfunction, including erection (73.0%), ejaculation (35.1%), firmness (8.10%) and desire (18.9%), were the most commonly used measurements to report sexual health in men. In women, lubrification/dryness (27.0%), desire (24.3%), orgasm (27.0%) and dyspareunia (29.7%) were the most commonly reported (Table 2).

#### Comparison of sexual dysfunction outcome by treatments and measurements

Thirty-three (89.2%) studies addressed sexual dysfunction following radical cystectomy, one (2.7%) following radical radiotherapy, one (2.7%) after cystoscopy, and two (5.4%) after other treatments for bladder cancer. There are no

**Table 2** Measures of reported sexual dysfunction by sex

| Sex | Measurement | Number of Studies (%) |
|---|---|---|
| **Men** | Erection | 27 (73.0%) |
| | Firmness | 3 (8.10%) |
| | Desire | 7 (18.9%) |
| | Ejaculation | 13 (35.1%) |
| **Women** | Lubrification / Dryness | 10 (27.0%) |
| | Desire | 9 (24.3%) |
| | Orgasm | 10 (27.0%) |
| | Dyspareunia | 11 (29.7%) |

studies looking at TURBT only. In four studies (10.8%), participants were treated with drug therapy for their sexual dysfunction. Twenty-one studies (56.8%) evaluated sexual dysfunction based on validated questionnaires, two (5.4%) with a non-validated questionnaire and 14 (37.8%) through interviewing participants.

### Patient and partners sexual satisfaction and mental wellbeing

Seven studies evaluated patient sexual satisfaction and mental wellbeing (Table 3). None of those included both patient and partner satisfaction and mental wellbeing. One study included sexual satisfaction for both patients and partners, but did not report on mental wellbeing [18]. Regarding mental wellbeing, perception of body image [20, 22, 24], worry about daily life [19], feeling of anxiety [23] and depression [22] were the most commonly reported outcomes. Six of those studies included patients with MIBC and one NMIBC. Six studies included patients in the age range of 50–65 years and two included patients 66–80 years old. Overall, radical cystectomy was found to be associated with negative feelings regarding patient's body image and consequently a negative effect in sexual satisfaction. Patients who underwent a bladder sparing technique had a better perception of their body and a better sexual satisfaction. There is no consistency in the measurements used for sexual satisfaction and/or mental wellbeing: interviews and semi-structured interviews, sexual function index questionnaire, QoL questionnaire (SHIM and IFSF) and a functional assessment of cancer therapy questionnaire.

## Discussion

Sexual dysfunction is a common phenomenon after bladder cancer treatment and yet sexual health is frequently overlooked. Of the 37 included studies included in our review, 15 studies included men only, 10 studies included women only and 12 studies included both sexes. Most studies included participants aged between 50 to 65 years. The majority of studies focused on patients with MIBC. The main outcomes measured in men were erection, ejaculation and desire and in women, lubrification/dryness, orgasm and dyspareunia. A broad range of measures were used in the studies including validated patient reported outcome tools, such as the SHIM and the IFSF questionnaire and interview-based studies.

One of the main observations following our systematic review is the heterogeneity in measurements used for sexual health. The SHIM tool is commonly used in prostate cancer and has also been most commonly used in the studies identified here. In female patients the available measurement tools are broader and less commonly implemented in practice. The most commonly used tool we found was the IFSF questionnaire. Both tools have been criticised for their lack of psychometric measures [25]. Indeed, the need for a robust measure of sexual function in bladder cancer that includes psychometric assessment is well recognised, but not yet developed [26]. Mohamed et al. (2014) identified unmet needs in MIBC patients and sexual function was a significant concern [8]. With no evidence of consistent clinical measures from practice, these findings are unsurprising. Patient and public involvement is needed to develop and include appropriate psychometrics measures in sexual health questionnaires. As previously noted by Peter Selby and Galina Velikova [27], patient input is essential, but the process is time consuming, sometimes quite expensive and can involve large numbers of patients or the general population to achieve meaningful results. Therefore, individuals and groups have tended to develop their own questionnaires which led to a lack of general consensus in the field and a confusing number of questionnaires.

Moreover, our systematic review highlights how sexual health may negatively impact on mental wellbeing and HRQoL – and hence indicates the need to address this gap for patients. As suggested by the definition of the WHO [4], sexual health has to be evaluated from a psychosocial perspective and not only the physical and physiological aspects. Although erectile dysfunction in men and physical and physiologic changes associated with cystectomy in women are the dominant factor driving sexual function, other causes of sexual dysfunction, such as depression or anxiety related to changed body image, distress regarding partner reaction to an altered body as well as the degree of problems that patients are experiencing due to their sexual function (bother), should be evaluated and managed.

Currently, HRQOL questionnaires like the Functional Assessment of Cancer Therapy – Bladder Cancer (FACT-BC) do include questions about interest in sex, while the Bladder Cancer Index (BCI) also includes questions about desire, arousal, sensation, and orgasm. Several EORTC questionnaires include a limited number of sexual functioning items. However, there is no single self-reported measure that covers the entire range of sexual health. Recently, the European Organization on Research and Treatment of Cancer (EORTC) developed an EORTC Sexual Health Questionnaire (EORTC SHQ-22) for assessing sexual health in cancer patients [28]. In addition to that, HRQOL assessment should target patient's current or very recent HRQOL status. This is of interest as (1) it has been suggested that patients overestimate their baseline HRQOL in the sexual function domains by 27% [29]; and (2) it would allow to better understand the degree of problems experienced by patients (measuring "bother"). It is also important to note that function and bother do not necessarily correlate as demonstrated by Letwin et al. [30] and that despite sexual health issues being an important concern to patients, they often experience difficulties in disclosing their complaints with health care providers or their partners. Lastly, as sexual wellbeing is closely

**Table 3** Patient and partner sexual satisfaction and mental wellbeing

| Study [ref] | Age range | Self-reported patient and partner satisfaction (if data available) | Mental wellbeing | Measurement |
|---|---|---|---|---|
| [18] | 50–65 | Participants were found to have frequent erectile dysfunction, ejaculation disorder, fear of hurting spouse/partner and leakage during sexual intercourse.<br>The participants' spouse/partner were found to have fear of hurting, decrease in sexual desire, inability to get pleasure/ orgasm and avoiding sexual intercourse. | No data. | Interview |
| [19] | 50–65 | 20% of participants were not sexually satisfied. No data regarding partner. | Among the patients, 42 (84%) of them were not feeling bad about their bladder tumors and 37 (74%) were not worrying about their daily lives. Moreover, 12 (24%) patients were not interested with sexuality. | International Sexual Function Index (IIEF-5) and Female Sexual Function Index (FSFI |
| [20] | 50–65 | TMT was associated with higher sexual quality of life. No data regarding partner. | Compared with RC, the patients treated with TMT reported significantly better perception of their body image. Patients who underwent TMT had significantly fewer concerns about their appearance and less life interference from their cancer diagnosis. Overall, the negative impact of cancer was significantly less for patients who had undergone TMT. | QoL questionnaire |
| [21] | 66–80 | 37.5% patients in the study agreed that treatment affected their sexual function. No data regarding partner. | At the time of diagnosis, patients of both sexes reported relatively high feelings of depression. | Semi-structured interviews. |
| [22] | 66–80 | Forty-six patients enrolled in the study. Of those, only 27 patients responded to the statement "I am satisfied with my sex life". Approximately the same number of patients agreed as disagreed, but the main response was neither to agree nor to disagree with this statement. Thirty-one patients responded to the statement "My sex life is not functioning". Most patients agreed with this statement. Only 23 patients responded to the statement "I am very happy with my sex life". Again, most patients neither agreed nor disagreed. No data regarding partner. | The patients were asked whether the change in their body appearance had resulted in psychological problems which had influenced their sex life. Twenty-five patients (61%) answered that this was not the case, whereas 11 (27%) answered that this was the case. | Female Sexual Function Index (FSFI) questionnaire |
| [23] | 50–65 | Radical cystectomy group, through the 4 measurements points, started, stayed and ended on a lower level than the case-control patients regarding overall sexual satisfaction. No data regarding partner. | The mean score for trait anxiety was similar in both groups (RC and CC). Only 5.6% of all RC patients had a high anxious personality compared to 20% in the CC group, but this was not statistically significant. | International Index of Erectile Function (FSFI) and International Index of Erectile Function (IIEF) |
| [24] | 50–65 | No data regarding sexual satisfaction. No data regarding partner. | Among patients who had undergone RC, 8.5% of the responders reported being unhappy with their body image, compared with the 5% reported by patients in BI group. | FACT-BL + additional concerns |

correlated with social interactions, patients' relationship status should also be considered when evaluating sexual wellbeing and its impact on HRQOL.

In our systematic review, most studies addressed sexual health in patients with MIBC who underwent radical cystectomy and only four studies focused on patients with NMIBC. This is potentially affecting the generalisibility of our observations as it is important to note that treatments for NMIBC and MIBC substantially differ, e.g. TURBT vs cystectomy. In a prospective study by Yoshimura et al. [31] on the impact of TURBT on QoL in patients with NMIBC, physical problems were found with the first TURBT, but when the fourth TURBT was performed, patients appeared to have adapted to frequent operations, although their general QoL remained affected. For cystectomy patients, it has been shown that although relationships with friends were unchanged, relationships with spouse or partner were disturbed by sexual problems [32]. Partner response to the presence of an external appliance, such as stoma, may also strain intimate relationships and contribute to a dysfunctional sex life. Nevertheless, these observations highlight that 1) the threat of recurrence, multiple cystoscopies, TURBT, and intravesical instillations make QoL assessment in superficial bladder cancer challenging; 2) the importance of looking at sexual function in patients with bladder cancer in a broader way is needed, i.e. including both the physical perspective as well as the patients' partner and relationships.

There are limitations of this study that warrant further discussion. The analysis of the included studies was unable to provide an extensive coverage of sexual health in NMIBC patients for which the impact of treatment in sexual health and consequently QoL may also be significative. Due to the nature of the methods used to measure sexual health and the lack of psychometric measures, further research is needed to better understand the role of bladder cancer treatment and psychosocial factors of sexual functioning.

## Conclusion

While recognition of the importance of the inclusion of psychometric measurements to assess sexual health is growing, this systematic review highlights the lack of consistent measures to assess sexual health in bladder cancer patients. With the focus on HRQoL arising in cancer survivorship, further studies are needed to develop, standardize and implement the use of sexual health questionnaires with appropriate psychometrics and social measures for bladder cancer patients.

## Appendix 1

**PROTOCOL:** Systematic literature review on sexual health for patients with bladder cancer.

**AIM:** To consolidate an overview of studies that address sexual health in bladder cancer patients

**Objectives**

- Assess the methodology used to evaluate sexual health in terms of coverage and validation after bladder cancer treatment,
- Understand the role of bladder cancer treatment and psychosocial factors of sexual functioning

**METHODS**

Reports of current systematic review protocol adhere to the Preferred Items for Systematic Reviews and Meta-Analysis Protocol (PRISMA-P) checklist. The systematic review itself will adhere to the PRISMA.

**Criteria for considering studies for this review.**

**Types of studies.**

Any study that investigated sexual function or sexual dysfunction; any study where sexual function/sexual dysfunction/sexual health were measured by self-reports or an interview. Studies were original full text report in English and were published in peer-reviewed journals.

**Types of participants.**

The population of interest will be bladder cancer patients. Demographic factors are no exclusion criteria except for age (< 18 years of age).

**Types of outcomes measures.**

For both primary and secondary outcome measures, there will be no exclusion based on length of follow-up.

**Primary outcomes.**

Sexual function or sexual dysfunction in bladder cancer patients.

**Secondary outcomes.**

Treatment and psychosocial factors of sexual functioning.

**SEARCH METHODS FOR IDENTIFICATION OF STUDIES.**

**Electronic searches.**

The following electronic databases will be searched from inception until the search date: the Cochrane Central Register of Controlled Trials (CENTRAL), MEDLINE (using the PubMed interface), Embase (using the embase.com interface) and PsychINFO.

**Data collection and analysis.**

**Selection of studies.**

All references found through the search process will be downloaded in a database created by reference management software (Endnote). After removing duplicates in Endnote, all references will be imported into Covidence for screening purposes. Obviously irrelevant studies, based on title and abstract, will independently be excluded by two review authors. After screening the titles and abstracts, two review authors will independently assess full-text reports for eligibility. Discrepancies will be discussed with a third review author. Reasons for exclusion of full-texts will be documented. Studies will be excluded if no full-text is available. Abstracts in any other language than English will be excluded. There will be no language restriction for full texts, and translations will be carried out if necessary. If studies have multiple publications with the same outcome(s) reported, manuscripts with the longest follow-up will be selected for inclusion.

**Data extraction.**

For each included study in the review, at least the following information will be extracted:

- General information: report title, report ID, authors' names, country, contact address, language of publication and year of publication.
- Population and setting: population description (from which study participants are drawn), setting when applicable (eg, inpatient, outpatient, hospital setting, home setting and combination) and inclusion and exclusion criteria.
- Methods: aim of study, design, start and end date and duration of participation.
- Participants: number of participants, received treatment.
- Outcomes: outcome name, time points measured and reported.
- Results: measurement of sexual function and sexual dysfunction, psychosocial factors measured.

**Dealing with missing data.**

If essential data are not available in the publication, we will first attempt to contact the study authors. If this is not possible, we will try to back-calculate from the data presented. If data will be obtained from other study authors, this will be reported in the review in a transparent manner. This way, we can keep in mind that these missing data obtained from study authors were not peer reviewed. Studies assessing lifestyle interventions may have issues with compliance. Therefore, reasons for missing data (eg, dropouts, losses to follow-up and withdrawals) will be carefully reported.

**Data synthesis.**

The findings from the included studies will be summarised in a table format.

**ETHICS AND DISSEMINATION.**

Ethics approval is not required, as no primary data will be collected. Results will be disseminated through a peer-reviewed publication.

The results of this systematic review could also have potential limitations in terms of biased results due to the nature of the patient reported outcomes.

## Appendix 2

**Search strategy**

PubMed.

"Urinary Bladder Neoplasms"[MESH] OR "Urinary Bladder/abnormalities"[MESH] OR "Urinary bladder/surgery"[MESH] OR "Carcinoma, Transitional Cell"[Mesh] OR "bladder cancer"[TIAB] OR "bladder cancers"[TIAB] OR "bladder carcinoma"[TIAB] OR "bladder carcinomas"[TIAB] OR "bladder malignancy"[TIAB] OR "bladder malignancies"[TIAB] OR "bladder neoplasm"[TIAB] OR "bladder neoplasms"[TIAB] OR "bladder tumor"[TIAB] OR "bladder tumors"[TIAB] OR "bladder tumour"[TIAB] OR "bladder tumours"[TIAB] OR "transitional cell carcinoma"[TIAB] OR "transitional cell carcinomas"[TIAB] OR "transitional cell cancer"[TIAB] OR "transitional cell cancers"[TIAB] OR "transitional cell malignancies"[TIAB] OR "transitional cell tumor"[TIAB] OR "transitional cell tumors"[TIAB] OR "transitional cell tumour"[TIAB] OR "transitional cell tumours"[TIAB]

**And**

"Sexual function" OR "sexual dysfunction" OR "wellbeing" OR "intimacy" OR "sexuality" OR "sexual physiology" OR "sexual physiopathology" "sexual heath"

**And**

"Cystectomy" OR "radical cystectomy" OR "partial cystectomy" OR "TURBT" OR "Transurethral resection of bladder tumour" OR "BCG" OR "chemotherapy" OR "Radiotherapy" OR "Bacillus Calmette–Guérin vaccine".

Cochrane Library.

"Urinary Bladder Neoplasms" OR "Urinary Bladder abnormalities" OR "Urinary bladder surgery" OR "Carcinoma, Transitional Cell" OR "bladder cancer" OR "bladder cancers" OR "bladder carcinoma" OR "bladder carcinomas" OR "bladder malignancy" OR "bladder malignancies" OR "bladder neoplasm" OR "bladder neoplasms" OR "bladder tumor" OR "bladder tumors" OR "bladder tumour" OR "bladder tumours" OR "transitional cell carcinoma" OR "transitional cell carcinomas" OR "transitional cell cancer" OR "transitional cell cancers" OR "transitional cell malignancies" OR "transitional cell tumor" OR "transitional cell tumors" OR "transitional cell tumour" OR "transitional cell tumours"

**And**

"Sexual function" OR "sexual dysfunction" OR "wellbeing" OR "intimacy" OR "sexuality" OR "sexual physiology" OR "sexual physiopathology"

**And**

"Cystectomy" OR "radical cystectomy" OR "partial cystectomy" OR "TURBT" OR "Transurethral resection of bladder tumour" OR "BCG" OR "chemotherapy" OR "Radiotherapy" OR "Bacillus Calmette–Guérin vaccine".

Embase.

Urinary Bladder Neoplasms OR Urinary Bladder abnormalities OR Urinary bladder surgery OR Carcinoma, Transitional Cell OR bladder cancer OR bladder cancers OR bladder carcinoma OR bladder carcinomas OR bladder malignancy OR bladder malignancies OR bladder neoplasm OR bladder neoplasms OR bladder tumor OR bladder tumors OR bladder tumour OR bladder tumours OR transitional cell carcinoma OR transitional cell carcinomas OR transitional cell cancer OR transitional cell cancers OR transitional cell malignancies OR transitional cell tumor OR transitional cell tumors OR transitional cell tumour OR transitional cell tumours

**And**

Sexual function OR sexual dysfunction OR sexual health OR wellbeing OR intimacy OR sexuality OR sexual physiology OR sexual physiopathology

**And**

Cystectomy OR radical cystectomy OR partial cystectomy OR TURBT OR Transurethral resection of bladder tumour OR BCG OR chemotherapy OR Radiotherapy OR Bacillus Calmette Guerin vaccine OR Intravesical therapy OR Systemic immunotherapy.

## Appendix 3

**Table 4** Treatment, measurement and outcome

| Study number [ref] | Patient profile | Treatment, preserving technique and/or urinary diversion | Measurement | Sexual function outcome |
|---|---|---|---|---|
| 1 [33] | Group 1 comprised 58 subjects (mean age 65 years) Group 2 comprised 50 subjects (mean age 61 years) Group 3 comprised 54 healthy subjects (mean age 63 years | Radical cystectomy compared in ileal conduit diversion, modified S-pouch and healthy subjects | Interviews | Erectile dysfunction was worse in groups 1 (who received ileal conduit diversion) (29%) and 2 (modified S-pouch neobladder) (35.5%) compared to group 3 (healthy subjects) (83.2%). The quality of erection (firmness) was similarly affected in groups 1 (17.7%) and 2 (22.2%) compared with group 3 (83.3%)<br><br>Sexual dysfunction was also evaluated for women and was not pronounced as in the men. Sexual desire was equally present in all groups and patients in group 1 expressed higher levels of dissatisfaction than the other two groups. |
| 2 [34] | Twenty men in each group (mean age 58 and 59 years) | Radical cystectomy with prostate capsule sparing or nerve sparing and neobladder urinary diversion | Sexual Health Inventory for Men questionnaire (SHIM) | Compared to baseline, sexual function decreased similarly for both groups. 55 and 65% of prostate capsule sparing and nerve sparing patients used aids or medications for erectile function, respectively. |
| 3 [18] | Twenty patients and their spouses/partners (mean age 59 and 58, respectively) | Cystectomy followed by urostomy | Interviews | Participants were found to have frequent erectile dysfunction, ejaculation disorder, fear of hurting spouse/partner and leakage during sexual intercourse.<br>The participants' spouse/partner were found to have fear of hurting, decrease in sexual desire, inability to get pleasure/orgasm and avoiding sexual intercourse. |
| 4 [35] | Ninety-one patients and 59 were included in the continent and incontinent group, respectively (mean age 55 and 59.5 years, respectively) | Radical cystectomy with orthopaedic neobladder or uretro-sigmoidostomy (continent group) or uretero-cutanoustomy or had ileal conduit (incontinent group) | Sexual Health Inventory for Men Questionnaire (SHIM) | Regarding sexual function, from 121 patients, 29 (23.9%) underwent nerve-sparing and 59 (48.7%) non nerve- sparing procedure. Erectile dysfunction affected 78.4% of them. There was a significant difference between both groups with lower degrees of erectile dysfunction in nerve-sparing group. After one year postoperatively, 19/29 (65.5%) patients who underwent nerve-sparing radical cystectomy demonstrated spontaneous complete tumescence, 6 (20.7%) achieved erections with the use of oral PDE5 inhibitors while 4 (13.8%) required intra-cavernosal injection therapy. All patients treated with non-nerve sparing RC required intra-cavernosal injection therapy to achieve erections. |
| 5 [36] | Hundred eighty-five men were included (mean age of 57 years) | Prostate sparing cystectomy | Interviews | In total, 136 patients (86.1%) maintained erectile function, of whom 27 (19.9%) successfully used sildenafil, and 6 patients (4.4%) used intra-cavernous injections. |
| 6 [19] | Forty-four men and 6 women (mean age 57.6 | Cystoscopy | International Sexual Function Index (IIEF- | Mild-moderate erectile dysfunction was found in men and sexual |

**Table 4** Treatment, measurement and outcome *(Continued)*

| Study number [ref] | Patient profile | Treatment, preserving technique and/or urinary diversion | Measurement | Sexual function outcome |
|---|---|---|---|---|
| | years) | | 5) and Female Sexual Function Index (FSFI) | dysfunction in women. |
| 7 [37] | Eleven men underwent conventional radical cystoprostatectomy and 14 patients had prostate-sparing cystectomy (mean age 61.55 and 57.5 years, respectively) | Orthotopic neobladder reconstruction after prostate-sparing cystectomy and conventional radical cystoprostatectomy | International Index of Erectile Function-5 (IIEF-5) | After surgery, IIEF-5 scores in conventional radical cystoprostatectomy and prostate-sparing cystectomy groups were 3.7 and 16.0, respectively. |
| 8 [38] | Sixty-three men and 4 women (mean age 63 years) | Robot-assisted radical cystoprostatectomy | Interview | With regard to sexual potency, twenty (43%) patients with neobladder reported spontaneous erections prior to surgery, 14 (29%) erectile dysfunction of some degree, and in 13 (28%) it is unknown. Of the 20 patients with normal sexual function prior to surgery, 90% had spontaneous erections that allowed them to have satisfactory sexual relations; of them, 3 managed it with the help of IPDE-5. Of the 14 patients who already reported some prior erectile dysfunction, 9 achieved satisfactory erections with IPD5. |
| 9 [20] | Hundred and nine patients underwent radical cystectomy and 64 patients underwent trimodality therapy (mean age 66 and 65, respectively) | Radical cystectomy and bladder-sparing trimodality therapy | QoL questionnaire | Male patients who had received trimodality therapy reported less difficulty gaining or maintaining an erection and decreased ejaculation problems compared with those who had undergone radical cystectomy. Patients who had undergone trimodality therapy also reported being less uncomfortable with being sexually intimate and less worried about contaminating their partner during sexual contact. |
| 10 [21] | Twenty-two men and 8 women (mean age 67 years) | Radical cystectomy and urinary diversion | Semi-structured interviews | Overall, 25 and 18.18% of younger and older patients, respectively, reported a discussion with the physician regarding changes in sexual function. Following surgery, younger patients were more likely to report problems with sexual dysfunction. |
| 11 [39] | Women between 20 and 28 years (mean 24 years) were 30.77%. Women of age range of 32–37 (mean 35 years) were 23.07% Women of age range of 40–54 (mean 49 years) were 48.5% | Radical cystectomy with preservation of genital organs and orthotopic ileal neobladder urinary diversion | Female Sexual Function Index (FSFI) questionnaire | Women who had reported good sexual function had DSFI score ranging from 20 to 32, which was reported by 84.61%. One woman had a score of 15, while another woman was not married and had no partner and she reported a score of zero. |
| 12 [22] | Seventy-one women (mean age of 67 years). | Radical cystectomy | Female Sexual Function Index (FSFI) questionnaire | Only 37% of the patients were sexually active post-surgery and those who were still sexually active tended to have less frequent sexual activity. A comparison of sexual desire before and after surgery found that 15 patients (37%) reported that this was unchanged, 22 patients (54%) that their desire for sex had decreased and one person that it had increased. Regarding ability to reach orgasm before and after surgery, 16 patients (39%) reported that this was unchanged and 18 (44%) that it was now harder to reach orgasm, while no |

**Table 4** Treatment, measurement and outcome *(Continued)*

| Study number [ref] | Patient profile | Treatment, preserving technique and/or urinary diversion | Measurement | Sexual function outcome |
|---|---|---|---|---|
| | | | | one reported that it was easier to reach orgasm. |
| 13 [40] | Sixty-eight men and 25 women (mean age 65 years) | Bacillus Calmette–Guérin (BCG) treatment | Semi-structured qualitative interviews | For those individuals who were sexually active, 60.0% of males experienced difficulty gaining or maintaining an erection and 43.1% of males had problems with ejaculation. Among sexually-active females, 62.5% experienced problems including vagi nal dryness. Nearly 50% of participants reported that it was very helpful to discuss concerns about sexual function with their partners. |
| 14 [34] | Forty patients (mean age 58 years) | Prostate capsule sparing and nerve sparing cystectomies | Sexual Health Inventory for Men Questionnaire (SHIM) | Average sexual function at 12 months compared with baseline decreased by 1 +/− 11 and 23 +/− 30 points for prostate capsule sparing and nerve sparing, respectively. Of patients with prostate capsule sparing and nerve sparing cystectomy, 55 and 65%, respectively, used aids or medication for erectile function. |
| 15 [23] | Eighteen patients undergoing radical cystectomy and 20 control (mean age 62.3 and 64.9 years, respectively) | Radical cystectomy | International Index of Erectile Function (FSFI) and International Index of Erectile Function (IIEF) | Regarding erectile dysfunction, intercourse satisfaction, orgasmic function, sexual desire and overall satisfaction—the radical cystectomy group started, stayed and ended on a lower level than the case control group throughout the study. No data reported for women. |
| 16 [41] | Fifteen women patients (mean age of 42 years) | Internal genitalia sparing cystectomy | Female Sexual Function Index (FSFI) | Sexual intercourse was regained after 6 weeks, a duration which is significantly shorter than in women without genital preservation. The mean FSFI scores in the study group were significantly higher than in cystectomy women without genital sparing. Similarly, there were significant differences in favour of genital sparing cases in all domains of FSFI. |
| 17 [42] | Seventy-eight men and 8 women (mean age 62 years) | Orthotopic neobladder | International Index of Erectile Function (IIEF-5) and visual analogue scale (VAS). | Most patients (88%) had a score of less than 10 points on IIEF-5, 5.3% of patients showed 10–14 points, 4% showed 15–19, and only 2.7% showed equal to or more than 20 points. Be cause evaluation by IIEF-5 had not been performed before surgery, we could not determine the precise influence of orthotopic neobladder on sexual function. |
| 18 [43] | Four men (mean age of 45 years) | Radical cystectomy | Interview | All patients reported adequate sexual function with normal erections and satisfactory intercourse similar to that reported before surgery. The erectile activity was regained within the first 5 months after surgery. Two patients (50%) preserved antegrade ejaculation the other two patients reported failure of ejaculation. |
| 19 [44] | Seven men (mean age of 40 years) | Radical cystectomy | Interview | Erectile function is normal in all patients with satisfactory sexual intercourse. Antegrade ejaculation was |

**Table 4** Treatment, measurement and outcome *(Continued)*

| Study number [ref] | Patient profile | Treatment, preserving technique and/or urinary diversion | Measurement | Sexual function outcome |
|---|---|---|---|---|
| | | | | documented in six cases. |
| 20 [45] | Four men and one woman (mean age 52.4 years) | Nerve sparing laparoscopic radical cystectomy | Female Sexual Function Index (FSFI) and International Index of Erectile Function score | Sexual function was preserved in the female patient and 2 of the 4 male patients. |
| 21 [24] | Eighty-two patients who had undergone radical cystectomy and 177 other therapy (mean age 64.4 years) | Radical cystectomy and other therapy | FACT-BL + additional concerns | Patients with their bladders preserved had more interest in sex when compared with patients who had their bladders removed. Twenty-one per cent of respondents who had their bladders preserved were not inter ested in sex as compared with 39% who underwent radical cystectomy. In the radical cystectomy group, about 89% of the respondents could not have and keep an erection, whereas in the bladder intact group only 32% of respondents could not have and keep an erection. |
| 22 [46] | Thirteen women (mean age 56.7 years) | Nerve sparing cystectomy with urethra and vaginal sparing | Female Sexual Function Index (FSFI | All 6 patients were sexually active 1 year after surgery. There is a significant vaginal dryness, a lack of arousal, and dyspareunia often led to discontinuation of sexual intercourse in the non-nerve-sparing group, with only 1 patient sexually active. |
| 23 [47] | Thirteen women (mean age 56.7 years) | Non nerve sparing and nerve sparing cystectomy | Female Sexual Function Index (FSFI | A reduction occurred in the mean score for desire, arousal, pain, and satisfaction. No change occurred in the mean score for orgasm or lubrication. One patient from the nerve-sparing group reported signifi cant dyspareunia after cystectomy that had resolved. All 6 patients had re sumed sexual activity at their 1-year follow-up visit. |
| 24 [48] | Twenty-nine women (mean age of 61 years) | Cystectomy and orthotopic ileal neobladder | Female Sexual Function Index (FSFI) | The 11 of 17 patients who remained sexually active after cystectomy even had slight improvement. Six patients ceased to be sexually active postoperatively due to erectile dysfunction or partner death. One patient with interstitial cystitis became sexually active following cystectomy due to the loss of pelvic pain. Another 12 patients remained sexually inactive postoperatively. |
| 25 (Nieuwenhuijzen, Meinhardt and Horenblas 2005) | Forty men (mean age of 56.9 years) | Prostate sparing cystectomy and neobladder | Interviews on erection and ejaculatory function and the international index of erectile function questionnaire | Erectile function could be determined in 40 patients, and potency was maintained in 77.5%, impaired in 12.5% and absent in 10%. |
| 26 [49] | Forty-nine men (mean age 57.8 years). | Nerve-sparing radical cystectomy, orthotopic diversion, conduit diversion and cutaneous continent diversion | Sexual Health Inventory for Men (SHIM) | Total mean SHIM score decreased after radical cystectomy. Of the 49 patients, 42 (86%) did not have erections sufficient for vaginal penetration. Of these 42 patients, 22 (52%) tried sildenafil citrate. Of these 22 patients, only 2 (9%) responded positively. Only 9 (14%) of 49 sexually |

**Table 4** Treatment, measurement and outcome *(Continued)*

| Study number [ref] | Patient profile | Treatment, preserving technique and/or urinary diversion | Measurement | Sexual function outcome |
|---|---|---|---|---|
| | | | | active men were potent after surgery. Of these 9 potent patients, 8 (89%) had undergone nerve-sparing radical cystectomy. |
| 27 [50] | Twenty-eight patients (mean age of 51.0 years). | Supra-ampullar cystectomy | Self-administered questionnaire | Potency was preserved in 26 patients (92.8%), reporting satisfactory sexual intercourses; 15 patients (53.5%) also maintained antegrade ejaculation allowing procreation in 3 cases. |
| 28 [51] | Twenty-seven women (mean age 54.79 years) | Radical cystectomy | Female Sexual Function Index (FSFI) | The total mean baseline Index of Female Sexual Function score decreased. The most common symptoms reported by the patients included diminished ability or inability to achieve orgasm in 12 (45%), decreased lubrication in 11 (41%), decreased sexual desire in 10 (37%), and dyspareunia in 6 patients (22%). Only 13 (48%) of the 27 patients were able to have successful vaginal intercourse, with 14 (52%) reporting decreased satisfaction in overall sexual life after radical cystectomy. Eight partners (30%) had a decrease in desire for sexual activity owing to apprehension after cancer diagnosis and treatment. |
| 29 [52] | Ten men and 3 women (mean age 55 years) | Cystectomy and neobladder | Structured interview | Erectile function was insufficient in 3 men. In 5 men ejaculation was antegrade, in 4 it was retrograde and 1 had each experience from time to time. In the women lubrication and orgasmic feeling was reported to be normal after surgery. |
| 30 [53] | Eighteen men (mean age 62.5 years) | Radical radiotherapy | Non-validated questionnaire | Eight out of 17 patients felt that their sex life was a lot worse since radiotherapy and four felt that their sex life was a little. Five patients felt that their sex life was unchanged. No patient felt their sex life had improved. Despite this, seven patients were unconcerned that their sex life had changed. Only eight of those 12 patients whose sex life had deteriorated were concerned about the decline in their sexual function and indeed only two noted great concern over the decline. |
| 31 [54] | Hundred-twelve men (mean age 63 years) | Radical cystectomy | Semi-structured interview | Of the men 20% were sexually inactive before cystectomy and 35% had at least mild erection problems. These percentages increased to 50 and 91, respectively, postoperatively. Most men who tried to reach orgasm after cystectomy could do so but 36% reported that they rarely or never had orgasms. About half of the men who were orgasmic after cystectomy complained that the intensity and pleasure of the sensation were reduced. However, the desire for sexual activity did not change as drastically as the ability to function. |
| 32 | Nine women (mean age 59 | Radical cystectomy | Interviews | For most couples postoperative sexual |

**Table 4** Treatment, measurement and outcome *(Continued)*

| Study number [ref] | Patient profile | Treatment, preserving technique and/or urinary diversion | Measurement | Sexual function outcome |
|---|---|---|---|---|
| [55] | years) | | | activity included intercourse, although 4 women experienced severe dyspareunia and the other 3 active women had mild discomfort at first. One couple was not able to have intercourse until a session of sexual counselling 20 months postoperatively helped the wife to relax. One woman still has not been able to tolerate vaginal penetration, although she can reach orgasm through noncoital stimulation.<br>Levels of sexual desire remained normal in 7 women but patient 9 continued to experience low sexual desire and patient 4 lost her desire for sexual activity. Of the 7 women who resumed sexual activity 6 have been able to overcome most or all of the dyspareunia that they experienced at first. The pain and discomfort included a sensation of vaginal tightness in 5 women, including 1 of the 2 whose vagina was repaired by turning the posterior wall downwards. Three women had trouble with vaginal dryness despite use of a water-based lubricant. Only 1 woman produced enough natural vaginal lubrication for comfortable intercourse. |
| 33 (Bergman, Nilson and Peterson 1979) | Forty-two men (mean age 62.3 years) | Cystectomy, prostatectomy and vesiculcctomy | Interviews<br>Most cases partners were also interviewed. | At the time of the interview, ten men had not attempted to resume sexual activity after the operation.<br>Only 3 patients were able to have penile erection after cystectomy. Although the remaining 24 patients were sexually active, they did not have a normal erection after the operation. Some of the men who achieved orgasm by masturbation reported a sensation of erection during orgasm. |
| 34 [56] | Seventy-three women (mean age 52.3 years) | Radical cystectomy with urinary diversion | Female Sexual Function Index (FSFI) | Sexual relations had ceased completely in 19 patients (26%), while it was maintained in 54 patients (74%). Among the postoperatively sexually active female various sexual dysfunctions were reported. Overall satisfaction among sexually active females was found to be the same as preoperatively in 14 patients (26%), it had worsened in 32 (59.2%) and was completely lost in eight patients (14.8%). |
| 35 [57] | Seventy-six men (mean age of 57 years) | Cystectomy and bladder substitution | Interview | After cystectomy, only 9% of all patients were still able to have an erection every second time or more often. Thirty-eight percent stated that they were still capable of orgasm, but a rather large proportion (21%) claimed that they did not know. Of the 29 patients with retained orgasmic function, 41% reported no decrease in quality. Only 11% of conduit patients had unchanged or some coital activity post- operatively, as compared to 35% of bladder substitute patients report |

**Table 4** Treatment, measurement and outcome *(Continued)*

| Study number [ref] | Patient profile | Treatment, preserving technique and/or urinary diversion | Measurement | Sexual function outcome |
|---|---|---|---|---|
| | | | | ing unchanged or some activity. |
| 36 [58] | Twenty-one men (mean age 59.4 years) | Cystectomy with or without urethrectomy | Interview | All had tactile sexual activity and preserved sexual desire. Around the 12 in whom the urethra was preserved, 4 had full and long lasting erection but of short duration. These 5 patients, all had erections that was satisfactory for vaginal penetration and intercourse and four were unable to achieve an erection. Among those whom the urethra was preserved, all but three could experience orgasm. Among the nine patients treated by cystectomy and urethral excision two reported that they had weak erections insufficient for vaginal penetration and intercourse. The remaining seven failed to achieve erection. Three patients in this group experienced orgasm, one patient with a weak erection and two of the seven patients who could not achieve an erection. |
| 37 [59] | 18 pre-menopausal women (mean age of 37.8 years) | Radical cystectomy | Female Sexual Function Index (FSFI) questionnaire | Fifteen patients had an unchanged sexual life, practicing sexual intercourse at a once-weekly average rate with normal orgasms. Three pa tients complained of dyspareunia that was managed with treatment. |

#### Abbreviations

BC: Bladder cancer; BCG: Bacillus Calmette–Guérin; QoL: Quality of life; NMIBC: Non-muscle invasive bladder cancer; MIBC: Muscle invasive bladder cancer; HRQoL: Health-related quality of life; EORTC : European Organisation for Research and Treatment of Cancer; EORTC SHQ-22: European Organisation for Research and Treatment of Cancer Sexual health questionnaire - 22; TURBT: Trans urethral resection of bladder tumour; IFSF: Index of Female Sexual Function; SHIM: Sexual Health Inventory for Men; WHO: World health organisation

#### Acknowledgements

Not applicable.

#### Authors' contributions

all authors have read and approved the manuscript. Conception and design: AB, RM, MVH. Acquisition of data: AB, RM. Analysis and interpretation of data: AB, RM, MVH. Drafting of the manuscript: AB. Critical revision of the manuscript for important intellectual content: CH, DE, SA, MK, FC, HW, SB, KC, SM, RN, PK, AH, SG, MN, KB, RT, MVH.

#### Competing interests

Not applicable.

#### Author details

[1]King's College London, School of Cancer and Pharmaceutical Studies, Translational Oncology & Urology Research (TOUR), TOUR, Guy's Hospital, 3rd Floor Bermondsey Wing, London SE1 9RT, UK. [2]The Royal Marsden, Department Urology, London, UK. [3]Department of Surgical Sciences, Uppsala University, Uppsala, Sweden. [4]Department of Biobank Research, Umeå University, Umeå, Sweden. [5]Department of Oncology, Guy's and St Thomas' NHS Foundation Trust, London, UK. [6]Department of Urology, Guy's and St Thomas' NHS Foundation Trust, London, UK.

#### References

1. The Prevalence and Types of Sexual Dysfunction in People With Cancer | HealthCentral n.d. https://www.healthcentral.com/article/the-prevalence-and-types-of-sexual-dysfunction-in-people-with-cancer (Accessed 11 Aug 2019).
2. Laumann EO, Paik A, Rosen RC. Sexual dysfunction in the United States. JAMA. 1999;281:537. https://doi.org/10.1001/jama.281.6.537.
3. Levin RJ. Critically revisiting aspects of the human sexual response cycle of masters and Johnson: correcting errors and suggesting modifications. Sex Relatsh Ther. 2008;23:393–9. https://doi.org/10.1080/14681990802488816.
4. WHO | Sexual health. WHO 2016.
5. Wettergren L, Kent EE, Mitchell SA, Zebrack B, Lynch CF, Rubenstein MB, et al. Cancer negatively impacts on sexual function in adolescents and young adults: the AYA HOPE study. Psychooncology. 2017;26:1632–9. https://doi.org/10.1002/pon.4181.
6. Basson R, Rees P, Wang R, Montejo AL, Incrocci L. Sexual function in chronic illness. J Sex Med. 2010;7:374–88. https://doi.org/10.1111/j.1743-6109.2009.01621.x.
7. Bhanvadia SK. Bladder Cancer survivorship. Curr Urol Rep. 2018;19:111. https://doi.org/10.1007/s11934-018-0860-6.
8. Mohamed NE, Chaoprang Herrera P, Hudson S, Revenson TA, Lee CT, Quale DZ, et al. Muscle invasive bladder cancer: examining survivor burden and unmet needs. J Urol. 2014;191:48–53. https://doi.org/10.1016/j.juro.2013.07.062.
9. Paterson C, Jensen BT, Jensen JB, Nabi G. Unmet informational and supportive care needs of patients with muscle invasive bladder cancer: a systematic review of the evidence. Eur J Oncol Nurs. 2018;35:92–101. https://doi.org/10.1016/J.EJON.2018.05.006.
10. Isharwal S, Konety B. Non-muscle invasive bladder cancer risk stratification. Indian J Urol. 2015;31:289–96. https://doi.org/10.4103/0970-1591.166445.
11. Jeong CW. Quality of Life in Bladder Cancer Patients. Bl. Cancer, Elsevier; 2018. p. 507–22. https://doi.org/10.1016/B978-0-12-809939-1.00028-X.
12. Bladder cancer: diagnosis and Bladder cancer: diagnosis and management management NICE guideline. 2015.

13. Pederzoli F, Campbell JD, Matsui H, Sopko NA, Bivalacqua TJ. Surgical factors associated with male and female sexual dysfunction after radical cystectomy: what do we know and how can we improve outcomes? Sex Med Rev. 2018;6:469–81. https://doi.org/10.1016/j.sxmr.2017.11.003.
14. EAU Guidelines | Uroweb n.d. https://uroweb.org/guidelines/ (Accessed 11 Aug 2019).
15. Moeen AM, Safwat AS, Gadelmoula MM, Moeen SM, Abonnoor AEI, Abbas WM, et al. Health related quality of life after urinary diversion. Which technique is better? J Egypt Natl Canc Inst. 2018;30:93–7. https://doi.org/10.1016/j.jnci.2018.08.001.
16. Bladder Cancer & Sexual Health | BladderCancer.net n.d. https://bladdercancer.net/living/sexual-health/ (Accessed 22 Sept 2019).
17. Sex life | Bladder cancer | Cancer Research UK n.d. https://www.cancerresearchuk.org/about-cancer/bladder-cancer/living-with/sex-life (Accessed 22 Sept 2019).
18. Kandemir D, Oskay Ü. Sexual problems of patients with Urostomy: a qualitative study. Sex Disabil. 2017;35:331–40. https://doi.org/10.1007/s11195-017-9494-8.
19. Bolat D, Celik S, Aydin ME, Aydogdu O, Gunlusoy B, Degirmenci T, et al. Assessment of the quality of life and sexual functions of patients followed-up for non-muscle invasive bladder cancer: preliminary results of the prospective-descriptive study. Türk Üroloji Dergisi/Turkish J Urol. 2018;44:393–8. https://doi.org/10.5152/tud.2018.30040.
20. Mak KS, Smith AB, Eidelman A, Clayman R, Niemierko A, Cheng J-S, et al. Quality of life in long-term survivors of muscle-invasive bladder Cancer. Int J Radiat Oncol. 2016;96:1028–36. https://doi.org/10.1016/J.IJROBP.2016.08.023.
21. Mohamed NE, Pisipati S, Lee CT, Goltz HH, Latini DM, Gilbert FS, et al. Unmet informational and supportive care needs of patients following cystectomy for bladder cancer based on age, sex, and treatment choices. Urol Oncol Semin Orig Investig. 2016;34:531.e7–531.e14. https://doi.org/10.1016/J.UROLONC.2016.06.010.
22. Booth BB, Rasmussen A, Jensen JB. Evaluating sexual function in women after radical cystectomy as treatment for bladder cancer. Scand J Urol. 2015; 49:463–7. https://doi.org/10.3109/21681805.2015.1055589.
23. Goossens-Laan CA, PJM K, JLHR B, De Vries J. Patient-reported outcomes for patients undergoing radical cystectomy: a prospective case-control study. Support Care Cancer. 2014;22:189–200. https://doi.org/10.1007/s00520-013-1946-9.
24. Allareddy V, Kennedy J, West MM, Konety BR. Quality of life in long-term survivors of bladder cancer. Cancer. 2006;106:2355–62. https://doi.org/10.1002/cncr.21896.
25. Forbes MK, Baillie AJ, Schniering CA. Critical flaws in the female sexual function index and the international index of erectile function. J Sex Res. 2014;51:485–91. https://doi.org/10.1080/00224499.2013.876607.
26. Modh RA, Mulhall JP, Gilbert SM. Sexual dysfunction after cystectomy and urinary diversion. Nat Rev Urol. 2014;11:445–53. https://doi.org/10.1038/nrurol.2014.151.
27. Selby P, Velikova G. Taking patient reported outcomes Centre stage in cancer research – why has it taken so long? Res Involv Engagem. 2018;4:25. https://doi.org/10.1186/s40900-018-0109-z.
28. Oberguggenberger AS, Nagele E, Inwald EC, Tomaszewski K, Lanceley A, Nordin A, et al. Phase 1-3 of the cross-cultural development of an EORTC questionnaire for the assessment of sexual health in cancer patients: the EORTC SHQ-22. Cancer Med. 2018;7:635–45. https://doi.org/10.1002/cam4.1338.
29. Litwin MS, McGuigan KA. Accuracy of recall in health-related quality-of-life assessment among men treated for prostate cancer. J Clin Oncol. 1999;17:2882–8. https://doi.org/10.1200/JCO.1999.17.9.2882.
30. Litwin MS, Hays RD, Fink A, Ganz PA, Leake B, Leach GE, et al. Quality-of-life outcomes in men treated for localized prostate cancer. JAMA. 1995;273:129–35. https://doi.org/10.1001/jama.273.2.129.
31. Yoshimura K, Utsunomiya N, Ichioka K, Matsui Y, Terai A, Arai Y. Impact of superficial bladder cancer and transurethral resection on general health-related quality of life: an SF-36 survey. Urology. 2005;65:290–4. https://doi.org/10.1016/j.urology.2004.09.050.
32. Månsson A, Johnson G, Månsson W. Psychosocial adjustment to cystectomy for bladder carcinoma and effects on interpersonal relationships. Scand J Caring Sci. 1991;5:129–34.
33. Protogerou V, Moschou M, Antoniou N, Varkarakis J, Bamias A, Deliveliotis C. Modified S-pouch neobladder vs ileal conduit and a matched control population: a quality-of-life survey. BJU Int. 2004;94:350–4. https://doi.org/10.1111/j.1464-410X.2004.04932.x.
34. Jacobs BL, Daignault S, Lee CT, Hafez KS, Montgomery JS, Montie JE, et al. Prostate capsule sparing versus nerve sparing radical cystectomy for bladder Cancer: results of a randomized, controlled trial. J Urol. 2015;193:64–70. https://doi.org/10.1016/J.JURO.2014.07.090.
35. Moeen AM, Safwat AS, Gadelmoula MM, Moeen SM, Abonnoor AEI, Abbas WM, et al. Health related quality of life after urinary diversion. Which technique is better? J Egypt Natl Canc Inst. 2018;30:93–7. https://doi.org/10.1016/J.JNCI.2018.08.001.
36. Voskuilen CS, Fransen van de Putte EE, Pérez-Reggeti JI, van Werkhoven E, Mertens LS, van Rhijn BWG, et al. Prostate sparing cystectomy for bladder cancer: a two-center study. Eur J Surg Oncol. 2018;44:1446–52. https://doi.org/10.1016/j.ejso.2018.05.032.
37. Chen PY, Chiang PH. Comparisons of quality of life and functional and oncological outcomes after Orthotopic Neobladder reconstruction: prostate-sparing cystectomy versus conventional radical Cystoprostatectomy. Biomed Res Int. 2017;2017. https://doi.org/10.1155/2017/1983428.
38. Kanashiro A, Gaya JM, Palou J, Gausa L, Villavicencio H. Robot-assisted radical cystoprostatectomy: Analysis of the complications and oncological and functional aspects. Actas Urológicas Españolas. 2017;41:267–73. https://doi.org/10.1016/j.acuroe.2017.03.006.
39. Wishahi M, Elganozoury H. Survival up to 5-15 years in young women following genital sparing radical cystectomy and neobladder: oncological outcome and quality of life. Single-surgeon and single-institution experience. Cent Eur J Urol. 2015;68:141–5. https://doi.org/10.5173/ceju.2015.475
40. Kowalkowski MA, Chandrashekar A, Amiel GE, Lerner SP, Wittmann DA, Latini DM, et al. Examining sexual dysfunction in non-muscle-invasive bladder cancer: results of cross-sectional mixed-methods research. Sex Med. 2014;2:141–51. https://doi.org/10.1002/sm2.24.
41. Ali-El-Dein B, Mosbah A, Osman Y, El-Tabey N, Abdel-latif M, Eraky I, et al. Preservation of the internal genital organs during radical cystectomy in selected women with bladder cancer: a report on 15 cases with long term follow-up. Eur J Surg Oncol. 2013;39:358–64. https://doi.org/10.1016/J.EJSO.2013.02.004.
42. Takenaka A, Hara I, Soga H, Sakai I, Terakawa T, Muramaki M, et al. Assessment of long-term quality of life in patients with orthotopic neobladder followed for more than 5 years. Int Urol Nephrol. 2011;43:749–54. https://doi.org/10.1007/s11255-010-9851-3.
43. Salem HK. Radical cystectomy with preservation of sexual function and fertility in patients with transitional cell carcinoma of the bladder: new technique. Int J Urol. 2007;14:294–8. https://doi.org/10.1111/j.1442-2042.2007.01607.x.
44. Salem HK. Preservation of ejaculatory and erectile function after radical cystectomy for urothelial malignancy. J Egypt Natl Canc Inst. 2005;17:239–44.
45. Lane BR, Finelli A, Moinzadeh A, Sharp DS, Ukimura O, Kaouk JH, et al. Nerve-sparing laparoscopic radical cystectomy: technique and initial outcomes. Urology. 2006;68:778–83. https://doi.org/10.1016/j.urology.2006.05.027.
46. Nandipati KC, Bhat A, Zippe CD. Neurovascular preservation in female orthotopic radical cystectomy significantly improves sexual function. Urology. 2006;67:185–6. https://doi.org/10.1016/J.UROLOGY.2005.07.024.
47. Bhatt A, Nandipati K, Dhar N, Ulchaker J, Jones S, Rackley R, et al. Neurovascular preservation in orthotopic cystectomy: impact on female sexual function. Urology. 2006;67:742–5. https://doi.org/10.1016/j.urology.2005.10.015.
48. Volkmer BG, Gschwend JE, Herkommer K, Simon J, Küfer R, Hautmann RE. Cystectomy and orthotopic ileal neobladder: the impact on female sexuality. J Urol. 2004;172:2353–7. https://doi.org/10.1097/01.ju.0000145190.84531.66.

49. Zippe CD, Raina R, Massanyi EZ, Agarwal A, Jones JS, Ulchaker J, et al. Sexual function after male radical cystectomy in a sexually active population. Urology. 2004;64:682–5. https://doi.org/10.1016/j.urology.2004.05.056.
50. Terrone C, Cracco C, Scarpa RM, Rossetti SR. Supra-ampullar cystectomy with preservation of sexual function and ileal orthotopic reservoir for bladder tumor: twenty years of experience. Eur Urol. 2004;46:264–70. https://doi.org/10.1016/j.eururo.2004.03.006.
51. Zippe CD, Raina R, Shah AD, Massanyi EZ, Agarwal A, Ulchaker J, et al. Female sexual dysfunction after radical cystectomy: a new outcome measure. Urology. 2004;63:1153–7. https://doi.org/10.1016/j.urology.2003.12.034.
52. Miyao N, Adachi H, Sato Y, Horita H, Takahashi A, Masumori N, et al. Recovery of sexual function after nerve-sparing radical prostatectomy or cystectomy. Int J Urol. 2001;8:158–64. https://doi.org/10.1046/j.1442-2042.2001.00274.x.
53. Little FA, Howard GCW. Sexual function following radical radiotherapy for bladder cancer. Radiother Oncol. 1998;49:157–61. https://doi.org/10.1016/S0167-8140(98)00109-1.
54. Schover LR, Evans R, Von Eschenbach AC. Sexual rehabilitation and male radical cystectomy. J Urol. 1986;136:1015–7. https://doi.org/10.1016/S0022-5347(17)45192-5.
55. Schove LR, Von Eschenbach AC. Sexual function and female radical cystectomy: a case series. J Urol. 2017;134:465–8. https://doi.org/10.1016/s0022-5347(17)47242-9.
56. El-Bahnasawy MS, Osman Y, El-Hefnawy A, Hafez A, Abdel-Latif M, Mosbah A, et al. Radical cystectomy and urinary diversion in women: impact on sexual function. Scand J Urol Nephrol. 2011;45:332–8. https://doi.org/10.3109/00365599.2011.585621.
57. Bjerre BD, Joh C. Sexological problems after cystectomy: bladder substitution compared with Ileal conduit diversion: a questionnaire study of male patients. Scand J Urol Nephrol. 1998;32:187–93. https://doi.org/10.1080/003655998750015557.
58. Tomić R, Sjödin JG. Sexual function in men after radical cystectomy with or without urethrectomy. Scand J Urol Nephrol. 1992;26:127–9.
59. Moursy EES, Eldahshoursy MZ, Gamal WM, Badawy AA. Orthotopic genital sparing radical cystectomy in pre-menopausal women with muscle-invasive bladder carcinoma: a prospective study. Indian J Urol. 2016;32:65–70. https://doi.org/10.4103/0970-1591.173112.

12

# Silodosin improves functional consequences of lower urinary tract obstruction secondary to benign prostate hypertrophy, a proof of concept study in the spontaneously hypertensive rat supplemented with testosterone

Rana Assaly[1,2], Julie Faugeroux[1,2], Miguel Laurin[1,2], Sandrine Compagnie[1,2], Laurent Alexandre[1], François Giuliano[1,2,3] and Delphine Behr-Roussel[1,2*]

**Abstract**

**Background:** The main purpose of this study is to investigate the effect of silodosin on the urodynamic consequences in a previously established model of lower urinary tract symptoms associated with benign prostate hyperplasia, the spontaneously hypertensive rats (SHR) supplemented with testosterone.

**Methods:** Three groups of animals (8-week-old; $n = 10$/group) were considered: Wistar Kyoto (control) rats (WKY), SHR supplemented with testosterone at 3 mg/kg/day and treated with either vehicle (SHR-T, $n = 10$) or silodosin at 0.1 mg/kg/day (SHR-T + silodosin, n = 10) by oral gavage for 6 weeks. Cystometry experiments were performed. The bladder was harvested, weighed and paraffin-embedded for morphometric analysis. The prostate was also harvested and weighed.

**Results:** The number of animals included in the analysis were $n = 10/10$ for WKY and $n = 7–8/10$ for each SHR rats supplemented with testosterone group. SHR-T displayed a significant decrease in the intercontraction interval, infused volume and mean flow rate whereas the frequency of non-voiding contractions was increased. Silodosin improved the voiding behavior of SHR-T by significantly increasing the intercontraction interval, the infused volume and the mean flow rate and decreasing the number of non-voiding contractions. SHR-T displayed a significant increase in prostate and bladder weights and a 15% increase in the detrusor wall area compared to WKY.

**Conclusions:** Chronic silodosin treatment relieved storage symptoms in SHR supplemented with testosterone and decreased the frequency of non-voiding detrusor contractions during the filling phase.

**Keywords:** Benign prostatic hyperplasia, Lower urinary tract obstruction, Bladder function, Silodosin, Experimental cystometry, Spontaneously hypertensive rats

* Correspondence: d.behr.roussel@pelvipharm.com
[1]Pelvipharm, Montigny-le-Bretonneux, France
[2]Université Paris-Saclay, UVSQ, Inserm, END-ICAP, Versailles, France

## Background

Lower urinary tract symptoms (LUTS) resulting from benign prostatic hyperplasia (BPH) are common problems in the aging male population [1]. These symptoms comprise two main components, the storage urinary symptoms also defined by the term overactive bladder and the voiding symptoms i.e. impairment of outflow.

According to guidelines and recommendations α1 receptor antagonists are first line drug treatment for patients with BPH/LUTS [2]. Among the subtypes of α1 receptors, it has been assumed that the 1A subtype is responsible for the dynamic component of BPH/LUTS and related voiding symptoms since it predominates in smooth muscle of prostate and proximal urethra [3]. Thus, the conventional mechanism of α1 receptor antagonists to relieve the symptoms is via relaxation of prostatic and urethral smooth muscle. In recent years, α1A receptor antagonists were reported to improve not only voiding but also storage symptoms. Indeed, several authors described changes in urodynamic parameters in BPH/LUTS patients suggesting a role for α1 receptor antagonists to decrease detrusor pressure at maximum urinary flow and to improve the degree of bladder outlet obstruction [4, 5]. Chapple et al [6] reported that silodosin, a uroselective α1A receptor antagonist, improved the International Prostate Symptom Subscores for both voiding and storage symptoms in LUTS/BPH patients. However, the mechanisms of action by which α1A receptor antagonists improve storage symptoms remain unclear. It has also been hypothesized the beneficial effects of α1A receptor antagonists may involve sites of action in addition to prostatic and urethral smooth muscle, such as the bladder and/or the spinal cord [7]. However bladder outlet obstruction remains a key pathophysiological feature in BPH/LUTS patients. In order to evaluate the effect of α1A receptor antagonists on voiding and storage symptoms associated with bladder outflow obstruction and to elucidate the corresponding mechanisms of action, it is important to use an animal model presenting urodynamic changes probably associated not only with mechanical obstruction caused by prostate enlargement but also with increase in urethral and prostate smooth muscle tone.

The present study was designed to investigate the effect of silodosin on the urodynamic consequences in a previously established model of LUTS related BPH [8], the spontaneously hypertensive rats (SHR) supplemented with testosterone. This model displays all key features of BPH/LUTS i.e. prostate enlargement, increased sympathetic tone of bladder outlet mimicking the static and the dynamic components of voiding symptoms related to BPH and signs of detrusor overactivity. In addition, correlation between bladder wall or detrusor wall thickness and bladder outlet obstruction and symptom severity has been reported in BPH/LUTS patients [9, 10], thus histological assessment of detrusor wall area, sandwiched between the mucosa and adventitia, was performed in this study.

## Methods

Adult 8-week-old male Wistar Kyoto rats (WKY, $n = 10$) and SHR rats (SHR, $n = 20$) (Janvier labs, France) were used in this study. The number of animals used is the minimum that is consistent with scientific integrity and regulatory acceptability, consideration having been given to the welfare of individual animals in terms of the number and extent of procedures to be carried out on each animal. The animals were housed 1 week prior to the beginning of the experiments at the animal facility with free access to standard chow (Chow M20, 841,201, SDS, UK) and water and maintained on inversed 12 h dark/light cycle (light off 10:00/22:00). Beginning with the acclimatization period and during the whole protocol, the rats were housed by 2 in a ventilated cage (Allentown Inc., USA). The rat environment was enriched with kraft paper fibers for nesting, polycarbonate square tunnel and gnawing material (*SERLAB, France*). All procedures were approved by the local ethical committee (CEE47) and performed in accordance with the legislation on the use of laboratory animals (NIH publication N°85–23, revised 1996) and Animal Care Regulations in force in France as of 1988 (authorization from competent French Ministry of Agriculture - Agreement No. B78–423-1, July 2017). After the acclimation period, SHR rats were identified with a unique identification number; then using random number table, they were randomly allocated to 2 experimental groups receiving either vehicle, methylcellulose 5% (SHR-T, $n = 10$, mean weight prior to treatment 269.9 ± 4.1 g) or silodosin at 0.1 mg/kg/day (SHR-T + silodosin, n = 10, mean weight prior to treatment 267.8 ± 3.9 g) by oral gavage for 6 weeks. Concomitantly, SHR rats received daily subcutaneous testosterone supplementation at 3 mg/kg/day to induce prostate growth. WKY rats (WKY, $n = 10$, mean weight prior to treatment 250.2 ± 5.5 g) received daily subcutaneous sesame oil and vehicle by oral gavage.

At the end of the treatment period, cystometry experiments were performed. Finally, the rats were anesthetized with isoflurane (2.0–2.5%, Centravet, France) and then euthanized by intraperitoneal injection of pentobarbital at 0.1 ml/100 g of body weight (Centravet, France) in accordance with Animal Care Regulations in force in France. The bladder was then harvested, weighed and paraffin-embedded for histological examination and measure of the bladder wall thickness. The prostate was also harvested and weighed.

### Intravesical catheter implantation

As described previously [8], an intravesical catheter was implanted in the bladder dome of each rat 2 days before the cystometry experiments. Briefly, the rats were anesthetized with isoflurane (1.5–2.0%, Centravet, France) and their temperature maintained at 37 °C using a homeothermic blanket. Then a polyethylene catheter (PE-50: 0.965 mm OD) prefilled with saline solution was inserted through the apex bladder dome exposed via a midline abdominal incision. The catheter was fixed with a 4-zero cotton purse-string suture and its free end was tunneled subcutaneously and exteriorized at the back of the neck. Each rat was maintained individually in a cage with food and water ad libitum until cystometry experiment.

### Cystometry experiments

Cystometric investigations were performed in conscious rats. As previously described [8], the rats were placed in metabolic cages and the free tip of the bladder catheter was connected to a pressure transducer for bladder pressure monitoring and to a syringe pump for bladder perfusion. The rats were allowed an acclimation period then the bladder was continuously perfused with saline at 50 µl/min. Weighing devices placed underneath the metabolic cages were used to quantify the micturition volumes. Once the bladder continuous perfusion started, a 60-min stabilization period was considered to ensure reproducible micturition cycles i.e., the variations in micturition volumes and in intervals between micturition did not exceed ±10%, before starting a 60-min evaluation period. During this evaluation period, intravesical pressure was recorded and the following parameters related to voiding contractions were measured: maximal amplitude, baseline intravesical pressure, micturition pressure threshold and intercontraction interval for reflex-evoked bladder micturition. Also, frequency of non-voiding contractions and the volume threshold to elicit non-voiding contractions for each cycle during the filling phase were measured (Fig. 1). Furthermore, the infused volume between two voiding contractions, index of the bladder capacity, and the voided volume of each voiding contraction were analyzed, and the mean urine flow rate was assessed.

### Histological examination of bladder wall hypertrophy

The rats were euthanized and the bladder was harvested, paraffin embedded and 5-µm sections were performed using a microtome (RM 2245®, Leica Biosystems, France). The sections were stained with hematoxylin-eosin using an automated multistainer (ST5020® &CV5030 Coverslipper® Leica Biosystems, France) for evaluation of detrusor wall area, the detrusor being sandwiched between the mucosa and adventitia. The acquisition of slides images was then performed using Aperio AT2 - Scanner for On-Screen Diagnosis® (Leica Biosystems, France). Then images were analyzed with NIS Elements Software (NIS elements, Nikon, France) to compute the detrusor wall area from each section by a blinded experimenter. For each animal, 4 transverse sections were analyzed and a mean area of sections per animal was then determined.

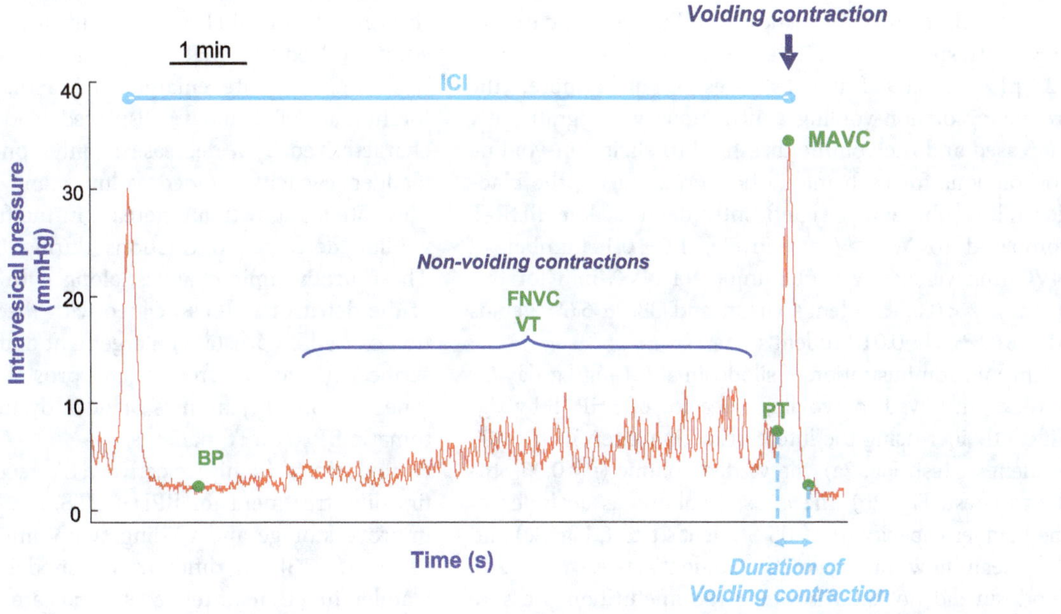


**Fig. 1** Illustration of the parameters computed for bladder voiding and non-voiding contractions during cystometry in a conscious of SHR-testosterone treated rat. MAVC: maximal amplitude of voiding contractions, BP: baseline intravesical pressure, PT: micturition pressure threshold, ICI: intercontraction interval. FNVC: frequency of non-voiding contractions, VT: volume threshold to elicit non-voiding contractions for each micturition cycle during the bladder filling phase

### Statistical analysis

All results are presented as mean ± SEM. The number of animals included in the analysis were $n = 10/10$ for WKY and $n = 7–8/10$ for each SHR rats supplemented with testosterone group i.e., SHR-T and SHR-T + silodosin. The cystometry data of some rats were not interpretable due to either technical problem or urine emission by dribbling during cystometry experiments.

$P$ values $< 0.05$ were considered significant. Statistical analyses were performed using Student's t-test.

### Drugs and chemicals

Silodosin was dissolved in 0.5% methylcellulose. Silodosin was provided by Recordati (Italy). All other drugs and chemicals were purchased from Sigma-Aldrich (France).

## Results

There was no statistical difference on maximal amplitude of voiding contractions and baseline intravesical pressure between WKY and SHR-T. Conversely, all other parameters characterizing the voiding contractions were significantly decreased in SHR-T compared to WKY, respectively, 5.8 ± 0.5 mmHg versus 8.4 ± 0.8 mmHg for pressure threshold, $p < 0.05$ Student's t-test; 615.4 ± 55.4 s versus 825.8 ± 67.7 s for intercontraction interval, $p < 0.05$ Student's t-test; 512.8 ± 46.1 µL versus 688.2 ± 56.4 µL for infused volume as an index of bladder capacity, $p < 0.05$ Student's t-test; and 19.5 ± 3.7 µL/s versus 35.8 ± 5.0 µL/s for mean urine flow rate, p < 0.05 Student's t-test. Only the decrease in voided volume in SHR-T did not reach statistical significance compared to WKY (respectively, 523.4 ± 56.2 µL versus 699.0 ± 72.5 µL, $p = 0.09$ Student's t-test). Furthermore, the frequency of non-voiding contractions was significantly increased and the volume threshold to elicit non-voiding contractions for each micturition cycle during the bladder filling phase was significantly decreased in SHR-T compared to WKY (respectively, 1.6 ± 0.1 number of NVC/min versus 1.2 ± 0.1 number of NVC/min for frequency, $p < 0.05$ Student's t-test; and 33.1 ± 6.6% versus 61.8 ± 6.8%, $p < 0.01$ Student's t-test).

Chronic administration of silodosin at 0.1 mg/kg/day for 6 weeks improved the voiding behavior of SHR-T by significantly increasing the intercontraction interval ($p < 0.05$ Student's t-test, Fig. 2a), the voided volume ($p < 0.05$ Student's t-test, Fig. 2b), the infused volume as an index of the bladder capacity ($p < 0.05$ Student's t-test, Fig. 2c) and the mean flow rate ($p < 0.05$ Student's t-test, Fig. 2d). Silodosin did not alter however the micturition pressure threshold. Compared to the vehicle-treated SHR-T, the silodosin-treated SHR-T showed a significantly lower number of non-voiding contractions (Fig. 2e) whereas the decrease in the volume threshold to elicit these non-voiding contractions did not reach statistical significance (Fig. 2f).

At a microscopic level, distinct layers were observed in bladder cross sections. The bladder lumen was lined by the urothelium that interdigitated with the lamina propria. The detrusor muscular area lied beneath the lamina propria and was surrounded by the most outer adventitia layer. Morphometric analysis showed a hypertrophy of the detrusor wall reflected by a 15% increase in the detrusor wall area of SHR-T compared to WKY ($p < 0.05$, Student's t-test). Daily oral gavage of silodosin at 0.1 mg/kg for 6 weeks did not alter the increased bladder detrusor area of SHR-T.

SHR-T displayed a significant increase in prostate and bladder weights compared to WKY, respectively, 310.9 ± 19.8 mg/100 g body weight versus 162.5 ± 10.2 mg/100 g body weight for prostate, $p < 0.001$ Student's t-test and 60.1 ± 2.9 mg/100 g body weight versus 48.4 ± 2.6 mg/100 g body weight for bladder $p < 0.01$ Student's t-test. Silodosin administered at 0.1 mg/kg/d for 6 weeks did not modify either organ weights.

## Discussion

The effect of chronic treatment with silodosin on the urodynamic consequences of testosterone supplementation in the SHR, a model of BPH has been investigated. Whether the beneficial effect of silodosin on urodynamic parameters could be related to a drug effect on detrusor histology has also been assessed.

The relevance of the SHR supplemented with testosterone as a model for lower urinary tract symptoms resulting from BPH [8] is confirmed by the present study. Indeed, the SHR supplemented with testosterone i) showed prostate enlargement, a diagnostic criterion for human BPH and ii) displayed bladder hyperactivity characterized by a decrease in intercontraction interval, bladder capacity, voided volume and average voiding flow rate along with an increase in the frequency of non-voiding detrusor contractions during the filling phase. These urodynamic changes, along with the hypertrophy of the detrusor wall associated with mechanical obstruction caused by prostate enlargement and a previously described increase in urethral and prostate smooth muscle tone in SHR [11] mimics bladder dysfunction in symptomatic BPH/LUTS patients.

Silodosin, a highly selective α1A receptor antagonist, first-line treatment for BPH/LUTS, has been reported to improve storage and voiding symptoms in clinical trials [5, 6, 12, 13]. In different rat models with abnormal bladder function unrelated to prostate enlargement i.e., the SHR [14–16] and the bladder outlet obstruction models [17–19], silodosin was found to exert a beneficial effect on bladder function. Although the size of the prostate is not a predictive factor for the severity of LUTS,

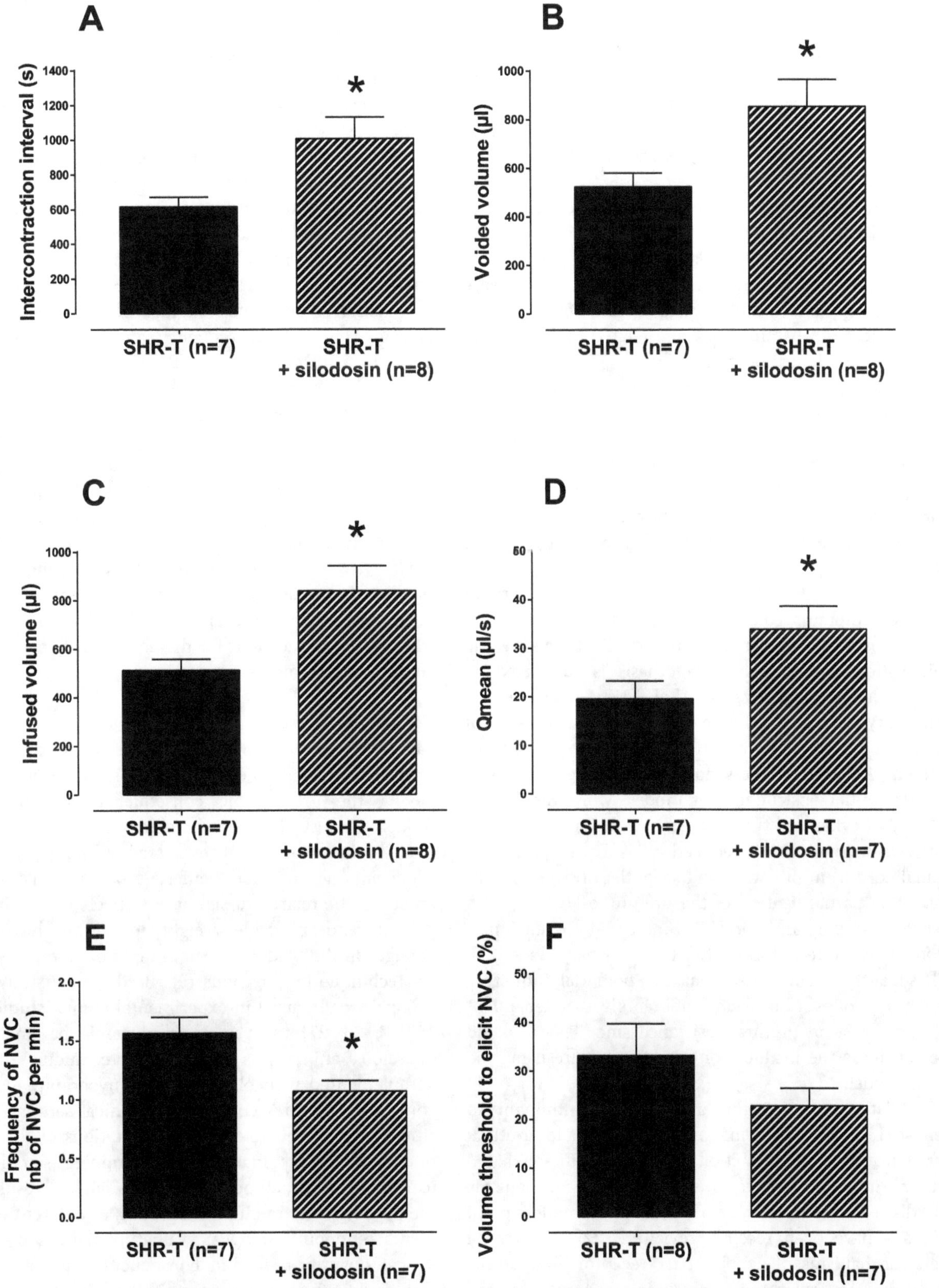


**Fig. 2** Cytometry parameters measured in conscious SHR supplemented by subcutaneous injections of testosterone that received by oral gavage once daily either vehicle (SHR-T) or silodosin at 0.1 mg/kg (SHR-T + silodosin) for 6 weeks. Data are expressed as mean ± SEM. *$p < 0.05$, Student's t-test

enlarged prostate is an important feature for a model of BPH/LUTS. Hence, it was important to investigate whether silodosin could improve bladder function in a model that displays key features of BPH i.e. prostate enlargement, increased sympathetic tone of bladder outlet mimicking the static and the dynamic components of BPH related voiding symptoms and detrusor overactivity.

Chronic silodosin treatment relieved storage symptoms in SHR-T as shown by the increased intercontraction interval and improved bladder capacity in silodosin-treated compared to vehicle-treated SHR-T. An increase in the voided volume and average voiding flow rate were also found, both parameters being related to the voiding phase of the micturition cycle.

Bladder hyperactivity is also characterized by non-voiding contractions, corresponding to non-voiding detrusor contractions during the filling phase [8, 14, 19]. Interestingly, silodosin decreased the frequency of non-voiding contractions in SHR-T. Such an effect of silodosin could neither be correlated to significant effects of the drug on prostate and/or bladder weight nor on any histological changes in the bladder.

We postulate that the beneficial effects of silodosin on storage symptoms could be due to an inhibitory effect by silodosin on bladder afferents activity triggering the micturition reflex. Such a hypothesis is supported by recent findings by Aizawa et al. [17], describing an inhibitory effect elicited by a 6-day constant infusion of silodosin on single–unit activities of mechanosensitive afferent Aδ- and C-fibers during the filling-phase in a bladder outlet obstruction rat model. Moreover, Yazaki et al., [20] evidenced that a constant infusion of silodosin for 2 weeks significantly reduced c-Fos expression in the spinal cord from rats with bladder outlet obstruction obtained by partial ligation of the urethra, c-Fos increased expression being an indicator of increased afferent input from mechanoreceptors in the lower urinary tract [21]. These authors concluded that the potential inhibitory effect of silodosin on bladder afferents was independent of a decrease in urethral resistance since silodosin did not decrease the bladder contraction pressure using the same model.

To date, α1A receptor antagonists are thought to relieve LUTS by reducing prostatic tone and urethral resistance via the inhibition of α1 receptor-mediated smooth muscle contractions. The molecular mechanisms of disease progression and bladder remodeling in humans have been recently reviewed [22] and several new mechanisms of action of α1 receptor antagonists, and more particularly of silodosin, an α1A receptor antagonist considered to have a higher uroselectivity than other α1A receptor antagonists, have been suggested. The impairment in bladder blood flow, subsequent to the bladder wall hypertrophy caused by bladder outlet obstruction, seems to play a key role in the natural history of BPH. The decrease in bladder blood flow due to ischemia coupled with an increased expression of mRNA of α1A receptors in bladder microvessels in a bladder outlet obstruction rat model [18] and SHR [16, 23] have been reported. Thus, silodosin could improve bladder blood flow in addition to its inhibitory effect on bladder afferents. Indeed, constant infusion of silodosin for 2 weeks improved bladder blood flow in a bladder outlet obstruction rat model while preventing an increase in voiding frequency [18]. Likewise, 6 weeks of silodosin oral delivered improved bladder blood flow while decreasing micturition frequency and voided volume in SHR [16, 23]. Masuda et al., [24] even suggested that the bladder ischemia induced by bladder outlet obstruction increases the generation of reactive oxygen species activating a signalling cascade leading to the stimulation of bladder afferent fibers. Finally, Goi et al., [25] suggested that silodosin may improve bladder blood flow and bladder contraction by preventing fibrosis of bladder smooth muscle in a model of atherosclerosis-induced chronic bladder ischemia. Thus, it would be interesting to investigate in future studies whether morphological remodeling by decreasing fibrosis of bladder smooth muscle in this model may account for the observed effect of silodosin on urodynamic parameters.

## Conclusions

This is a proof-of concept experimental study that described the beneficial effect of silodosin treatment on relieving the urodynamic consequences in an animal model, the testosterone supplemented SHR, a model of LUTS related BPH, suggesting an inhibitory effect of silodosin on the bladder afferent pathway. This effect could not be related to significant effects of the drug on prostate and/or bladder weight nor on any histological changes in the bladder. It should be noted, the cystometry technique in conscious rats used in this study, even though broadly used in experimental animal studies [14, 15, 17, 26, 27] to evaluate urodynamic parameters in conscious animals, is an invasive technique and not complemented with bladder electromyography test, two contrasting features compared to clinical setting. Future studies are needed to fulfill the limitations of this proof of concept study mainly (i) determining sample size using statistical method based on the current results and the expected loss of study individuals in different experimental endpoints and (ii) evaluating fibrosis by histological quantification and consequently futures studies would allow to investigate the effect of silodosin on morphological remodeling and fibrosis of bladder smooth muscle in this model of SHR supplemented with testosterone.

### Abbreviations

SHR: Spontaneously hypertensive rat; WKY: Wistar Kyoto rat; SHR-T: Spontaneously hypertensive rat supplemented with testosterone; SHR-T + silodosin: Spontaneously hypertensive rat supplemented with testosterone that received chronic silodosin treatment; LUTS: Lower urinary tract symptoms; BPH: Benign prostate hyperplasia; MAVC: Maximal amplitude of voiding contractions; BP: Baseline intravesical pressure; PT: Micturition pressure threshold; ICI: Intercontraction interval; NVC: Non-voiding contractions; FNVC: Frequency of non-voiding contractions; VT: Volume threshold to elicit non-voiding contractions for each micturition cycle during the bladder filling phase

### Acknowledgements

Not applicable.

### Authors' contributions

RA, FG and DBR conceived the design of the study. The experimental work, data collection compilation and analysis were performed by RA, JF, ML, SC and DBR. RA drafted the manuscript. FG and DBR edited the manuscript. All authors read and approved the final manuscript.

### Competing interests

F Giuliano is a lecturer for Recordati, other authors declare that they have no conflict of interest.

### Author details

[1]Pelvipharm, Montigny-le-Bretonneux, France. [2]Université Paris-Saclay, UVSQ, Inserm, END-ICAP, Versailles, France. [3]AP-HP, Neuro-Uro-Andrology, Department of Physical Medicine and Rehabilitation, Raymond Poincaré Hospital, Garches, France.

### References

1. Gacci M, Eardley I, Giuliano F, Hatzichristou D, Kaplan SA, Maggi M, et al. Critical analysis of the relationship between sexual dysfunctions and lower urinary tract symptoms due to benign prostatic hyperplasia. Eur Urol. 2011; 60(4):809–25.
2. Gravas S, Cornu JN, Gacci C, et al. EAU guidelines on Management of non-neurogenic male lower urinary tract symptoms (LUTS), incl. Benign prostatic obstruction (BPO). Edn. presented at the EAU Annual congress Barcelona. Arnhem: EAU Guidelines Office; 2019.
3. Michel MC, Vrydag W. Alpha1-, alpha2- and beta-adrenoceptors in the urinary bladder, urethra and prostate. Br J Pharmacol. 2006;147(Suppl 2):S88–119.
4. Creta M, Bottone F, Sannino S, Maisto E, Franco M, Mangiapia F, et al. Effects of alpha1-blockers on urodynamic parameters of bladder outlet obstruction in patients with lower urinary tract symptoms suggestive of benign prostatic enlargement: a review. Minerva Urol Nefrol. 2015.
5. Fusco F, Palmieri A, Ficarra V, Giannarini G, Novara G, Longo N, et al. alpha1-blockers improve benign prostatic obstruction in men with lower urinary tract symptoms: a systematic review and meta-analysis of urodynamic studies. Eur Urol. 2016;69(6):1091–101.
6. Chapple CR, Montorsi F, Tammela TL, Wirth M, Koldewijn E, Fernandez FE. Silodosin therapy for lower urinary tract symptoms in men with suspected benign prostatic hyperplasia: results of an international, randomized, double-blind, placebo- and active-controlled clinical trial performed in Europe. Eur Urol. 2011;59(3):342–52.
7. Michel MC, Schafers RF, Goepel M. Alpha-blockers and lower urinary tract function: more than smooth muscle relaxation? BJU Int. 2000;86(Suppl 2):23–8.
8. Oudot A, Oger S, Behr-Roussel D, Caisey S, Bernabe J, Alexandre L, et al. A new experimental rat model of erectile dysfunction and lower urinary tract symptoms associated with benign prostatic hyperplasia: the testosterone-supplemented spontaneously hypertensive rat. BJU Int. 2012;110(9):1352–8.
9. Kessler TM, Gerber R, Burkhard FC, Studer UE, Danuser H. Ultrasound assessment of detrusor thickness in men-can it predict bladder outlet obstruction and replace pressure flow study? J Urol. 2006;175:2170–3.
10. Oelke M, Hofner K, Jonas U, de la Rosette JJ, Ubbink DT, Wijkstra H. Diagnostic accuracy of noninvasive tests to evaluate bladder outlet obstruction in men: detrusor wall thickness, uroflowmetry, postvoid residual urine, and prostate volume. Eur Urol. 2007;52:827–34.
11. Maggi CA, Manzini S, Giuliani S, Meli A. Infravesical outflow obstruction in rats: a comparison of two models. Gen Pharmacol. 1989;20(3):345–9.
12. Kawabe K, Yoshida M, Homma Y. Silodosin, a new alpha1A-adrenoceptor-selective antagonist for treating benign prostatic hyperplasia: results of a phase III randomized, placebo-controlled, double-blind study in Japanese men. BJU Int. 2006;98(5):1019–24.
13. Marks LS, Gittelman MC, Hill LA, Volinn W, Hoel G. Rapid efficacy of the highly selective alpha1A-adrenoceptor antagonist silodosin in men with signs and symptoms of benign prostatic hyperplasia: pooled results of 2 phase 3 studies. J Urol. 2009;181(6):2634–40.
14. Jin LH, Andersson KE, Kwon YH, Park CS, Yoon SM, Lee T. Substantial detrusor overactivity in conscious spontaneously hypertensive rats with hyperactive behaviour. Scand J Urol Nephrol. 2009;43(1):3–7.
15. Patra PB, Thorneloe KS. Enhanced sensitivity to afferent stimulation and impact of overactive bladder therapies in the conscious, spontaneously hypertensive rat. J Pharmacol Exp Ther. 2011;338(1):392–9.
16. Inoue S, Saito M, Tsounapi P, Dimitriadis F, Ohmasa F, Kinoshita Y, et al. Effect of silodosin on detrusor overactivity in the male spontaneously hypertensive rat. BJU Int. 2012;110(2 Pt 2):E118–24.
17. Aizawa N, Watanabe D, Fukuhara H, Fujimura T, Kume H, Homma Y, et al. Inhibitory effects of silodosin on the bladder mechanosensitive afferent activities and their relation with bladder myogenic contractions in male rats with bladder outlet obstruction. Neurourol Urodyn. 2018.
18. Goi Y, Tomiyama Y, Yokoyama A, Tatemichi S, Maruyama K, Kobayashi M, et al. Effect of silodosin, a selective alpha(1A)-adrenoceptor antagonist, on voiding behavior and bladder blood flow in a rat model of bladder outlet obstruction. Eur J Pharmacol. 2015;764:489–96.
19. Persson K, Pandita RK, Spitsbergen JM, Steers WD, Tuttle JB, Andersson KE. Spinal and peripheral mechanisms contributing to hyperactive voiding in spontaneously hypertensive rats. Am J Phys. 1998;275(4 Pt 2):R1366–73.
20. Yazaki J, Aikawa K, Shishido K, Yanagida T, Nomiya M, Ishibashi K, et al. Alpha1-adrenoceptor antagonists improve bladder storage function through reduction of afferent activity in rats with bladder outlet obstruction. Neurourol Urodyn. 2011;30(3):461–7.
21. Seki S, Erickson KA, Seki M, Nishizawa O, Igawa Y, Ogawa T, et al. Elimination of rat spinal neurons expressing neurokinin 1 receptors reduces bladder overactivity and spinal c-fos expression induced by bladder irritation. Am J Physiol Renal Physiol. 2005;288(3):F466–73.
22. Fusco F, Creta M, De NC, Iacovelli V, Mangiapia F, Li MV, et al. Progressive bladder remodeling due to bladder outlet obstruction: a systematic review of morphological and molecular evidences in humans. BMC Urol. 2018;18(1):15.
23. Saito M, Shimizu S, Ohmasa F, Oikawa R, Tsounapi P, Dimitriadis F, et al. Characterization of silodosin and naftopidil in the treatment of bladder dysfunction in the spontaneously hypertensive rat. Neurourol Urodyn. 2013; 32(4):393–8.
24. Masuda H, Kihara K, Saito K, Matsuoka Y, Yoshida S, Chancellor MB, et al. Reactive oxygen species mediate detrusor overactivity via sensitization of afferent pathway in the bladder of anaesthetized rats. BJU Int. 2008;101(6): 775–80.
25. Goi Y, Tomiyama Y, Maruyama I, Tatemichi S, Maruyama K, Kobayashi M, et al. Silodosin, an alpha(1A)-Adrenoceptor antagonist, may ameliorate ischemia-induced bladder denervation and detrusor dysfunction by improving bladder blood flow. Pharmacology. 2016;97(3–4):161–70.
26. Uvin P, Everaerts W, Pinto S, Alpízar YA, Boudes M, Gevaert T, et al. The Use of Cystometry in Small Rodents: A Study of Bladder Chemosensation. J Vis Exp. 2012;66:e3869. https://doi.org/10.3791/3869.
27. Andersson KE, Soler R, Füllhase C. Rodent models for urodynamic investigation. Neurourol Urodynam. 2011;30:636–46.

# 13

# Anti-TNF agents and potential effects on male fertility: Are men being counseled?

Lauren Folgosa Cooley, James Wren, Mary Kate Keeter, Isaac Lam, Nelson Bennett and Robert E. Brannigan*

**Abstract**

**Background:** Adult men with autoimmune conditions are commonly prescribed anti-tumor necrosis factor (anti-TNF) agents; however, there is a paucity of quality evidence as to their effect on male fertility (e.g. semen parameters and sperm quality). Our objective was to determine if men with autoimmune conditions are being counseled regarding the unknown reproductive effects of anti-TNF agents prior to initiation of therapy.

**Methods:** A retrospective analysis of 1010 male patients age 18–45 who were prescribed an anti-TNF agent were assessed for (1) receipt of counseling regarding potential reproductive effects; (2) screening for anatomic or laboratory abnormalities associated with infertility; (3) election for sperm cryopreservation.

**Results:** Only 10.3% of men received counseling, and this was not associated with age ($p = 0.77$). Those who received counseling were significantly more likely to have a genitourinary exam performed, be assessed for presence of a varicocele, be asked about or endorse low libido or erectile dysfunction, have a testosterone, LH, FSH, or prolactin level checked, and have a semen analysis performed (all, $p < 0.0001$). Rates of sperm cryopreservation were low, but statistically higher in men who received counseling (5.77% (+) counseling, 1.10% (–) counseling) ($p = 0.002$).

**Conclusions:** The limited current literature lacks a consensus regarding the short- and long-term male reproductive effects of anti-TNF therapy. Despite this lack of clarity, rates of pre-initiation counseling were low. Rates of sperm cryopreservation, while improved in the counseled group remained low, suggesting prescribing physicians may be unaware of this option for patients.

**Keywords:** Infertility, Counseling, Anti-TNF, Sperm cryopreservation, Autoimmune

## Background

Tumor necrosis factor (TNF) blockade has revolutionized the treatment of autoimmune conditions such as inflammatory joint and bowel disease, helping to reduce disease-associated morbidity and mortality [1]. However, the impact of these agents on male fertility is unclear based on the limited current literature. While the role of TNF in male spermatogenesis is still under investigation, the basic science literature suggests TNF plays critical role in spermatogenesis and maintaining the blood-testis barrier [2–4]. TNF is produced by germ cells and acts as a paracrine cytokine, binding to both Sertoli and Leydig cells [2–4]. Suominen et al. demonstrated that TNF is important in regulating germ cell apoptosis by promoting germ cell survival, which is blocked by infliximab (a TNF antagonist) [5]. Furthermore, sperm production was found to be reduced by 54% in a TNF-related-to-apoptosis-inducing ligand (TRAIL) deficient mouse model in whom TNF signaling is impaired [6]. While TNF is integral to spermatogenesis, if unregulated, high levels of TNF can also be detrimental by leading to testicular inflammation [7]. Therefore, maintaining an adequate equilibrium is essential.

The effect of TNF blockade on human fertility is poorly understood. While two small studies have shown no deleterious effect of anti-TNF agents on semen

* Correspondence: r-brannigan@northwestern.edu
Department of Urology, Northwestern University Feinberg School of Medicine, 676 N. St. Clair St. Arkes 23-015, Chicago, IL 60611, USA

quality, spermatogenesis, production of anti-sperm antibodies, and testosterone levels [8, 9], others have demonstrated increased risk for asthenospermia (decreased sperm motility) [10–12] and impaired sperm morphology [12, 13]. In the rheumatology literature, concern has been raised of cases where sperm counts were significantly reduced following initiation of an anti-TNF agent [14]. Despite the "very low level of evidence" for the effects of anti-TNF agents on male fertility, a review of drug effects on male fertility by Semet et al. states that sperm cryopreservation and discontinuation of treatment for fertility concerns is not necessary for males initiating anti-TNF therapy [15].

Given the discordant research regarding specific reproductive effects, our objective was to ascertain if men prescribed anti-TNF agents are being: (1) counseled regarding potential for adverse reproductive effects; (2) screened for anatomic or laboratory abnormalities associated with infertility; and (3) electing for sperm cryopreservation.

## Methods

We performed an IRB-approved (STU00205946), retrospective chart review of 1010 male patients between the ages of 18 and 45 from January 2006 to September 2017 seen at a single academic medical center. Additional inclusion criteria included having never been prescribed an anti-TNF agent prior to the study period and being prescribed only one anti-TNF agent during the study period. Men prescribed multiple anti-TNF agents during the study period were excluded from analysis. Anti-TNF agents prescribed in this study were adalimumab, infliximab, etanercept, golimumab, and certolizumab.

Counseling was defined as a documented discussion (for example, office visit note or documented telephone encounter) between the patient and prescribing provider that the prescribed agent may pose a risk to reproduction or fertility. The counseling must have occurred prior to starting treatment. To assess if men were screened for anatomic or laboratory abnormalities associated with infertility, we determined if men received (1) a genitourinary exam, (2) screening for varicocele, (3) diagnosis or assessment for low libido, (4) testosterone, FSH, LH, and/or prolactin level, (5) semen analysis (separate from cryopreservation), and (6) sperm cryopreservation. Genitourinary examination was confirmed by a documented assessment of the penis, meatus, and/or testes. Varicocele screening must have included a documentation of absence of varicocele or a grading score and laterality of assessed varicocele by palpation. Sperm cryopreservation included only men who elected cryopreservation. All six parameters may have occurred at the initial visit when the anti-TNF agent was prescribed or during their course of treatment (not necessarily by prescribing provider). Demographic information including marital status, race, and ethnicity were determined from the medical record. Patient diagnosis was defined as prescribing clinician diagnosis entered in the medical record at the time the anti-TNF agent was prescribed.

Each pharmaceutical approved for use in the United States by the Food and Drug Administration (FDA) has a corresponding highlights of prescribing information sheet, which includes information regarding known impact of a drug on fertility. Highlights of prescribing information sheets were assessed for statements and literature references regarding impact of each anti-TNF agent on male fertility (Table 2).

Data was analyzed using GraphPad Prism. Categorical variables and proportion of events between those that did or did not receive counseling were compared using chi-square test. Means with standard deviation were compared using Student's *t*-test after determining normal distribution (Shapiro-Wilk test). A $p$ value ≤0.05 was considered significant.

## Results

### Demographics

A total of 1010 men met inclusion criteria for this study. Demographic information for included patients is provided in Table 1. In summary, average age was 32.4 years and mean duration of treatment was 832 days (2.3 years). The cohort was predominantly white (67.62%) and non-Hispanic (76.44%). The majority of participants were single (non-married) (58.51%). Men in this study were most likely to be diagnosed with psoriasis or psoriatic arthritis (35.05%), inflammatory bowel disease (Crohn's [21.10%] and ulcerative colitis [17.62%]), or ankylosing spondylitis (10.99%). The most common prescribers were dermatologists, gastroenterologists, and rheumatologists.

### Evaluation of anti-TNF agent prescribing information to consumers and clinicians

FDA prescribing information sheets for anti-TNF agents assessed in this study were evaluated for discussion of impact of each medication on male fertility (Table 2). The prescribing information for the three most common prescribed agents in this study, adalimumab, infliximab and etanercept, stated the impact of these agents on fertility is unknown [16–18]. While animal studies have been performed to evaluate fertility following use of golimumab and certolizumab, there is no reference, study results, or study methods provided for critical review [19, 20].

### Men prescribed anti-TNF agents rarely receive counseling regarding potential impact on fertility

Prior to starting an anti-TNF agent for the first time, 10.3% of men received counseling regrading potential impact on fertility (Table 3). Men who received

**Table 1** Demographics of study patients

| | Adalimumab | Etanercept | Infliximab | Golimumab | Certolizumab | Total |
|---|---|---|---|---|---|---|
| **Number of patients** | 600 | 161 | 219 | 8 | 22 | 1010 |
| **Age** (years) | 32.8 ± 7.5 | 33.0 ± 6.9 | 30.9 ± 7.4 | 33.9 ± 7.5 | 31.8 ± 7.1 | 32.4 ± 7.5 |
| **Duration of treatment** (days) | 799 ± 700 | 958 ± 878 | 853 ± 850 | 794 ± 725 | 669 ± 466 | 832 ± 806 |
| **Race** | **n %** | **n %** | **n %** | **n %** | **n %** | **n %** |
| American Indian | 1 (0.17) | 0 (0.00) | 2 (0.91) | 0 (0.00) | 0 (0.00) | 3 (0.30) |
| Asian | 16 (2.67) | 5 (3.11) | 9 (4.10) | 0 (0.00) | 0 (0.00) | 30 (2.97) |
| Black | 29 (4.83) | 4 (2.48) | 27 (12.32) | 0 (0.00) | 0 (0.00) | 60 (5.94) |
| Hispanic | 1 (0.17) | 1 (0.62) | 2 (0.91) | 0 (0.00) | 0 (0.00) | 4 (0.40) |
| Pacific Islander | 1 (0.17) | 0 (0.00) | 0 (0.00) | 0 (0.00) | 0 (0.00) | 1 (0.01) |
| White | 404 (67.33) | 99 (61.5) | 153 (69.86) | 8 (100) | 19 (86.36) | 683 (67.62) |
| Declined | 78 (13.00) | 36 (22.4) | 9 (4.10) | 0 (0.00) | 0 (0.00) | 123 (12.18) |
| Other | 70 (11.67) | 16 (9.94) | 17 (7.76) | 0 (0.00) | 3 (13.64) | 106 (10.50) |
| **Ethnicity** | **n %** | **n %** | **n %** | **n %** | **n %** | **n %** |
| Hispanic | 29 (4.83) | 10 (6.21) | 13 (5.93) | 0 (0.00) | 0 (0.00) | 52 (5.15) |
| Not Hispanic/Latino | 465 (77.50) | 103 (63.98) | 177 (80.82) | 8 (100) | 19 (86.36) | 772 (76.44) |
| Declined | 106 (17.67) | 48 (29.81) | 29 (13.24) | 0 (0.00) | 3 (13.64) | 186 (18.41) |
| **Marital Status** | **n %** | **n %** | **n %** | **n %** | **n %** | **n %** |
| Single | 342 (57.00) | 77 (47.83) | 153 (69.86) | 6 (75.00) | 13 (59.09) | 591 (58.51) |
| Married | 205 (34.17) | 71 (44.10) | 64 (29.22) | 2 (25.00) | 9 (40.91) | 351 (34.75) |
| Divorced | 4 (0.67) | 3 (1.86) | 0 (0.00) | 0 (0.00) | 0 (0.00) | 7 (0.69) |
| Other | 49 (8.17) | 10 (6.21) | 2 (0.91) | 0 (0.00) | 0 (0.00) | 61 (6.04) |
| **Diagnosis** | **n %** | **n %** | **n %** | **n %** | **n %** | **n %** |
| Ankylosing spondylitis | 61 (10.16) | 42 (26.09) | 7 (3.19) | 0 (0.00) | 1 (4.55) | 111 (10.99) |
| Behcet's | 2 (0.33) | 0 (0.00) | 1 (0.46) | 0 (0.00) | 0 (0.00) | 3 (0.29) |
| Blau Syndrome | 2 (0.33) | 0 (0.00) | 0 (0.00) | 0 (0.00) | 0 (0.00) | 2 (0.20) |
| Crohn's | 107 (17.83) | 0 (0.00) | 90 (41.09) | 3 (37.50) | 13 (59.09) | 213 (21.10) |
| Hidradenitis suppurativa | 25 (4.17) | 1 (0.62) | 1 (0.46) | 0 (0.00) | 0 (0.00) | 27 (2.67) |
| Psoriasis ± arthritis | 256 (42.67) | 83 (51.55) | 11 (5.02) | 2 (25.00) | 2 (9.09) | 354 (35.05) |
| Rheumatoid arthritis | 24 (4.00) | 20 (12.42) | 18 (8.22) | 0 (0.00) | 1 (4.55) | 63 (6.24) |
| Sarcoidosis | 2 (0.33) | 0 (0.00) | 12 (5.48) | 0 (0.00) | 0 (0.00) | 14 (1.39) |
| Seronegative arthritis | 28 (4.67) | 11 (6.83) | 0 (0.00) | 0 (0.00) | 1 (4.55) | 40 (3.96) |
| Sjogren's | 1 (0.17) | 2 (1.24) | 2 (0.91) | 0 (0.00) | 0 (0.00) | 5 (0.49) |
| Ulcerative Colitis | 92 (15.33) | 2 (1.24) | 77 (35.16) | 3 (37.50) | 4 (18.18) | 178 (17.62) |

All participants were male and prescribed a single anti-TNF agent (adalimumab, etanercept, infliximab, golimumab, or certolizumab). Duration of treatment is presented as average ± standard deviation. Race and ethnicity categories reflect the options available for data insertion in Epic Systems

counseling were significantly more likely to have a genitourinary exam performed, be screened for a varicocele, be asked about concerns with libido or sexual function, have a testosterone, LH, FSH or prolactin level checked, have a semen analysis performed, and elect for sperm cryopreservation (Table 3). Men who received counseling were significantly more likely to elect for sperm cryopreservation, but rates of cryopreservation were low in both groups (5.77% (+) counseling, 1.10% (−) counseling). Age was not a statistically significant factor related to likelihood to receive counseling ($p = 0.77$).

## Discussion

Anti -TNF agents are commonly prescribed to young adult men with autoimmune conditions on a long-term basis. While it is known on a molecular level that TNF is required for optimal spermatogenesis, the literature currently lacks large cohort, randomized, prospective evidence to adequately answer this question. Furthermore, according to the FDA highlights of prescribing information for each anti-TNF agent evaluated in this study, the majority stated the impact of the agent on fertility was unknown. Those that reported no risk did not

**Table 2** Impact of anti-TNF agents on fertility from FDA prescribing information

| Anti-TNF agent (Generic / Brand name) | Prescribing information |
|---|---|
| Adalimumab / Humira© | "Long-term animal studies of HUMIRA have not been conducted to evaluate the carcinogenic potential or its effect on fertility" [16]. |
| Infliximab / Remicade© | "It is not known whether infliximab can impair fertility in humans" [17]. |
| Etanercept / Enbrel© | "Long-term animal studies have not been conducted to evaluate the carcinogenic potential of etanercept or its effect on fertility" [18]. |
| Golimumab / Simponi© | "A fertility study conducted in mice using an analogous anti-mouse TNFα antibody showed no impairment to fertility" [19]. |
| Certolizumab / Cimzia© | "The cTN3 PF (TNFα pegylated Fab fragment) had no effects on the fertility and general reproductive performance of male and female rats at intravenous doses up 100 mg/kg, administered twice weekly" [20]. |

FDA prescribing information for each anti-TNF agent listed was analyzed for discussion of impact of each agent on male fertility

provide literature or study reference to allow for evaluation of their data (Table 2). Despite this lack of quality of evidence, the recommendations found in the literature suggest sperm cryopreservation or discontinuation of anti-TNF therapy for male fertility concerns is not necessary [15]. This discordant information available to prescribers in the literature may help to explain why only 10.3% of over 1000 men prescribed an anti-TNF agent in our study cohort received counseling as to potential adverse effects on fertility. This suggests that patients and clinicians may be unaware of this knowledge gap or may not be documenting the fertility aspect of their discussion.

Furthermore, men prescribed anti-TNF agents are a unique population in that their primary disease (e.g. inflammatory bowel disease (IBD) or ankylosing spondylitis) can affect sexual function and desire, which could also impact their fertility. Men with IBD, for example, have been shown to have increased rates of hypogonadism, reduced sexual interest, difficulty achieving or maintaining erection, and higher rates of depression compared to age matched controls [21–24]. Additionally, men with ankylosing spondylitis suffer from debilitating arthritis, spinal stiffness, and loss of spinal mobility which has been associated with impaired erectile function, arousal, and sexual satisfaction [25]. Our study demonstrated that the majority of men were not asked about libido or sexual function, which is a common problem that can significantly impact quality of life. Furthermore, while hypogonadism has been associated with increased systemic inflammatory markers and risk of autoimmune conditions in men, restoration of eugonadism has not been demonstrated to our knowledge with control of underlying autoimmune disease [26]. For example, Cutolo et al. demonstrated that use of anti-TNF agents did not change systemic levels of sex androgens in men with rheumatoid arthritis [27].

We found that if men received counseling regarding potential for adverse reproductive effects when taking anti-TNF agents, they were significantly more likely to be screened for anatomic abnormalities (e.g. meatal stenosis, varicocele, small testis volume) and have laboratory tests associated with infertility (e.g. testosterone level, semen analysis) performed. While this is only an association, it suggests that discussion of fertility may prompt further examination and workup to screen for other

**Table 3** Men with pre-initiation counseling are more likely to undergo reproductive assessment and sperm cryopreservation

| Counseling | Received | | Did not receive | | p |
|---|---|---|---|---|---|
| | 104/1010 | (10.3%) | 906/1010 | (89.7%) | < 0.0001 |
| **Components of history and examination** | | | | | |
| GU Exam | 83/104 | (79.8%) | 267/906 | (29.4%) | < 0.0001 |
| Varicocele | 26/104 | (25.0%) | 17/906 | (1.9%) | < 0.0001 |
| Libido/Sexual Function | 46/104 | (44.2%) | 108/906 | (11.9%) | < 0.0001 |
| **Laboratory Assessment** | | | | | |
| Serum Hormone Testing | 29/104 | (27.9%) | 28/906 | (3.1%) | < 0.0001 |
| Semen Analysis | 18/104 | (17.3%) | 26/906 | (2.9%) | < 0.0001 |
| **Sperm Cryopreservation** | 6/104 | (5.7%) | 10/906 | (1.1%) | 0.002 |

104 men received counseling compared to 906 men who did not receive counseling. $p < 0.05$ considered significant

factors that may affect fertility. Lastly, rates of sperm cryopreservation were significantly higher in men who received counseling but were very low overall (< 6%). This suggests that clinicians may not be aware of this option or how best to approach the topic with patients, which has been demonstrated in other patient populations, such as men diagnosed with cancer [28, 29].

This study is limited by its retrospective nature, reliance on documentation by providers, and being a single institution study. Our data suggests that the impact of anti-TNF agents on male fertility is largely unknown as reported by the FDA prescribing information for each agent. Furthermore, it suggests rates of counseling regarding this topic are low. Given our study is from a single center only, we cannot generalize our findings to education received by all men who are started on anti-TNF therapy. Additionally, information available to providers and practice patterns may have changed over the timeline of this study (2006–2017). Until further research delineates the effect of anti-TNF agents on male fertility, we urge clinicians to counsel patients about this lack of evidence and discuss the option of fertility preservation measures, out of an abundance of caution, prior to starting treatment.

## Conclusions

The impact of anti-TNF agents on human male fertility is unclear, with the basic science and clinical literature published to date lacking conclusive evidence on the short and long term reproductive effects of anti-TNF therapy. Despite this lack of clarity, our data suggests that men are not being counseled regarding the potential for adverse reproductive outcomes. Furthermore, rates of sperm cryopreservation and discussion of sexual history in this population were low. A large, prospective study assessing the impact of anti-TNF agents on semen parameters, sexual health, and overall fertility outcomes is needed in order to better identify impacts of therapy, so physicians can more effectively counsel patients.

#### Abbreviations

IBD: Inflammatory bowel disease; FDA: Food and Drug Administration; FSH: Follicle stimulating hormone; LH: Luteinizing hormone; TNF: Tumor necrosis factor; TRAIL: TNF-related-to-apoptosis-inducing ligand

#### Acknowledgements

Not applicable.

#### Authors' contributions

LFC was involved in study conceptual design, data gathering, data analysis and interpretation, and was a major contributor to manuscript writing and editing. JW was involved in study conceptual design, manuscript writing and editing. MKK was involved in data gathering, manuscript writing and editing. IL was involved in data gathering, data analysis, and manuscript editing. NB was involved in study conceptual design, manuscript writing and editing. REB was involved in study conceptual design, data analysis and interpretation, manuscript writing and editing. All authors read and approved the final manuscript.

#### Authors' information

*LFC, Cooley MD PhD, Urology Resident
*JW, Wren MD, Assistant Professor of Urology
*MKK, Keeter MPH, Senior Research Program Coordinator
*IL, Lam BS, Medical Student
*NB, Bennett MD, Associate Professor of Urology
*REB, Brannigan MD, Chief of Male Reproductive Medicine and Men's Health and Professor of Urology

#### Competing interests

The authors declare that they have no competing interests.

#### References

1. Li P, Zheng Y, Chen X. Drugs for autoimmune inflammatory diseases: from small molecule compounds to anti-TNF agents. Front Pharmacol. 2017;8:1–12.
2. Ricciolo A, Starace D, D'Alessio A, Starace G, Padula F, De Cesaris P, et al. TNF-a and IFN-y regulate the expression and function of the Fas system in the seminiferous epithelium. J Immunol. 2000;165:743–9.
3. Li MW, Xia W, Mruk DD, Wang CQ, Yan HH, Siu MK, et al. Tumor necrosis factor (alpha) reversibly disrupts the blood testis barrier and impairs Sertoli-germ cell adhesion in the seminiferous epithelium of adult rat testes. J Endocrinol. 2006;190:313–29.
4. Loveland KL, Klein B, Puescl D, Indumathy S, Bergmann M, Loveland BE, et al. Cytokines in male fertility and reproductive pathologies: immunoregulation and beyond. Front Endocrinol. 2017;8:1–16.
5. Suominen JS, Yanyan W, Kaipia A, Toppari J. Tumor necrosis factor-alpha (TNF-a) promotes cell survival during spermatogenesis, and this effect can be blocked by infliximab, a TNF-a antagonist. Eur J Endocrinol. 2004;151: 629–40.
6. Lin Y, Richburg JH. Characterization of the role of tumor necrosis factor apoptosis inducing ligand (TRAIL) in spermatogenesis through the evaluation of Trail gene-deficient mice. PLoS One. 2014;9:e93926.
7. O'Bryan MK, Hedger MP. Inflammatory networks in the control of spermatogenesis: chronic inflammation in an immunologically privileged tissue? Adv Exp Med Biol. 2008;636:92–114.
8. Villiger PM, Caliezi G, Cottin V, Forger F, Senn A, Ostensen M. Effects of TNF antagonists on sperm characteristics in patients with spondyloarthritis. Ann Rheum Dis. 2010;69:1842–4.
9. Micu MC, Micu R, Surd S, Girlovanu M, Bolboaca SD, Ostensen M. TNF-α inhibitors do not impair sperm quality in males with ankylosing spondylitis after short-term or long-term treatment. Rheumatology. 2014;53:1250–5.
10. Montagna GL, Malesci D, Buono R, Valentini G. Asthenoazoospermia in patients receiving anti-tumour necrosis factor (alpha) agents. Ann Rheum Dis. 2005;64:1667.
11. Mahadevan U, Terdiman JP, Aron J, Jacobsohn S, Turek P. Infliximab and semen quality in men with inflammatory bowel disease. Inflamm Bowel Dis. 2005;11:395–9.
12. Serghini M, Fekih M, Karoui S, Ben Mustapha N, Kallel L, Matri S, et al. Fertility and inflammatory bowel diseases. Tunis Med. 2010;88:623–8.
13. Mahadevan U. Fertility and pregnancy in the patient with inflammatory bowel disease. Gut. 2006;55:1198–206.
14. Wildi LM, Haraoui B. Reversible male infertility under treatment with an anti-TNFa agent: a case report. Ann Rheum Dis. 2012;71:473–4.
15. Semet M, Paci M, Saias-Magnan J, Metzler-Guillermian C, Boissier R, Lejeune H, et al. The impact of drugs on male fertility: a review. Andrology. 2017;5: 640–63.
16. FDA highlights of prescribing information: Humira. Revised 2011. [Internet. Accessed November 1, 2018.] Available from: https://www.accessdata.fda.gov/drugsatfda_docs/label/2011/125057s0276lbl.pdf.
17. FDA highlights of prescribing information: Remicade. Revised 2013. [Internet. Accessed November 1, 2018.] Available from: https://www.accessdata.fda.gov/drugsatfda_docs/label/2013/103772s5359lbl.pdf.
18. FDA highlights of prescribing information: Enbrel. Revised 2012. [Internet. Accessed November 1, 2018.] Available from: https://www.accessdata.fda.gov/drugsatfda_docs/label/2012/103795s5503lbl.pdf

19. FDA highlights of prescribing information: Simponi. Revised 2011. [Internet. Accessed November 1, 2018.] Available from: https://www.accessdata.fda.gov/drugsatfda_docs/label/2011/125289s0064lbl.pdf.
20. FDA highlights of prescribing information: Cimzia. Revised 2017. [Internet. Accessed November 1, 2018.] Available from: https://www.accessdata.fda.gov/drugsatfda_docs/label/2017/125160s270lbl.pdf.
21. Blotiere PO, Rudant J, Barre A, Racine A, Weill A, Peyrin-Biroulet L, et al. Conditions of prescription of anti-TNF agents in newly treated patients with inflammatory bowel disease in France (2011-2013). Dig Liver Dis. 2016;48: 620–5.
22. Curtis JR, Singh JA. The use of biologics in rheumatoid arthritis: current and emerging paradigms of care. Clin Ther. 2011;33:679–707.
23. Knowles SR, Gass C, Macrae F. Illness perceptions in IBD influence psychological status, sexual heath and satisfaction, body image, and relational functioning: a preliminary exploration using structural equation modeling. J Chrons Colitis. 2013;7:e344–50.
24. Timmer A, Bauer A, Kemptner D, Furst A, Rogler G. Determinants of male sexual function in inflammatory bowel disease: a survey-based cross sectional analysis in 280 men. Inflamm Bowel Dis. 2007;13:1236–43.
25. Liu Y, Dong H, Chen Z, Wang Y, Tu SH. Impact of ankylosing spondylitis on sexual function: a systemic review and meta analysis. Exp Ther Med. 2015;9: 1501–7.
26. Baillargeon J, Snih SA, Raji MA, Urban RJ, Sharma G, Sheffield-Moore M, et al. Hypogonadism and the risk of rheumatic autoimmune disease. Clinc Rheumatol. 2016;35(12):2983–7.
27. Cutolo M, Sulli A, Capellino S, Villaggio B, Montanga P, Pizzorni C, et al. Anti-TNF and sex hormones. Ann N Y Acad Sci. 2006;1069:391–400.
28. Osterberg S, Ramasamy R, Masson P, Brannigan RE. Current practices in fertility preservation in male cancer patients. Urol Ann. 2014;6:13–7.
29. Vindrola-Padros C, Dyer K, Cyrus J, Lubker IM. Healthcare professionals' views on discussing fertility preservation with young cancer patients: a mixed method systemic review of the literature. Psychooncology. 2017;26: 4–14.

# 14

# A case report of primary upper urinary tract signet-ring cell carcinoma and literature review

Zhaohua Ye, Qiwu Mi*, Daosheng Luo, Zhixiong Li and Jiexin Luo

**Abstract**

**Background:** Upper tract urothelial carcinoma with pure non-urothelial histology is an exception but variants are present in ~ 25% of cases. Primary upper urinary tract signet -ring cell carcinoma is extremely rare.

**Case presentation:** We report the case of a 65-year-old male diagnosed primary upper urinary tract signet-ring cell carcinoma while underwent percutaneous nephrolithotomy. Radical nephroureterectomy and adjuvant chemotherapy were performed sequentially. The patient is now recovering well with a regular follow-up for more than 1 year.

**Conclusions:** The upper urinary tract malignancy often appears as a high grade, high stage tumor and has a uniformly poor prognosis, but a timely multimodal management can bring a good outcome.

**Keywords:** primary upper urinary tract signet ring cell carcinoma, calculi, percutaneous nephrolithotomy, radical nephroureterectomy

## Background

Upper tract urothelial carcinoma (UTUC) with pure non-urothelial histology is an exception but variants are present in ~25% of cases [1, 2], including squamous cell carcinoma and adenocarcinoma. Among the cases mentioned above, upper urinary tract signet ring cell carcinoma (SRCC) is rare [3, 4]. The upper urinary tract malignancy often appears as a high grade, high stage tumor and has a uniformly poor prognosis [5]. Radical nephroureterectomy (RNU) with bladder cuff removal has been the standard treatment for UTUC [6]. But there is no standard perioperative therapeutic strategy exists for upper urinary tract SRCC because of their rarity.

## Case presentation

A 65-year-old male presented to our hospital with a 30 years history of right flank pain. His pain is a mild and intermittent dull pain, without radiation pain, gross hematuria, fever, urinary frequency or urgency and dysuria. The physical examination was unremarkable. Laboratory examinations showed Serum creatinine was 167umol/L (normal range 57-111umol/L), CEA, CA-199, and CA72-4 were normal. Abdominal CT demonstrated significant dilatation of the right renal pelvis and the right upper and mid-ureter with multiple calculi. The walls of the renal pelvis and the upper and mid-ureter were thickened with hyperdense soft tissue lesion. (Figure 1)

After three negative urinary cytology examinations, the patient underwent ureteroscopic examination, which showed middle ureteral wall was rough and stenosis with soft tissue mass, but biopsy specimens from this area were non-diagnostic. We tried to insert a double J stent to provide drainage but it failed. Then we recommended a right-sided radical nephroureterectomy but the families refused. They strongly required to the treatment of urinary calculi only. Then a right-side percutaneous nephrolithotomy (PCNL) was performed. Renal access was achieved using B-US guidance with 22-Fr Amplatz sheath. A large amount of white gelatinous material were found in the renal pelvis and taken out for histopathology examination. The calculi were either removed intact or fragmented using a pneumatic lithoclast. A 20-Fr Foley catheter was kept as a nephrostomy tube and

* Correspondence: mqw175@163.com
Department of Urology, Dongguan People's Hospital, Dongguan 523000, China

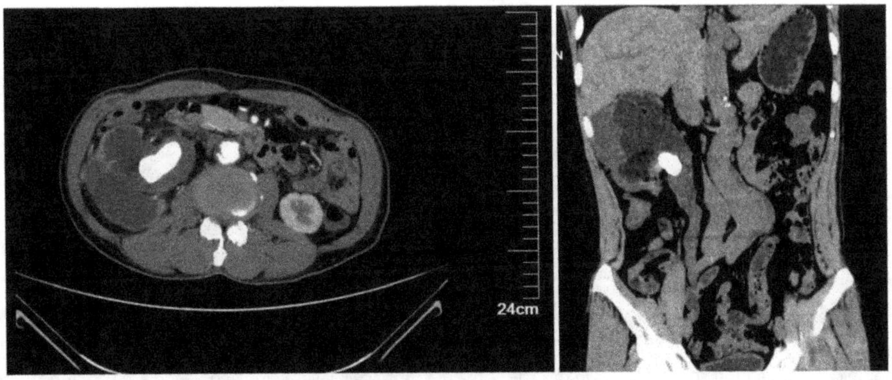


**Fig. 1** Abdominal CT demonstrated significant dilatation of the right renal pelvis and the right upper ureter with multiple calculi. The walls of the renal pelvis and the upper and mid-ureter were thickened with hyperdense soft tissue lesion

the catheter balloon was injected with 10ml saline and pulled to compress the nephrostomy tract (Figure 2). The histopathological examination showed the tumor cells containing intracellular mucin-filled vacuole displacing the hyperchromatic nucleus to one side suggestive of signet ring cell carcinoma (Figure 3). Immunohistochemical examination showed: CK, CK7, CK20, CEA, CDX2 (+), Villin (small +), Vim, GATA3, P53 (-), Ki-67 (about 60% +).Post-operative PET/CT (18F-FDG8.6mCi as the tracer) showed there was no evidence of further primary malignancy or metastases. Therefore, we considered the tumor as primary upper urinary tract signet ring cell carcinoma. A right-sided RNU with bladder cuff and nephrostomy tract sinus removal were performed subsequently (Figure 4). Histopathology examination found signet-ring cell invaded the renal pelvis, upper ureter and the surrounding adipose tissue through the muscle, the focal nerve and vessels were also involved. Part of the renal pelvis epithelium was presented with obvious intestinal metaplasia and atypical hyperplasia, suggesting the tumor originated from the kidney. Six weeks after the surgery, he received 3 cycles chemotherapy (Gemcitabine 1000mg/m2 on days 1 and 8, every 21 days) as adjuvant therapy. 16 months postoperatively, clinical examinations and CT scans showed normal results without metastasis or localized recurrence.

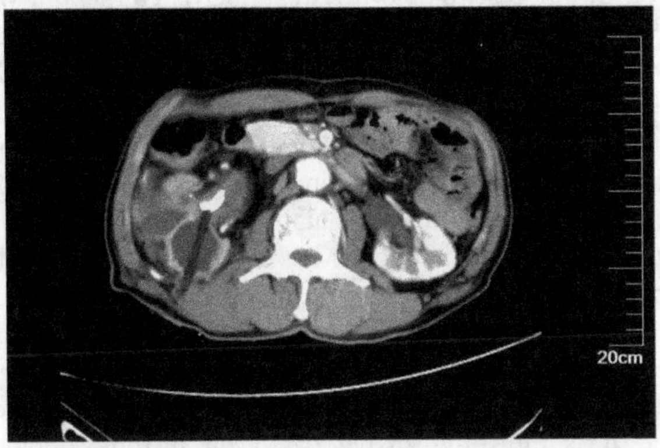


**Fig. 2** A 20-Fr Foley catheter was kept as a nephrostomy tube and the catheter balloon was pulled to compress the nephrostomy tract

## Discussion and conclusion

Urothelial carcinomas (UCs) are the fifth most common tumors [7], with the UTUC accounting for only 5-10% [8, 9]. Approximately 60% of UTUC are invasive at the time ofdiagnosis. The peak incidence of upper tract urothelial carcinoma occurs in the age from 70 to 90 years old, and the ratio of male to female is about 3:1 [10, 11]. Cases of histologically non-urothelial carcinoma are rare. Among these special cases, squamous cell carcinoma is most frequently reported, and there are variants such as micropapillary carcinoma, sarcomatoid carcinoma, SRCC, etc. Primary SRCC of the urinary tract is a relatively rare. Since primary SRCC of urinary bladder was first described by Saphir in 1955 [12], over 300 cases of urinary tract SRCC have been reported in the English literature, but the report about primary upper urinary tract SRCC is extremely rare. The first example of this variant had been documented by Ekfors and Nurmi in 1988 [13] and there are less than 10 cases so far. SRCC is most commonly found in the gastrointestinal tract. The pathogenesis of SRCC in the urothelium is not yet clear. Referring to the SRCC of urinary bladder, the current hypothesis holds that the signet-ring cell arising from the glandular metaplasia is caused by chronic inflammation or secondary to the stone stimulation [14–17] or from the totipotential urothelium by direct transition [18–20]. More scholars now support the first hypothesis. For this patient, a history of chronic stone stimulation did exist. Hematuria and flank pain could be the most common symptom at presentation, while a palpable abdominal mass indicates a late stage of the disease. However, it is difficult to distinguish stone

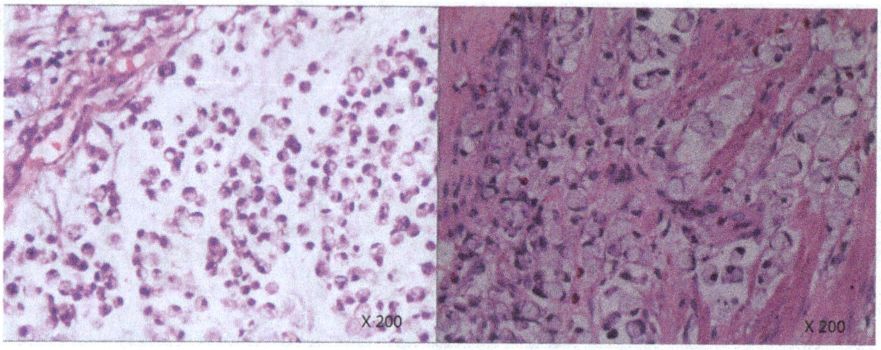


**Fig. 3** The histopathological examination showed the tumor cells containing intracellular mucin-filled vacuole displacing the hyperchromatic nucleus to one side suggestive of signet ring cell carcinoma

from tumors only by symptoms and physical examination. Moreover, patients may be asymptomatic [21]. Although hematological oncology examinations are negative in most cases, including our case, abnormality could still be detected from CT scan. Fojecki G et al. concluded that CTU including corticomedullary phase (CMP) is the preferred imaging modality in the diagnostic workup of UTUC [22]. Histopathology is the golden standard for diagnosing UTUC, but there is no consensus which biopsy method is the best to achieve representative samples [23]. Urinary cytology and URS biopsy were negative neither for this patient. Two studies including 762 UTUC patients reported that the percentage of abnormal urothelial cells from preoperative cytology were found in the urine was only about 39% [24, 25]. Ureteroscopy is used to visualise the upper urinary tract and biopsy suspicious lesions. Flexible ureteroscopy is more useful with novel digital technology and biopsy device. However, Margolin et al. [26] obtained that the likelihood of missing invasion on URS biopsy was significantly increased when the diameter of biopsy fragments was smaller than 1 mm. That might be the reason for the false negative diagnosis of this case. This patient was finally diagnosed with upper urinary tract malignancy through PCNL. We had informed the risk and possible complications of PCNL, but the patient's families insisted on kidney-sparing surgery. Admittedly, PCNL is not the most appropriate treatment for this patient, but we had taken the following strategies to avoid the spread of the tumor. Tract dilation was performed in a one-step method rather than a step-by-step method. The pressure and the flow rate of the irrigation fluid were under strict control. The total intraoperative time was 30 mins and the Foley catheter was used as a nephrostomy tube while the balloon was pulled tightly to compress the nephrostomy tract. The histopathological analysis of the specimens from renal pelvis revealed signet-ring cell components. Thus, a secondary SRCC or a rare variant of primary upper urinary tract SRCC was suspected. It is reported that histopathology is one of the method of identification. Stearns et al. described a case of a metastatic, undifferentiated gastric carcinoma, and stated that it grew mainly in adventitial or periureteral tissue without mucosal involvement [27]. Hes O et al. observed that metastatic cell usually grow in a dissociated manner [28]. In our case, part of the renal pelvis epithelium was presented with obvious intestinal metaplasia and atypical hyperplasia, suggesting the tumor originated from the kidney. Whether immunohistochemical analysis can be useful is still controversial. Singh J et al. described that immunohistochemical staining using CK7 and CK20 could also be helpful in evaluating the cancer's primary origin [29] while Lendorf ME et al. observed that the immunoprofiles of primary urinary SRCC and SRCC arising from the gastrointestinal tract are overlap, including CK7, CK20, CEA, epithelial membrane antigen, CDX2, villin and E-cadherin [30]. Suh N et al. believed that it is indistinguishable based on histomorphology and immunohistochemistry [31]. Thus, upper gastrointestinal endoscopy and colonoscopy should be

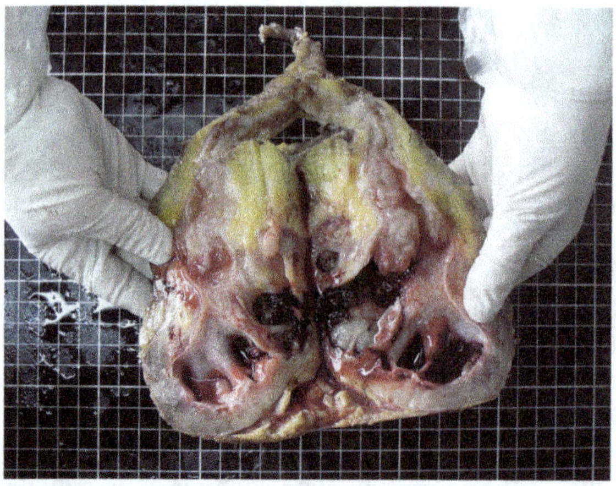

**Fig. 4** A right-sided radical nephroureterectomy with bladder cuff and nephrostomy tract sinus removal were performed

performed to rule out any eventual primary site. Since the patient refused invasive examination, a PET/CT was performed instead and it showed no evidence of further primary malignancy. Dong MJ et al. reported a case of the false negative $^{18}$F-FDG PET images of gastric SRCC with right adnexa metastasis. They observed that false negative $^{18}$F-FDG PET in malignant tumor may be correlated with the pathologic type, differentiation degree and the lesion size [32]. However, there is no case of symptoms of metastatic urinary tract SRCC appearing earlier than those of primary tumors and there is only one case of melanoma where symptoms of ureteral metastasis preceded the recognition of the primary neoplasm [33]. As we are writing, more than one year has passed since the diagnosis, and the patient is well without recurrence or metastasis. Although the follow-up time is not very long, in our opinion an occult primary tumor is unlikely. The RNU with bladder cuff and nephrostomy tract sinus removal and postoperative adjuvant chemotherapy (AC) was performed subsequently. Perioperative administration of chemotherapeutic agents has been explored for a long time. A phase 3 RCT from multi-institutional collaboration in the UK (POUT study), revealed that AC significantly improves disease-free survival and metastasis-free survival compared to surveillance and chemotherapy given at relapse in patients with UTUC [34]. Cobo-Dols M et al. [35] and El Ammari JE et al. [36] had respectively reported a success case of primary SRCC of bladder treated with radical cystectomy followed by systemic AC with cisplatin and gemcitabine. Considering there is no standard AC strategy for upper urinary tract SRCC, we referenced the chemotherapy for SRCC of urinary bladder. Meanwhile, the loss of renal function limited the use of platinum-based drugs, leading us to the administration of gemcitabine alone. According to the follow-up for more than one year after surgery, the prognosis of the patient is favorable. According to the TNM classification 2017 for urothelial carcinoma of the upper urinary tract, the pT3 category renal pelvis tumors are defined as the primary tumor invades beyond muscularis into peripelvic fat or renal parenchyma. Although there is no grading classification for upper urinary tract SRCC, it should be treated as high-grade disease. Thus, a long-term follow-up is still needed for this patient.

Patients with a long history of urinary calculi must be recognized the possibility of urinary tumors and regular workup should be done in order to diagnose the tumor in its early stage. Radiologic findings have a certain effect but non-specific. CTU including CMP is recommended. Histopathological examination is still the golden standard in the diagnosis of tumor occurs. Upper urinary tract SRCC is a rare tumor with a very poor prognosis that requires multimodal management. To plan the optimal therapeutic strategy, it is necessary to rule out a primary malignance outside the urinary tract. Treatment should be performed expeditiously given the aggressive nature of this disease and should include a combination of radical surgery and adjuvant chemotherapy. Prognosis is best predicted by pathologic grade and stage. Continued research is necessary to reveal the severity of this disease and standardize the diagnostic work-up and therapeutic strategy of upper urinary tract SRCC.

**Abbreviations**

SRCC: Signet ring cell carcinoma; PCNL: Percutaneous nephrolithotomy; UTUC: Upper tract urothelial carcinoma; UCs: Urothelial carcinomas; RNU: Radical nephroureterectomy; CTU: Computed tomography urography; AC: Adjuvant chemotherapy

**Acknowledgements**

Zhaohua Ye would like to thank Miss Li Jiaying for her valuable comments.

**Authors' contributions**

YZ collected the patient data, analyzed and interpreted the data and wrote the first draft. LZ assisted in data collection and interpretation. MQ, LD and LJ reviewed the manuscript and were involved in its critical revision before submission. All authors read and approved the final manuscript.

**Competing interests**

None of the authors has any conflict of interest to disclose.

**References**

1. Rink M, Robinson BD, Green DA, et al. Impact of histological variants on clinical outcomes of patients with upper urinary tract urothelial carcinoma. J Urol. 2012;188(2):398–404. https://doi.org/10.1016/j.juro.2012.04.009.
2. Masson-Lecomte A, Colin P, Bozzini G, et al. Impact of micropapillary histological variant on survival after radical nephroureterectomy for upper tract urothelial carcinoma. World J Urol. 2014;32(2):531–7. https://doi.org/10.1007/s00345-013-1141-0.
3. Olgac S, Mazumdar M, Dalbagni G. Urothelial carcinoma of the renal pelvis: a clinicopathologic study of 130 cases. Am J Surg Pathol. 2004;28(12):1545–52.
4. Perez-Montiel D, Wakely PE, Hes O, et al. High-grade urothelial carcinoma of the renal pelvis: clinicopathologic study of 108 cases with emphasis on unusual morphologic variants. Mod Pathol. 2006;19:494–503. https://doi.org/10.1038/modpathol.3800559.
5. Delahunt B, Nacey JN, Meffan PJ. Signet ring cell adenocarcinoma of the ureter [J]. Brit J Urol. 1991;68(5):555–6.
6. Rouprет M, Babjuk M, Comperat E, et al. European association of urology guidelines on upper urinary tract urothelial carcinoma: 2017 update. Eur Urol. 2018;73(1):111–22.
7. Siggel RL, Miller KD. Cancer statitics, 2016. CA Cancer J Clin. 2016;66:7–30.
8. Siggel RL, Miller KD. Cancer statitics, 2015. CA Cancer J Clin. 2015;65:5–29.
9. Munoz JJ, et al. Upper tract urothelial neoplasms: incidence and survival during the last 2 decades. J Urol. 2000;164:1523.
10. Shariat SF, et al. Gender differences in radical nephroureterectomy for upper tract urothelial carcinoma. World J Urol. 2011;29:481.
11. Lughezzani G, Sun M, Perrotte P, et al. Gender-related differences in patients with stage I to III upper tract urothelial carcinoma: results from the surveillance, epidemiology, and end results database. Urology. 2010;75:321–7. https://doi.org/10.1016/j.urology.2009.09.048.
12. Grignon DJ, Ro JY, Ayala AG, Johnson DE. Signet-ring cell carcinoma of the urinary bladder. Am J Pathol. 1955;31:223–31.
13. Ekfors TO. Primary signet-ring cell carcinoma of the ureter. A case report. APMIS. 1988;96:471–4.
14. Brawer MK, Waisman J. Papillary adenocarcinoma of ureter. Urology. 1982;19:205–9.

15. Nocks BN, Heney NM, Daly JJ. Primary adenocarcinoma of the urinary bladder. Urology. 1983;21:26–9.
16. Thomas DG, Ward AM, Williams JL. A study of 52 cases of adenocarcinoma of the bladder. Br J Urol. 1971;43:4–15.
17. Ward AM. Glandular neoplasia within the urinary tract. The aetiology of adenocarcinoma of the urothelium with a review of the literature. I. Introduction: the origin of glandular epithelium in the renal pelvis, ureter and bladder. Virchows Arch A Pathol Pathol Anat. 1971;352:296–311.
18. Braun EV, Majid A, Fayemi A, Beaugard E. Primary signet-ring cell carcinoma of the urinary bladder: Review of the literature and report of a case. Cancer. 1981;47:1430–5.
19. Choi H, Lamb S, Pintar K, Jacobs SC. Primary signet-ring cell carcinoma of the urinary bladder. Cancer. 1984;53:1985–90.
20. DeTure FA, Dein R, Hackett RL, Drylie DM. Primary signet-ring cell carcinoma of bladder exemplifying vesical epithelial multipotentiality. Urology. 1975;6: 240–4.
21. Abbas M, Kramer MW, Spieker T, Herrman TR, Merseburger AS, Müller KM, Kuczyk MA, Becker JU, Kreipe HH. Primary mucinous adenocarcinoma of the renal pelvis with carcinoma in situ in the ureter. J Egypt Natl Canc Inst. 2014;26:51–4.
22. Fojecki G, Magnusson A, Traxer O, et al. Consultation on UTUC, Stockholm 2018 aspects of diagnosis of upper tract urothelial carcinoma. World J Urol. 2019;37:2271–8. https://doi.org/10.1007/s00345-019-02732-8.
23. Skolarikos A, et al. Cytologic analysis of ureteral washings is informative in patients with grade 2 upper tract TCC considering endoscopic treatment. Urology. 2003;61(6):1146–50.
24. Kobayashi Y, Saika T, Miyaji Y, et al. Preoperative positive urine cytology is a risk factor for subsequent development of bladder cancer after nephroureterectomy in patients with upper urinary tract urothelial carcinoma. World J Urol. 2012;30:271–5. https://doi.org/10.1007/s00345-011-0731-y.
25. Tanaka N, Kikuchi E, Kanao K, et al. The predictive value of positive urine cytology for outcomes following radical nephroureterectomy in patients with primary upper tract urothelial carcinoma: a multi-institutional study. Urol Oncol. 2014;32:48.e19–26. https://doi.org/10.1016/j.urolonc.2013.07.003.
26. Margolin EJ, Matulay JT, Li G, et al. Discordance between Ureteroscopic biopsy and final pathology for upper tract Urothelial carcinoma. J Urol. 2018;199:1440–5. https://doi.org/10.1016/j.juro.2018.02.002.
27. STEARNS DB, FARMER DA. Ureteral metastasis secondary to gastric carcinoma: case report. J Urol. 1958;80:214–7.
28. Hes O, Curík R, Mainer K. Urothelial signet-ring cell carcinoma of the renal pelvis with collagenous spherulosis: a case report. Int J Surg Pathol. 2005;13: 375–8.
29. Singh J, Zherebitskiy V, Grynspan D, et al. Metastatic signet ring cell adenocarcinoma of the bladder. Can Urol Assoc J. 2013;6:E15–9.
30. Lendorf ME,Dohn LH,Á Dunga B,et al. An updated review on primary signet-ring cell carcinoma of the urinary bladder and report of a case. Scand J Urol 2018;52:87–93.DOI:https://doi.org/10.1080/21681805.2017.1418020.
31. Suh N, Yang XJ, Tretiakova MS, Humphrey PA, Wang HL. Value of CDX2, villin, and alpha-methylacyl coenzyme a racemase immunostains in the distinction between primary adenocarcinoma of the bladder and secondary colorectal adenocarcinoma. Mod Pathol. 2005;18:1217–22.
32. Dong MJ, Lin XT, Zhao J, et al. Malignant tumor with false negative 18F-FDG PET image. Zhonghua Zhong Liu Za Zhi. 2006;28:713–7.
33. JUDD RL. Melanoma of the ureter: a case report. J Urol. 1962;87:805–7.
34. Birtle AJ, Chester JD, Jones RJ, et al. Results of POUT: A phase III randomised trial of perioperative chemotherapy versus surveillance in upper tract urothelial cancer (UTUC). J Clin Oncol. 2018;36(6_suppl):407.
35. Cobo-Dols M, Alcaide J, Gutiérrez V, et al. Primary signet-ring cell adenocarcinoma of the urinary bladder: a case report. Oncología (Barc). 2006;29:177–80.
36. El Ammari JE, Ahsaini M, Riyach O, et al. Primary signet-ring cell carcinoma of the urinary bladder successfully managed with cisplatin and gemcitabine: a case report. J Med Case Rep. 2013;7:37. https://doi.org/10.1186/1752-1947-7-37.

# 15

# Anatomical and functional outcomes after hysterectomy and bilateral sacrospinous ligament fixation for stage IV uterovaginal prolapse

Tilemachos Kavvadias[1,2*], Birgitt Schoenfisch[1], Sara Yvonne Brucker[1] and Christl Reisenauer[1]

## Abstract

**Background:** Aim of this study is to examine pelvic floor symptoms, anatomical results and patients' satisfaction after sacrospinous vaginal fixation for stage 4 pelvic organ prolapse.

**Methods:** All patients with stage 4 pelvic organ prolapse were treated with vaginal hysterectomy, native tissue cystocele and rectocele repair and bilateral sacrospinous vaginal fixation. Anatomical and functional outcomes according to the POPq classification system and the German version of the Australian pelvic floor questionnaire were assessed. Changes between baseline, first follow-up and second follow-up were assessed by the paired Wilcoxon rank test using R, version 3.5.1.

**Results:** 20 patients were included in the study. Scores in all four domains of the pelvic floor symptom questionnaire (bladder, bowel, prolapse, sexual function) were significantly improved at 6 and 12-months follow-up. One patient presented with a symptomatic stage 3 cystocele that needed a second surgical intervention and two patients needed surgery due to a de novo stress urinary incontinence. There were no perioperative adverse events and all patients reported full satisfaction after surgery.

**Conclusions:** The vaginal approach with hysterectomy, native tissue repair and bilateral sacrospinous vaginal fixation seems to be a safe and effective method for the treatment of advanced stage POP, offering excellent relief in all pelvic floor symptoms.

**Keywords:** Native tissue repair; Pelvic organ prolapse; Bilateral sacrospinous ligament fixation

* Correspondence: tilemachos.kavvadias@usb.ch
[1]Department of Obstetrics and Gynecology, University Hospital Tübingen, Calwerstrasse 7, 72076 Tübingen, Germany
[2]Department of Gynecology and Obstetrics, University Hospital Basel, Spitalstrasse 21, 4031 Basel, Switzerland

## Background

Pelvic organ prolapse (POP) is defined as a 'downward displacement' of the uterus and /or the vaginal compartments and their neighbouring organs such as bladder, rectum and bowel, causing bothersome symptoms and affecting a woman's quality of life [1]. It has been reported that in a general population 40% of women aged between 45 and 85 years have an objective POP on examination, but only 12% of these women are symptomatic [2]. Conservative treatment with a pessary is often considered as first line therapy, with surgery reserved for patients who decline or fail management of POP with a pessary. While the choice of procedure depends on severity of POP, patients' goals and surgeons' expertise, vaginal native tissue repair without using synthetic mesh or graft materials is considered as appropriate surgical treatment option for most women with primary POP [3, 4]. Furthermore, it is very common that surgical treatments for anterior, posterior and apical pelvic floor support loss are combined, in order to achieve optimal results [4, 5].

Apical support is of great importance for the stability of the pelvic floor. There is a growing understanding that adequate vaginal apex support is essential for a durable surgical repair in women with advanced prolapse [6]. Moreover, surgical correction of the anterior and posterior wall may fail unless the apex is adequately supported [7]. Vaginal sacrospinous ligament fixation (SSLF) is one of the most common procedures performed for the restoration of apical support loss and is considered effective and safe. It shows a subjective success rate of 84–99% and an objective success rate of 67–93% [8]. SSLF can be performed unilaterally or bilaterally and it has the advantage that no synthetic material or graft is needed. The bilateral approach however has been criticized for insufficient midline support, leaving the central part of the apex without support and vulnerable to intra-pelvic pressure on the genital hiatus, although this is more of an objective outcome and may not affect subjective outcomes [8]. Furthermore, additional midline support may be provided by concomitant anterior and posterior repair, but the existing evidence is sparse, mainly observational, and retrospective. It is only limited to anatomical results and only few of the included patient in previous studies on the efficacy of SSLF had advanced POP (stage IV) [6].

The aim of this pilot study is to prospectively evaluate the efficacy of vaginal bilateral sacrospinous ligament fixation for POPQ stage IV and to examine the impact on patients' symptoms at six and twelve months follow-up after surgery.

## Methods

The study protocol was approved by the Ethics Committee at the University Hospital of Tübingen (Ethikkommission Universitätskliikum Tübingen) (ref. number: 130/2017BO2) and was registered with ClinicalTrials.gov (NCT 02998216).

This prospective interventional pilot, single centre, non-randomized study was conducted at the Department of Obstetrics and Gynecology Tübingen in the period from March 2017 to March 2018. All women suffering from symptomatic uterovaginal POP stage IV (Fig. 1), according to the Pelvic Organ Prolapse Quantification (POP-Q) system [1], were included in the study.

Exclusion criteria were previous POP or incontinence surgeries, age < 18 and > 75 years, participation in other clinical trials, active malignant disease and inability to understand the purpose of the study and sign the informed consent. The exclusion of women over 75 was made on the basis of recruiting a homogenous group of women who would profit from the procedure and would not require or prefer an obliterative procedure for the correction of their prolapse. We also had to provide an upper cut-off age in our inclusion criteria for anesthesiological reasons, to avoid including fragile and multimorbid patients.

The primary outcome measure was the improvement of the pelvic floor symptoms and the secondary outcome measure was the anatomical correction of prolapse.

Pelvic floor symptoms were assessed using the self-administered, validated German version of the Australian female pelvic floor questionnaire. Questions are grouped according to the physiological functions of the pelvic floor, i.e. bladder function, bowel function,

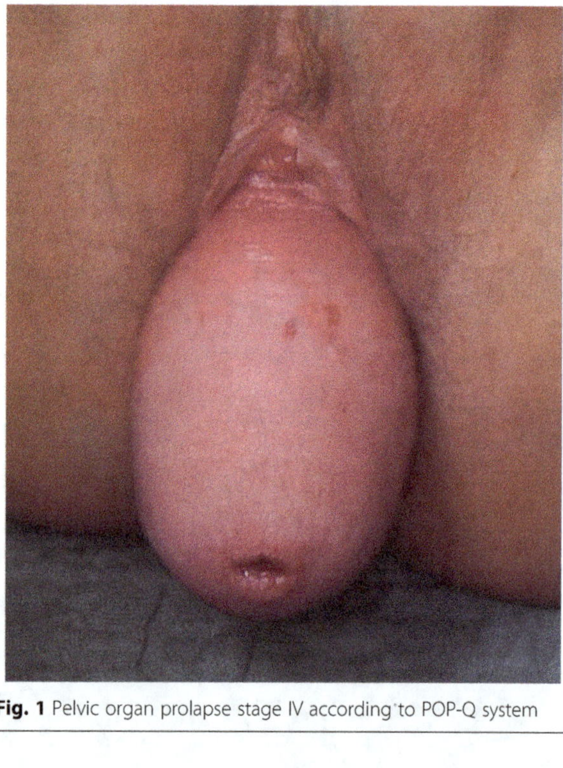

**Fig. 1** Pelvic organ prolapse stage IV according to POP-Q system

prolapse symptoms, and sexual function domains. The scores are then calculated on a 0 to 10 scale on each domain, ranging from less to most severe and giving a potential final overall score of maximum 40 [9, 10]. Patients were asked to answer the female pelvic floor questionnaire before, as well as 6 and 12 months after surgery. Additionally, a complete staging using the POP-Q system was performed using a standard measurement tape and patients' health condition was measured on 5-point Likert scales (1 = much worse, 5 = much better). The POP-Q quantification was not performed by the surgeon, in order to avoid bias. Epidemiological data, such as age, parity, comorbidities and medication, as well as duration of surgery, intra- and postoperative complications were recorded.

### Surgical intervention

All patients had a vaginal hysterectomy, anterior and posterior vaginal wall repair and bilateral sacrospinous ligament fixation of the vaginal cuff. No concomitant incontinence surgery was performed. Vaginal hysterectomy was done in a standard manner. The peritoneal closure was followed by anterior colporrhaphy. After a posterior midline colpotomy a blunt dissection of the pararectal space on both sides was performed. After visualisation of the sacrospinous ligament (SSL) and palpation of the ischial spine, two PDS 0 (Ethicon, LLC) absorbable sutures were placed in the middle third of the SSL, between the sacrum and the ischial spine on each side, without the use of a suture placing device (Fig. 2a). We used three Breisky retractors (at 12, 4 and 8 o'clock axis) to visualise the area and the neddle was passed through the ligament under sight using a long needle holder. No additional lightning was used. Then, the sutures were passed through the full thickness of the vaginal fornices. The vaginal cuff was closed transversely to avoid narrowing the upper vagina and compressing the rectum (Fig. 2b). After a levator ani myorrhaphy was performed, the 4 sutures were tied over the vaginal mucosa so that the vaginal cuff is in contact with the right and left SSL. This was followed by the perineorraphy as last step. All surgeries were performed by the same experienced gynaecologist (CR).

### Statistical analysis

Approximately normally distributed variables were characterized by mean ± standard deviation whereas for other continuous variables median and [minimum to maximum] were given. For the decision on normality, a Shapiro-Wilk test was used. Categorical data were described by numbers and percentages. The changes in POP-Q stages and pelvic floor questionnaire scores between baseline, first follow-up and second follow-up were assessed by the paired Wilcoxon rank test as these variables were considered ordinal respectively were not normally distributed. A significance level of 5% was chosen. All statistical analyses were done using R, version 3.5.1 (R Foundation for Statistical Computing, Vienna, Austria).

## Results

Between March 2016 and March 2017, 21 women with POP stage IV were screened and one was excluded because of other health issues. Twenty women with uterovaginal POP stage IV were included in the study. All of them had a vaginal hysterectomy, an anterior and posterior colporrhaphy and a bilateral SSLF between March 2016 and March 2017. At the time of the surgery, the patients were 68.0 ± 6.3 years old. Their mean body mass index (BMI) ranged from 17.7 kg/m$^2$ to 34.3 kg/m$^2$ with a mean of 24.6 ± 4.3 kg/m$^2$.

Fourteen out of 20 women had up to two vaginal deliveries, five women had three and one patient had four deliveries. Only one patient smoked, while three women suffered from diabetes mellitus and another one suffered from asthma bronchiale. Median operating time was 114 [90 to 240] minutes, median blood loss was 100 [50 to 150] ml. The postoperative course was uneventful for all patients, and no patient reported excessive buttock pain after surgery. No one required suture removal,

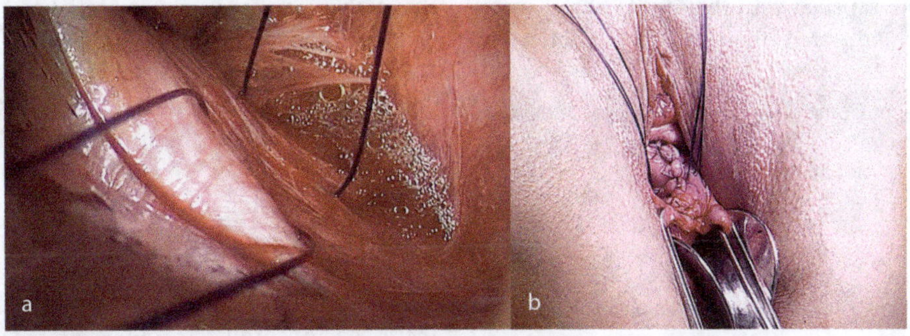

**Fig. 2** Sacrospinous ligament fixation technique: (**a**) - two PDS 0 (Ethicon, LLC) absorbable sutures were placed in the middle third of the sacrospinous ligament, (**b**) - the sutures passes through the full thickness of the vaginal fornices, the vaginal cuff was closed transversely

while all of them took a course of diclofenac in standard dosage for 5–7 days. No serious adverse events were reported for the duration of the study. Two patients asked for a treatment before the first study follow-up because of an exacerbation of their stress urinary incontinence and received a retropubic tension-free vaginal tape (TVT). The first six-month follow-up was performed after a median of 182.4 [157 to 272] days, the second twelve-month follow-up took place after a median of 366 [342 to 456] days.

Table 1 shows the anatomical outcomes. According to the POP-Q system, the POP stage was significantly improved at six and twelve months after surgery when compared to baseline ($p < 0.001$). All women were asymptomatic at both follow-up visits after surgery and had either a stage 0 or stage I POP, with exception of one woman. The latter presented at the first follow-up visit with a stage III symptomatic cystocele and received an anterior vaginal repair using an anterior mesh.

Total vaginal length was significantly shorter at first and second follow-up when compared to baseline (median 9 cm vs 7 cm, $p = 0.008$, vs 8 cm, $p = 0.005$). Likewise, the genital hiatus was shorter (median 5 cm vs 2 cm, $p = 0.001$, vs 2 cm, $p < 0.001$) and the perineal body was longer (median 3 cm vs 3 cm, $p = 0.116$, vs 4 cm, $p = 0.033$) (Table 2).

The total score and all four subdomains of the pelvic floor questionnaire showed significant improvement at the first follow-up visit and remained significantly better than baseline at the second follow-up visit (all $p \leq 0.006$), except sexual function ($p = 0.097$ resp. $p = 0.100$).

Total median scores of the pelvic floor questionnaire were also improved at first follow-up visit when compared to baseline and further improved at the second follow-up (12.8 vs 0.8 vs 0.0) (Fig. 3). Patients who were sexually active before surgery ($n = 8$), continued to be so at the twelve-month follow-up with the exception of one patient due to her husband's illness. One woman, who was sexually inactive before surgery due to her prolapse, reported a satisfying sexual function after surgery.

All patients were satisfied with the results of the surgical intervention and rated their health condition as "much better" on the Likert scale, both at first and second follow-up visits.

**Table 1** Anatomical outcome six and twelve months after vaginal hysterectomy, native tissue cystocele and rectocele repair and bilateral sacrospinous ligament fixation for stage IV pelvic organ prolapse treatment

| Number of patients | POP-Q Stage | | | | | n |
|---|---|---|---|---|---|---|
| | 0 | I | II | III | IV | |
| Baseline | 0 | 0 | 0 | 0 | 20 | 20 |
| First follow-up (6 months) | 10 | 4 | 0 | 1 | 0 | 15 |
| Second follow-up (12 months) | 11 | 6 | 0 | 0 | 0 | 17 |

## Discussion

The aim of this prospective case series was to assess the pelvic floor symptoms and anatomical results after vaginal hysterectomy with anterior and posterior vaginal wall repair, combined with bilateral SSLF for the primary treatment of uterovaginal POP stage IV. Scores in all four domains of the pelvic floor symptom questionnaire (bladder, bowel, prolapse, sexual function) were significantly improved at both follow-ups ($p < 0.001$). According to the POP-Q system, the POP stage was significantly improved at six and twelve months after surgery when compared to baseline ($p < 0.001$). All women were asymptomatic at both follow-up visits after surgery and had either a stage 0 or stage I POP, with exception of one woman. The latter presented at the first, six-month follow-up visit with a stage III symptomatic cystocele and received an anterior vaginal repair using an anterior mesh. The patient has had a previous accident with pelvic ring fracture. Whether this might have compromised the stability of the pelvic floor, or the recurrence represents a simple failure of surgery is not clear. The patient was completely asymptomatic after the second, twelve-months follow-up.

The surgical treatment of POP stage IV is challenging. Advanced POP is often combined with vaginal wall ulcerations so that the use of synthetic material becomes a risk factor or completely inappropriate. Furthermore, the excessive lengthening of the vagina may impose difficulties in an abdominal approach as the vaginal cuff may reach the fixation point (e.g. promontorium) and lead to unsatisfactory anatomical results. Abdominal hysterectomy and concomitant sacral colpopexy could lead to further increase of the total vaginal length [11]. Abdominal concomitant total hysterectomy and sacrocolpopexy increases operating time and costs and is associated with more complications [1, 12].

Another important factor in the conceptualisation of this study is the increasing trend of moving away from the use of synthetic graft material for the treatment of primary POP. After the US Food and Drug Administration (FDA) released two public health notifications regarding the potential complications of transvaginal POP repair with synthetic mesh in 2008 and 2011, transvaginal surgical meshes showed a substantial decline. In England, the number of SSLFs grew more than 3 times over the years, whereas sacrocolpopexy remained stable during the considered period of time (2005–2016) [13]. Furthermore, patients' information through media has increased. According to published data, more than two thirds of patients with POP are informed about their condition and treatment options. In many cases, they

**Table 2** Vaginal length, genital hiatus and perineal body at baseline, at six and twelve months after vaginal hysterectomy, native tissue cystocele and rectocele repair and bilateral sacrospinous ligament fixation for stage IV pelvic organ prolapse treatment

| Median [minimum to maximum] | Vaginal length (cm) | Genital hiatus (cm) | Perineal body (cm) |
|---|---|---|---|
| Baseline | 9 [7 to 15] | 5 [2 to 9] | 3 [2 to 6] |
| First follow-up (6 months) | 7 [6 to 10] | 2 [1 to 4] | 3 [3 to 5] |
| Second follow-up (12 months) | 8 [6 to 10] | 2 [1 to 3.5] | 4 [3 to 5] |
| Difference between Baseline and First follow-up | 1 [−1 to 5] | 2.5 [0 to 5] | −1 [−2 to 3] |
| Difference between Baseline and Second follow-up | 1 [−1 to 5.5] | 2.5 [0.5 to 5.5] | −1 [−2 to 3] |
| Difference between First and Second follow-up | 0 [0 to 1] | 0 [−1 to 1] | 0 [−1 to 0] |

reject any treatment, which involves synthetic materials [14, 15]. Hence, there is an emerging need to offer patients with advanced prolapse, who need apical support, efficient treatment options.

Traditionally, SSLF is performed unilaterally, mostly on the right side of the patient. Although it was initially meant as a treatment for post-hysterectomy vaginal vault prolapse, it is now a common procedure performed concomitant to vaginal hysterectomy for uterovaginal prolapse [16]. As treatment of posthysterectomy vault prolapse, Hewson reported a high initial overall satisfaction rate of approximately 90%, and this rate was maintained at 80%, after 4 years [17]. Reports that are more recent show distinctively modest results. Barber et al. in the OPTIMAL randomised trial reported a surgical success rate after SSLF of 60.5%, at 2 years postoperative [18]. Five years postoperative, the estimated surgical failure rate was 70.3% in the SSLF group [19]. The SSLF procedure, performed unilaterally was a modification of the Michigan 4-wall technique.

Arguing for a bilateral and against a unilateral approach, some authors claimed that a bilateral suspension provided a symmetrical and better support of the vaginal vault, while previous concerns of increased morbidity and an abnormal 'stretching' of the upper vaginal walls have not been confirmed [20]. However, available data for the bilateral SSLF and specifically for the impact on pelvic floor symptoms is still sparse. Febbraro et al. included 34 patients with POP stage III and IV (according to the American Urogynecologic Society classification, 1996), 24 with and 10 women without uterus, in a feasibility study using a stapler for the fixation of the vaginal cuff on the SSL. After an average of nineteen-month follow-up (range 9 to 32), the authors showed a perfect anatomic result in 77% of cases, one vaginal cuff prolapse recurrence, one cystocele stage II and three patients with vaginal shortening (< 6 cm), while there was one case of a rectal injury through the staple branch, and in 2 patients a small rectal laceration occurred. No postoperative constipation was noted [21]. A more recent report from Mothes et al. in 2015 presents results of 110 women who received a modified, minimal tension, bilateral SSLF [22]. The follow-up was at approximately 14 months and the authors report a 94.5% objective and 96% subjective cure respectively. They also report a 5.5% (6 out of 110 women) apical prolapse and 8.3% (9 out of 110 women) anterior compartment recurrence rate, while only 2/110 and 6/110 patients

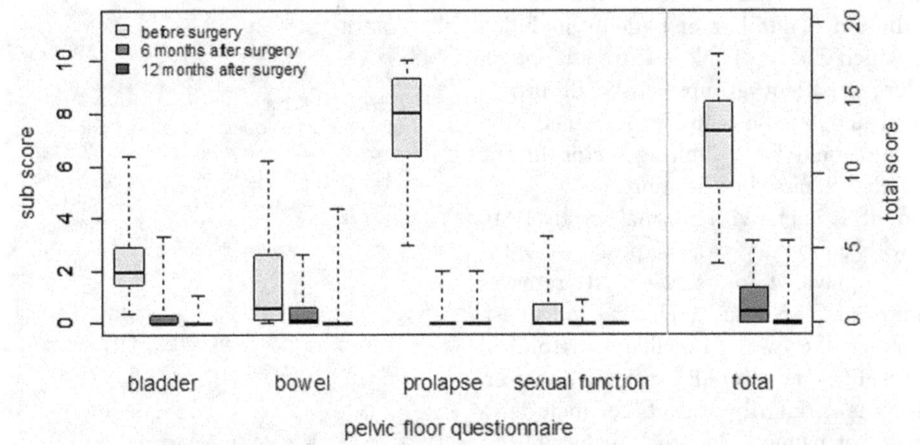


**Fig. 3** Total scores and subscores of the pelvic floor questionnaire at baseline (before surgery), at the first follow-up (six months after surgery) and at the second follow-up (twelve months after surgery)

respectively needed surgical treatment. Despite the very satisfying results at 14 months follow-up, the authors' approach remains difficult to reproduce due to the mainly subjective suture placement and it does not address the tissue bridging issues and possible insufficient support due to the lack of contact between vaginal wall and ligament tissue. Salvatore et al. in 2018 presented data from a small cohort of patients, who received bilateral SSLF after a second recurrence of prolapse and he showed that at twelve months follow-up, 90% of the patients were cured and reported significant improvement in quality of life and sexual function [23]. The authors used a suturing device and combined absorbable and non-absorbable sutures, while maintaining the classical approach of the SSLF, in contrast to the method of Mothes et al.

Our approach consisted of traditional native tissue repair with absorbable sutures for the SSLF, trying to prevent local foreign body reaction. We also used no suturing device but preferred the visualisation of the ligament for the placement of the sutures, in order to fully control their exact positioning and avoid device related complications such as rectum or nerve injury. As far as the symptoms of the patients in our cohort are concerned, the most important findings, except for the somewhat anticipated improvement of the prolapse scores are the overall recovery in all domains, the great patients' satisfaction and the consistency of the improvement over the follow-up time. In addition, the anatomical results in our patients were excellent. There was only one symptomatic cystocele five months after the initial treatment, which required surgical intervention with an anterior mesh, while all patients at second follow-up presented with POP-Q Stage either 0 or I.

Obviously, there are limitations to our study. The follow-up time of 12 months is considered short and long-term efficacy could be evaluated. Also, the interpretation of the results should be made with caution, mainly due to the small number of patients included in the analysis, which does not allow extrapolation of the results in larger patient groups. Also, all procedures were performed by the same experienced surgeon, so clustering could be a limiting factor in the interpretation of the results. Furthermore, our patient cohort consisted of women with normal mean BMI, who presented with a primary case of prolapse, without any previous pelvic floor surgery. It remains unknown, if more complex cases, including more risk factors would show the same excellent anatomical and functional results. One should consider, however, that this study was primarily meant to include a homogenous group of patients, in order to be able to objectify the results of a surgical intervention, which has been poorly investigated.

## Conclusion

The results presented in this paper indicate that bilateral SSLF combined with vaginal hysterectomy, native tissue cystocele and rectocele repair is a safe and effective choice for the treatment of an advanced uterovaginal prolapse in women with no previous pelvic floor surgery. Taking into consideration important knowledge from previously published studies, which also showed low morbidity and high satisfaction rates and symptom improvement, this method could be offered as an option to patients, who do not wish the use of alloplastic material in primary prolapse treatment. Nonetheless, long-term effectiveness should be rigorously explored.

### Abbreviations

POP: Pelvic organ prolapse; SSLF: Sacrospinous ligament fixation

### Acknowledgements

Not applicable.

### Authors' contributions

TK conception and design, acquisition of data, analysis and data interpretation, drafting of the manuscript. BS conception and design, statistical analysis, drafting of the manuscript. SB analysis and data interpretation, drafting of the manuscript. CR conception and design, acquisition of data, analysis and data interpretation, drafting of the manuscript. All authors have read and approved the manuscript.

### Competing interests

The authors declare that they have no competing interests.

### References

1. Haylen BT, Maher CF, Barber MD, Camargo S, Dandolu V, et al. International Urogynecological association (IUGA) / international continence society (ICS) joint report on the terminology for pelvic organ prolapse. Int Urogynecol J. 2016;27(2):165–94.
2. Slieker-ten Hove M, Pool-Goudzwaard A, Eijkemans M, Steegers-Theunissen R, Burger C, Vierhout ME. Prediction model and prognostic index to estimate clinically relevant pelvic organ prolapse in a general female population. Int Urogynecol J. 2009;20:1013–21.
3. Committee on Practice Bulletins - Gynecology, American Urogynecologic Society. Practice bulletin no. 185: pelvic organ prolapse. Obstet Gynecol. 2017;130(5):e234–50.
4. Jha S, Cutner A, Moran P. The UK National Prolapse Survey: 10 years on. Int Urogynecol J. 2018;29:795–801.
5. Shkarupa D, Kubin N, Pisarev A, Zaytseva A, Shapovalova E. The hybrid technique of pelvic organ prolapse treatment: apical sling and subfascial colporrhaphy. Int Urogynecol J. 2017;28:1407–13.
6. Barber MD, Maher C. Apical prolapse. Int Urogynecol J. 2013;24:1815–33.
7. Rooney K, Kenton K, Mueller ER, FitzGerald MP, Brubaker L. Advanced anterior vaginal wall prolapse is highly correlated with apical prolapse. Am J Obstet Gynecol. 2006;195:1837–40.
8. Petri E, Ashok K. Sacrospinous vaginal fixation - current status. Acta Obstet Gynecol Scand. 2011;90(5):429–36.
9. Baessler K, O'Neill SM, Maher CF, Battistutta D. A validated self-administered female pelvic floor questionnaire. Int Urogynecol J. 2010;21(2):163–72.
10. Baessler K, Kempkensteffen C. Validation of a comprehensive pelvic floor questionnaire for the hospital, private practice and research. Gynakol Geburtshilfliche Rundsch. 2009;49(4):299–307.
11. De La Cruz JF, Myers EM, Geller EJ. Vaginal versus robotic hysterectomy and concomitant pelvic support surgery: a comparison of postoperative vaginal length and sexual function. J Minim Invasive Gynecol. 2014;21(6):1010–4.

12. Maher C, Feiner B, Baessler K, Schmid C. Surgical management of pelvic organ prolapse in women. Cochrane Database Syst Rev. 2013;30(4): CD004014. https://doi.org/10.1002/14651858.CD004014.pub5.
13. Zacche MM, Mukhopadhyay S, Giarenis I. Trends in prolapse surgery in England. Int Urogynecol J. 2018;29(11):1689–95.
14. Tenggardjaja CF, Moore CK, Vasavada SP, Li J, Goldman HB. Evaluation of patients' perceptions of mesh usage in female pelvic medicine and reconstructive surgery. Urology. 2015;85(2):326–31.
15. Brown LK, Fenner DE, Berger MB, Delancey JOL, Morgan DM, et al. Defining patients' knowledge and perceptions of vaginal mesh surgery. Female Pelvic Med Reconstr Surg. 2013;19(5):282–7.
16. Chendrimada KM, Hashim H. Surgery for pelvic organ prolapse. Eur Urol Suppl. 2018:119–25.
17. Hewson AD. Transvaginal sacrospinous colpopexy for posthysterectomy vault prolapse. Aust NZJ Obstet Gynecol. 1998;38:318324.
18. Barber MD, Brubaker L, Burgio KL. Comparison of two transvaginal surgical approaches and perioperative behavioral therapy for apical vaginal prolapse: the OPTIMAL randomized trial. JAMA. 2014;311(10):1023–34.
19. Jelovsek JE, Barber MD, Brubaker L, Norton P, Gantz M, et al. Effect of uterosacral ligament suspension vs sacrospinous ligament fixation with or without perioperative behavioral therapy for pelvic organ vaginal prolapse on surgical outcomes and prolapse symptoms at 5 years in the OPTIMAL randomized clinical trial. JAMA. 2018;319(15):1554–65.
20. Shull BL, Capen CV, Riggs MW, Kuehl TJ. Bilateral attachment of the vaginal cuff m 16. Iliococcygeus fascia: an effective method of cuff suspension. Am J Obstet Gynecol. 1993;168:1669–77.
21. Febbraro W, Beucher G, Von Theobald P, Hamel P, Barjot P, et al. Feasibility of transvaginal bilateral fixation to the sacrospinous ligament with a stapler: prospective study of the first 34 cases. J Gynecol Obstet Biol Reprod. 1997; 26(6):815–21.
22. Mothes AR, Wanzke L, Radosa MP, Runnebaum IB. Bilateral minimal tension sacrospinous fixation in pelvic organ prolapse: an observational study. Eur J Obstet Gynecol Reprod Biol. 2015;188:1–5.
23. Vitale SG, Laganà AS, Noventa M, Giampaolino P, Zizolfi B, et al. Transvaginal bilateral sacrospinous fixation after second recurrence of vaginal vault prolapse: efficacy and impact on quality of life and sexuality. Biomed Res Int. 2018 Article ID:5727165.

16

# Spontaneous bilateral renal pelvis rupture during CT in the absence of urinary tract obstruction

Zongchen Li[1*] and Joey Chan Yiing Beh[2]

**Abstract**

**Background:** Atraumatic renal pelvis rupture without pre-existing renal or ureteric pathology is an uncommon event. It is reported in the setting of acute urinary tract obstruction, most often secondary to ureteric calculi. Typical symptoms include acute flank pain and nausea, mimicking pyelonephritis or other causes of acute abdomen. Spontaneous rupture occurring bilaterally without identifiable urinary tract obstruction is exceedingly rare, and has yet to be reported in current English literature. Possible contributing pathophysiological mechanisms can be postulated from reported cases of rupture with observed obstruction.

**Case presentation:** A 58-year-old woman undergoing multiphasic computed tomography (CT) for evaluation of asymptomatic microscopic haematuria developed on-table bilateral renal pelvis rupture seen only after contrast administration, on the delayed phase. There was no significant past medical history of note. The patient remained asymptomatic throughout and after the study, and was managed conservatively. Follow-up radiographical imaging over a month showed resolution of urinoma and no further contrast extravasation. No complications or recurrence was subsequently noted.

**Conclusions:** Spontaneous rupture of the renal pelvis can be a rare complication of intravenous contrast administration even in cases without identifiable urinary tract obstruction, and it can occur bilaterally. Cases can uncommonly be asymptomatic but typical symptoms should prompt evaluation of the kidneys, particularly when they are not included in the initial study or no delayed phase is protocolled. Interval imaging for resolution of urinoma and contrast extravasation is clinically relevant to monitor for and avoid infective sequelae.

**Keywords:** Spontaneous renal pelvis rupture, Forniceal rupture, Pyelosinus backflow, Contrast-induced osmotic diuresis, Case report

* Correspondence: lizongchen27@hotmail.com
[1]National University Hospital, Singapore, Singapore
Full list of author information is available at the end of the article

## Background

Spontaneous renal pelvis rupture, also known as forniceal rupture or pyelosinus backflow, is an uncommon complication of acute urinary tract obstruction. In the context of intravenous urography during acute renal colic, Schwartz et al. defined a rupture as ‘spontaneous’ if it occurred in the absence of trauma, abdominal compression, destructive renal lesion or prior surgical and endoscopic intervention [1].

It is thought to occur as a result of rapidly increasing intraluminal pressure [2] presumably overwhelming slower reactive mechanisms that act to reduce urine output, as seen in chronic hydronephrosis. Typical symptoms mimic those of acute abdomen or pyelonephritis, with unilateral flank pain and nausea [3]. This event has been reported most frequently in association with obstructive ureteric calculi, with other aetiologies such as extrinsic ureteric compression or bladder outlet obstruction following distantly behind [4].

Asymptomatic spontaneous rupture occurring bilaterally in the absence of urinary tract obstruction is hence extremely unusual. To the best of the authors’ knowledge, this has not been described in current English literature. We report one such case precipitated by CT urography and discuss possible pathophysiological mechanisms.

## Case presentation

A 58-year-old woman with no significant past medical history was referred to the outpatient urology clinic for asymptomatic microscopic haematuria noted incidentally on urinalysis. Routine CT urography was performed in the pre-contrast, nephrographic and delayed phases. A total of 75 mL of iodinated contrast agent (300 mg I/mL concentration) was administered, and no diuretics were given.

On the pre-contrast and nephrographic phases, a 2 mm non-obstructive renal calculus was noted on the right but the kidneys were otherwise unremarkable. No calculus was seen in the ureters and urinary bladder (Fig. 1). The latter was well-distended from voluntary retention of urine in preparation for the study. No perinephric fluid collection was noted at this point.

On the excretory phase performed at 6 min 13 s post-contrast, peripelvic contrast extravasation was observed bilaterally - suggestive of acute rupture (Fig. 2). No other site of urinoma was observed. A further delayed phase was performed at 50 min post-contrast to evaluate the

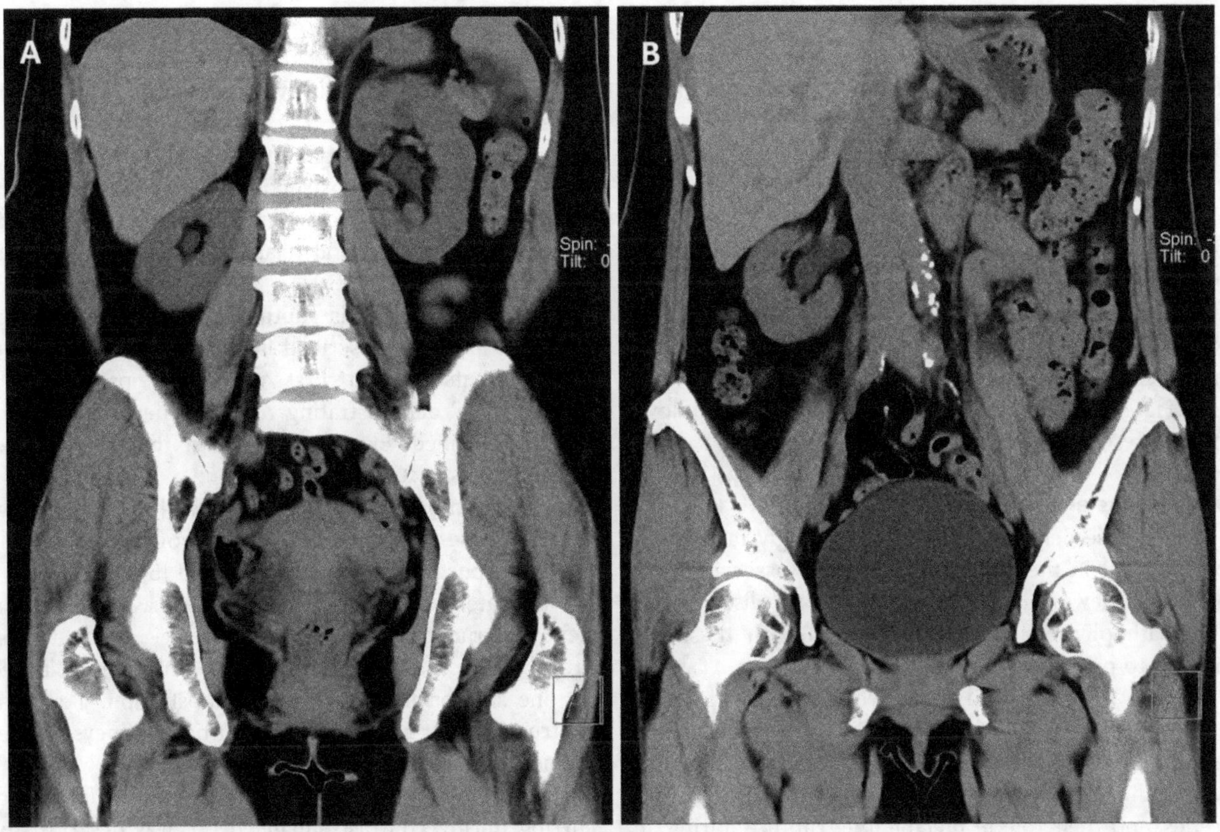


**Fig. 1** Non-contrast phase of the CT urogram showing no hydronephrosis or hydroureter bilaterally (**a**), and a well-distended urinary bladder (**b**). No ureteric or bladder calculus was seen

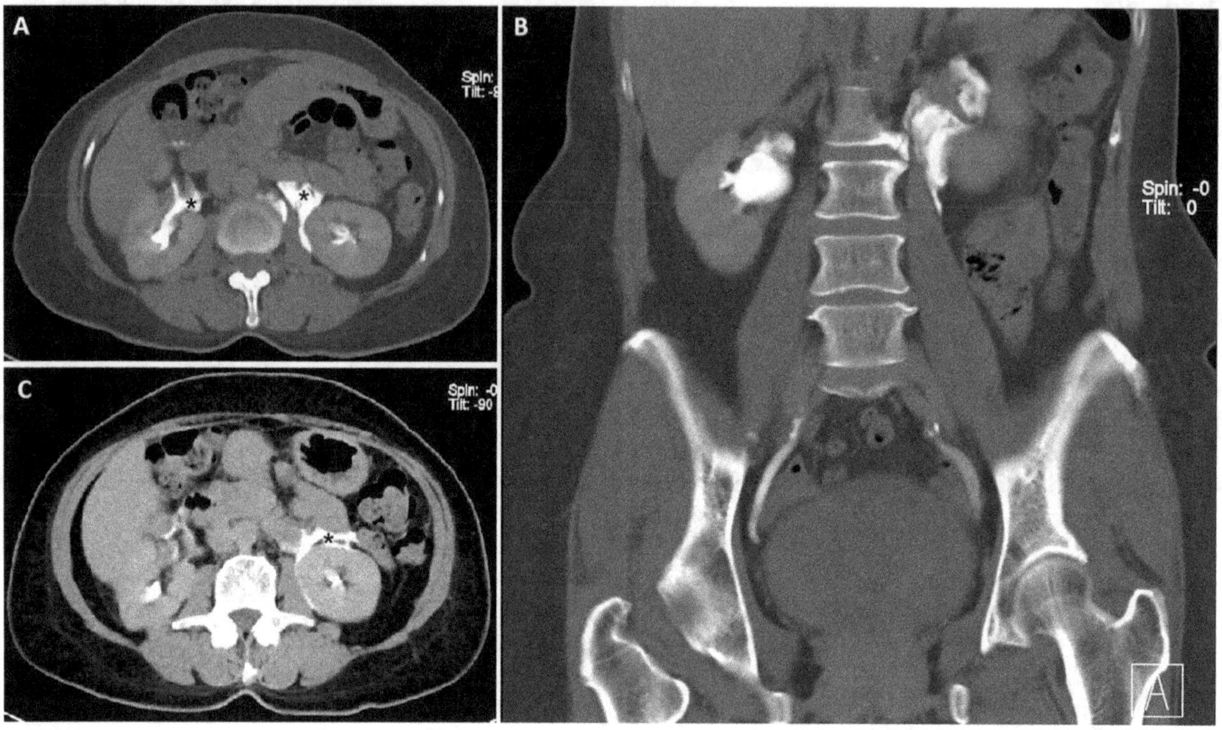


**Fig. 2** Initial delayed phase of the CT urogram (**a**, **b**) with peripelvic contrast extravasation marked with asterisks. Further delayed phase performed at 50 min (**c**) showing tracking of contrast

extent of urinoma, which showed tracking of contrast along the retroperitoneum without further peripelvic extravasation.

Throughout the study, no flank pain or other symptom was reported; the patient remained asymptomatic even after the event was observed acutely on-table. No abdominal or flank tenderness was elicited on examination.

She was managed conservatively and a radiograph performed the next day revealed no persistent contrast pooling. Follow-up intravenous urography performed a month after showed no recurrence of contrast extravasation (Fig. 3). Thereafter, she was discharged from follow-up after resolution of microscopic haematuria.

## Discussions and conclusions

This is a case demonstrating an exceedingly rare radiological event in the absence of classically associated risk factors. Reviewing related case reports, we discuss possible pathophysiological mechanisms though these are difficult to prove with a single case alone.

Rupture is reported to occur when intra-pelvic pressures exceed 25 to 75 mmHg and is seen most frequently at the fornices [5], possibly where the walls are the thinnest. Iodinated contrast agents are potent osmotic diuretics, and their role in precipitating rupture during an acute obstruction is clear. An early prospective study by Bernardino et al. demonstrated a positive relationship between the administered dose of intravenous contrast and the incidence of peripelvic contrast extravasation in patients with acute renal colic [2].

However, osmotic diuresis alone is an insufficient factor in the absence of obstruction. The primary mechanism is nonetheless likely dependent on this diuretic effect, given the temporal relationship between contrast administration and onset.

Unilateral renal pelvis rupture in the absence of obstruction has been described in the emergency care setting. Patients present first with flank pain, with a following CT demonstrating rupture where no obstruction is identified. Eken et al. suggest that unwitnessed transient obstruction, such as from a passed calculus, may be the most plausible mechanism [6]. Though that reported case had no known history of urinary calculi, another reported by Pampana et al. did [5].

The bilateral nature of rupture in this case makes transient obstruction by a passing ureteric calculus less probable. Moreover, a calculus was only demonstrated on one side prior to contrast administration. Transient obstruction more distally can affect both kidneys and remains a possible mechanism.

One other report of bilateral renal pelvis rupture occurring during contrast-enhanced CT was described by Chien et al. [7]. The case occurred during CT venography of the iliac veins, where a total of 170 mL of

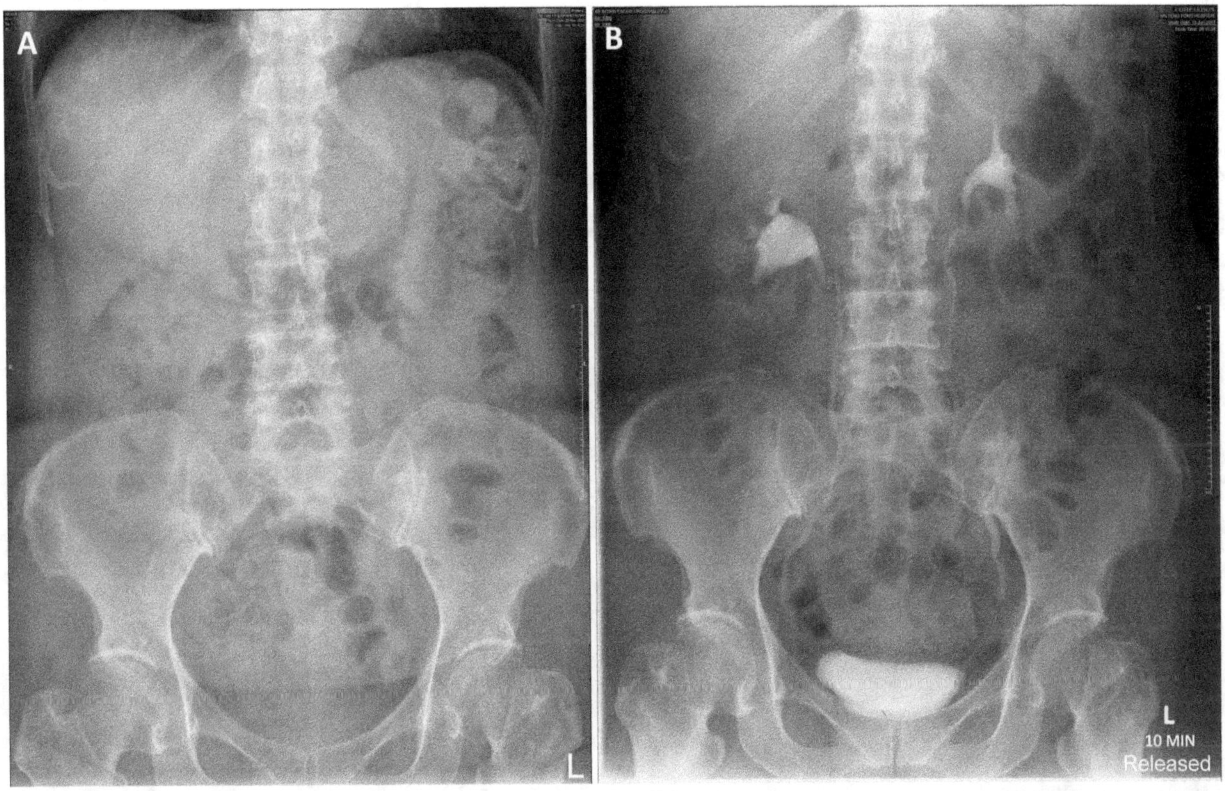


**Fig. 3** Interval plain radiograph performed the following day (**a**). Follow-up intravenous urography performed a month later (**b**). Both show no further contrast extravasation or persistent contrast pooling

intravenous contrast was administered and post-rupture catheterization drained a urine volume in excess of 1 l. A background of bladder outlet obstruction from prostatomegaly was reported, and the authors attribute it as the cause of rupture. Acute flank pain during the scan first alerted radiological staff of this complication.

Notably, the case we report did not manifest flank pain. There was also no known history or symptom of urinary obstruction, though the bladder did appear distended on CT. It is plausible that voluntary urinary retention acted as a form of transient 'obstruction' at the bladder outlet.

Even so, majority of patients with a filled bladder do not develop this complication. The initial presentation of microscopic haematuria in this specific case may hence be relevant. Urinary calculi predispose to urinary tract rupture, with one postulated mechanism of urothelial injury during passage [8]. As no urothelial mass was identified in this case, the cause of haematuria could have been recent asymptomatic passage of calculi. We postulate that this could have additionally predisposed to rupture.

In the case reported by Chien et al., the patient was also treated conservatively. Interval imaging and urinalysis showed resolution of both microscopic haematuria and contrast extravasation. Serial imaging is of value, as large or persistent urinomas carry a risk of infection and loss of renal function [9]. Other modalities such as sonography can be considered as well [5]. Existing literature suggests that such a conservative approach is appropriate in the absence of complications (e.g. superimposed infection, kidney injury), risk factors for complications (e.g. sizeable urinoma 100 mL or larger) or a solitary kidney [10–12]. The detection of further contrast extravasation or unresolving urinoma in this case would have prompted consideration of drainage and urinary diversion.

In conclusion, spontaneous rupture of the renal pelvis is a potential (albeit rare) complication of intravenous contrast administration in the absence of urinary tract obstruction, and it can occur bilaterally. Although cases can uncommonly be asymptomatic, typical symptoms such as flank pain following contrast injection behoove physicians to evaluate the kidneys – particularly when they are not included in the initial study or no delayed phase is protocolled. A missed or untreated complication (i.e. large urinoma), could become a nidus for intra-abdominal infection and damage the urinary tract by fibrosis and granuloma formation. Rupture should also prompt physicians to actively evaluate for underlying causes. Interval follow-up imaging for resolution is clinically relevant to monitor for and avoid such infective sequelae through radiological-guided drainage or urological intervention.

**Abbreviation**
CT: Computed tomography

**Acknowledgements**
Not applicable.

**Authors' contributions**
LZ wrote the case report and performed literature review. BJCY identified the case, provided its details and reviewed the draft manuscripts. Both authors have read and approved the final manuscript.

**Competing interests**
The authors declare that they have no competing interests.

**Author details**
[1]National University Hospital, Singapore, Singapore. [2]Ng Teng Fong General Hospital, Singapore, Singapore.

**References**

1. Schwartz A, et al. Spontaneous renal extravasation during intravenous urography. Am J Roentgenol. 1966;98(1):27–40. American Roentgen Ray Society. https://doi.org/10.2214/ajr.98.1.27.
2. Bernardino ME, Clennan BL. High dose urography: incidence and relationship to spontaneous peripelvic extravasation. Am J Roentgenol. 1976;127(3):373–6. American Roentgen Ray Society. https://doi.org/10.2214/ajr.127.3.373.
3. Yanaral, Fatih et al. "Spontaneous rupture of the renal pelvis due to obstruction of pelviureteric junction by renal stone: a case report and review of the literature". Urol Ann, vol 9, no. 3, 2017, p. 293. Medknow, doi: https://doi.org/10.4103/ua.ua_24_17.
4. Gershman B, et al. Causes of renal forniceal rupture. BJU Int. 2011;108(11): 1909–11. Wiley. https://doi.org/10.1111/j.1464-410x.2011.10164.x.
5. Pampana, E. et al. "Spontaneous ureteral rupture diagnosis and treatment". Case Rep Radiol, vol 2013, 2013, pp. 1-4. Hindawi Limited, doi:https://doi.org/10.1155/2013/851859.
6. Eken A, et al. Spontaneous rupture of the ureter. Singapore Med J. 2015; 56(02):e29–31. Singapore Medical Journal. https://doi.org/10.11622/smedj.2015029.
7. Chien JC-W, et al. Bilateral spontaneous peripelvic urinary extravasation. Kidney Int. 2014;86(2):448. Elsevier BV. https://doi.org/10.1038/ki.2013.514.
8. El-Boghdadly SA. Spontaneous rupture of the ureter proximal to ureteric stone. J Royal Soc Med. 1985;78(3):255–6. SAGE Publications. https://doi.org/10.1177/014107688507800316.
9. Goldwasser J, et al. Urinoma: prompt diagnosis and treatment can prevent abscess formation, hydronephrosis, and a progressive loss of renal function. Case Rep Emerg Med. 2018;2018:1–3. Hindawi Limited. https://doi.org/10.1155/2018/5456738.
10. Setia SA, et al. Renal forniceal rupture in the setting of obstructing ureteral stones: an analysis of stone characterization and urologic intervention pattern. J Endourol. 2020;34(3):373–8. Mary Ann Liebert Inc. https://doi.org/10.1089/end.2019.0706.
11. Sultan MF, et al. Spontaneous forniceal rupture: can it be treated conservatively? Urol Ann. 2017;9, 41. Medknow(1). https://doi.org/10.4103/0974-7796.198883.
12. Morgan TN, et al. Renal forniceal rupture: is conservative management safe? Urology. 2017;109:51–4. Elsevier BV. https://doi.org/10.1016/j.urology.2017.07.045.

17

# Primary vaginal calculus in a woman with urogenital sinus anomaly

Qiong Xu and Yu Zou*

**Abstract**

**Background:** Primary vaginal calculus is rare and often misdiagnosed due to its low incidence. The formation of primary vaginal calculus is mainly due to the pooling and stasis of urine within the vagina, and associated with urogenital tract abnormalities.

**Case presentation:** We present a case of a 23-year-old woman with urogenital sinus anomaly who presented with a vaginal calculus. The patient was not suspected of a calculus in the vagina until the patient suffered amenorrhea and dyspareunia. Pelvic computed tomography (CT) and magnetic resonance imaging (MRI) confirmed the patient had urogenital sinus anomaly with vaginal calculus. For the reason, the calculus was removed by surgery, and the reconstruction of vagina and urethra was performed. The postoperative recovery and follow-up were uneventful.

**Conclusions:** Although vaginal calculus and urogenital sinus anomaly are extremely rare in literature, the radiologist should be familiar with the imaging appearance of urogenital sinus anomaly, and be aware of the possibility of vaginal calculus.

**Keywords:** Urogenital sinus, Vaginal calculus, Computed tomography, Magnetic resonance imaging

## Background

Primary vaginal calculi are rare disorder which has been reported in association with urogenital tract abnormalities such as urogenital sinus anomaly, urethrovaginal fistulas, vaginal outlet obstruction and bladder exstrophy [1–5]. This report describes of a primary vaginal calculus caused by urogenital sinus anomaly.

## Case presentation

A 23-year-old woman was referred to our hospital because of recurrent abdominal pain for 7 years, amenorrhea and dyspareunia. The patient's mental state and movement ability was normal. She had a history of fracture of both legs and skin injury of pubic caruncle caused by trauma about 20 years ago.

Gynecological examination showed the patient had a single orifice on the urogenital region located where the urethra would be expected. There is a normally located anal perineal orifice. When forced urination, urine flowed out of the single orifice on the urogenital region. The urethral catheter was inserted about 70 mm through the single orifice, and no urine flowed out.

Pelvic CT scan showed a large calculus and a urethral catheter in the vagina (Fig. 1a, b, c). Pelvic MRI scan demonstrated the urethra and the vagina merged into a common channel about 3.45 cm long (Fig. 2b, c), and a large calculus about 7.8 cm × 6.8 cm × 7.7 cm in size lodging in the upper vagina, the uterus was moved upward (Fig. 2a,b,c); a urethral catheter entered the vagina through the opening on the urogenital region; both ovaries and bladder were normal and no other congenital malformation was noted (Fig. 2a). Transabdominal sonography imaging revealed a vaginal stone, and normal two kidneys, the bladder, uterus, cervix, and adnexa.

Under general anesthesia, entering the urogenital tract through the median perineum approach and a 2-cm incision was performed (Fig. 3a). A hard grayish-yellow

* Correspondence: zouyuzju@zju.edu.cn
Department of Radiology, Women's Hospital School of Medicine Zhejiang University, Hangzhou 310006, Zhejiang province, China

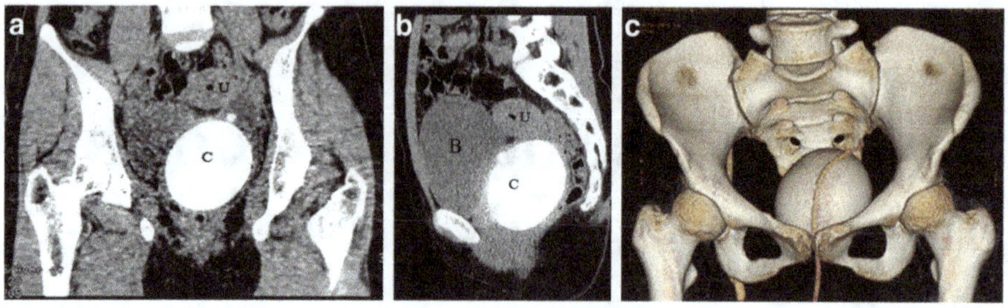


**Fig. 1** The multiple planar reconstruction (MPR) (**a**, **b**) and volume rendering (VR) (**c**) of pelvic CT, showing a large calculus in the vagina. B, bladder; U, uterus; C, calculus

abnormal mass was observed in the vaginal cavity (Fig. 3b), and there was no adhesion to the surrounding mucosa. The tissue around the calculus was carefully separated and the calculus was completely removed.

During the exploration after lithotomy, the common channel formed by vagina and urethra was detected, and the orifice of urethra was about 3 cm from the anterior vault of the vagina. The urethral catheter was inserted about 20 mm through the orifice of urethra, the urine flow was observed. Therefore, the estimated length of the urethra was about 2 cm. Hysteroscopic insertion of the vagina revealed thin endometrium and normal cervix, no other abnormality was found. The patient was diagnosed with a vaginal stone, urogenital sinus anomaly and thin endometrium.

Vaginal reconstruction (vaginoplasty) and urethra reconstruction (urethroplasty) were performed. The mucosa near the urethral orifice was taken and wrapped by 20 fr Foley's catheter, forming a urethra about 4 cm and neourethral meatus. The vaginal mucosa was pulled down and intermittently sutured with the perineal skin to form a vagina about 8 cm that could hold two fingers.

After the operation, the patient received the treatment of estrogen and progesterone, and menarche appeared 20 days later. One month after the operation, the patient recovered well, and could urinate by himself. After 8 months of follow-up, the patient had normal menstruation and urination. The patient is married and ready to conceive.

## Discussion and conclusion

Vaginal calculi are extremely rare and are classified as primary and secondary. The cause of primary vaginal calculi is probably caused by the pooling and stasis of urine within the vagina. In the literature, primary vaginal calculi are more frequently associated with urogenital tract abnormalities [1–5]. In our case, the urogenital sinus was undoubted the underlying cause of calculi formation. Urine flowed back into the vagina from the common channel, and was prone to stagnation, which seemed to help the formation of calculi.

In most cases, the clinical manifestations of patients are not specific. Most of the symptoms are caused by enlarged stones in the vagina, including infections, vaginal pain, dyspareunia, urinary incontinency [2, 5–8]. In our study, the patient presented with recurrent abdominal pain, amenorrhea and dyspareunia. At the beginning of

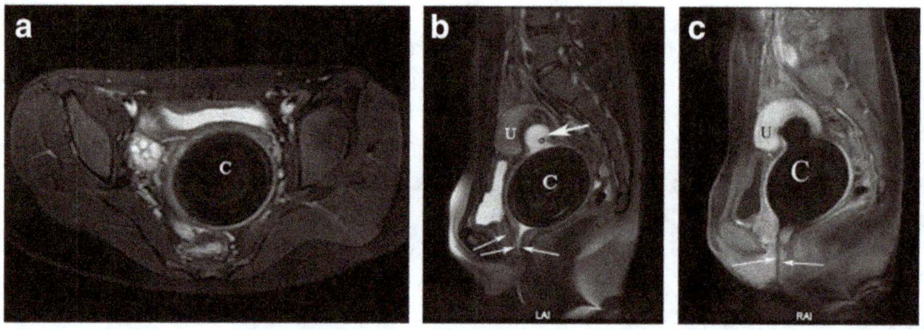


**Fig. 2** **a** Axial and **b** Sagittal T2-weighted imaging with fat saturation of pelvis, showing a large, extremely low-signal intensity mass (**c**) in the vagina that caused the uterus moved upward. A balloon catheter shadow (thick arrow) can be seen above the mass. The urethra and vagina form a common channel (arrow). **c** Sagittal contrast-enhancement T1-weighted imaging with fat saturation of pelvis, showing the mass has no enhancement

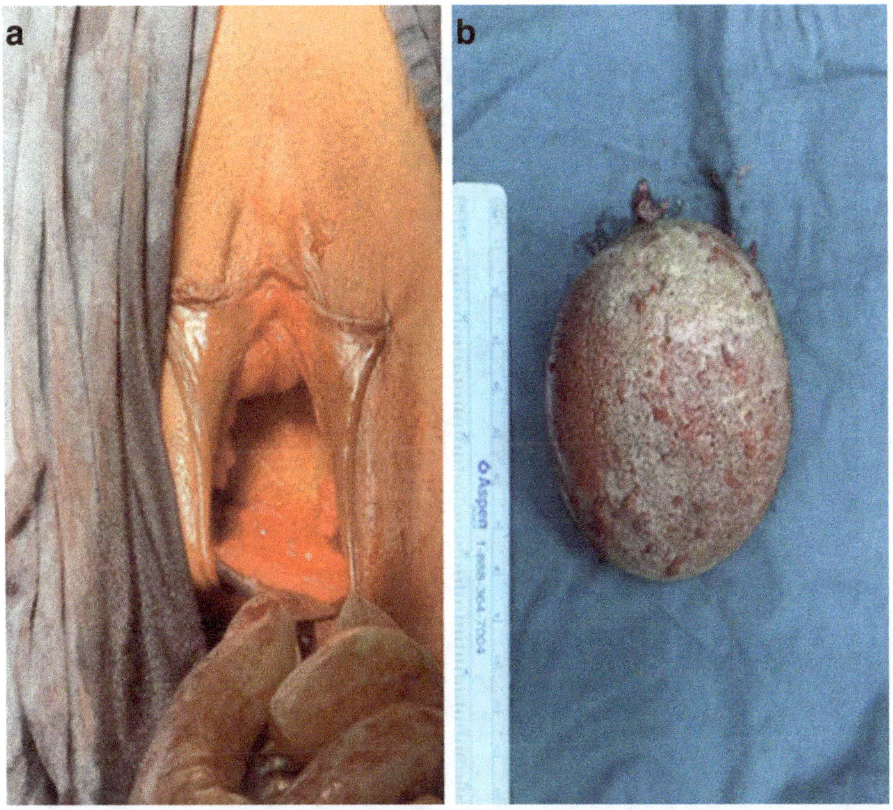


**Fig. 3 a** Vaginal calculus is seen through the median perineum incision in the vagina during its removal; **b** Image of the vaginal calculus removed during surgery

the treatment, the patient was not considered to have stone in the vagina until US, CT and MRI examinations.

B ultrasound and X-ray examinations of the pelvis are helpful to confirm the diagnosis of calculi, but it is difficult to determine the specific location of calculi by X-ray examination, and difficult to determine the relationship between large calculi and the pelvic organs by B ultrasound. Pelvic CT can show the exact position, structure and density of the calculi. Pelvic MRI can clearly show the location of the calculi, the structure of vagina and urethra as well as the endometrium and muscle layers. Therefore, CT and MRI examinations have strong advantages in distinguishing pelvic stones and correctly diagnosing vagina stones. In our study, multiple examinations such as gynecologic examination, CT, and MRI examinations can be used to accurately diagnose urogenital sinus with vaginal calculus.

The patient was amenorrhea, and hysteroscopy found that the patient's endometrium was thin. There are many reasons for the formation of thin endometrium and amenorrhea, including age, drugs, mechanical damage and so on. In our study, we believe that thin endometrium was the main cause of amenorrhea. Urine retained in the vagina was easy to enter the uterine cavity, stimulating and inhibiting endometrial hyperplasia. After the operation, the menstruation of the patient recovered after the treatment of estrogen and progesterone.

To our knowledge, only one case has been previous reported of vaginal calculus associated with an isolated urogenital sinus anomaly [1]. In the case, the patient was a 3-year-old girl who successfully completed endoscopic intracorporeal lithotripsy, and reconstructive surgery was postponed until puberty. In our study, the patient underwent open surgery to remove the calculus completely and reconstruct the vagina and urethra. The prognosis was good.

### Abbreviations

CT: Computed tomography; MRI: Magnetic resonance imaging; MPR: Multiple planar reconstruction; VR: Volume rendering; US: ultrasonic

### Acknowledgements

There is no acknowledgment.

### Authors' contributions

QX collected patient data and drafted the manuscript. QX, and YZ designed and organized this report and participated in writing the manuscript. YZ reviewed and approved the final manuscript. All authors read and approved the final manuscript.

**Competing interests**

The authors declare that they have no competing interests.

**References**

1. Ranawaka RS, Goyal A, Shabani A, Hennayake S, Dickson AP, Cervellione RM. Novel approach to vaginal calculus in a girl with urogenital sinus anomaly. J Pediatr Surg. 2015;S0022–3468(12)00546–5.
2. Wei D, Xie Y, Niu X. Vaginal stones caused by urethrovaginal fistula: A case report. Medicine (Baltimore). 2019;98:e18003.
3. Malhotra N, Kumar S, Roy KK, Agarwal R, Verma V. Vaginal calculus secondary to vaginal outlet obstruction. J Clin Ultrasound. 2004;32:204–6.
4. Plaire JC, Snodgrass WT, Grady RW, Mitchell ME. Vaginal calculi secondary to partial vaginal outlet obstruction in pediatric patients. J Urol. 2000;164:132–3.
5. Tavakkoli M, Ghoreifi A. Large vaginal and bladder calculi in a woman with previous operation of bladder exstrophy: a case report. Nephrourol Mon. 2013;6:e13637.
6. Ikeda Y, Oda K, Matsuzawa N, Shimizu K. Primary vaginal calculus in a middle-aged woman with mental and physical disabilities. Int Urogynecol J. 2013;24:1229–31.
7. Zilberlicht A, Feiner B, Haya N, Auslender R, Abramov Y. Surgical removal of a large vaginal calculus formed after a tension-free vaginal tape procedure. Int Urogynecol J. 2016;27:1771–2.
8. Ho TC, Lin IL. Primary vaginal stone in a young active woman. Taiwan J Obstet Gynecol. 2008;47:457–9.

# 18

# Lower urinary tract symptoms in men: Challenges to early hospital presentation in a resource-poor health system

Ikenna I. Nnabugwu[1*], Ijeoma L. Okoronkwo[2] and Chinwe A. Nnabugwu[2]

**Abstract**

**Background:** The point at which men seek medical care for lower urinary tract symptoms (LUTS) varies between individuals. Presentation to hospital with complications beyond LUTS appears prevalent in our setting. The aim of this survey is to assess from the community perspective in southeast Nigeria, the challenges to early presentation for medical evaluation for LUTS by men.

**Methods:** A questionnaire-based cross-sectional survey of randomly-selected men ≥40 years. The questionnaire captured respondent's age; presence, duration and severity of LUTS; access to health information; wealth-index; and when (and why) medical care for LUTS was sought. Analysis was with SPSS® version 20.

**Results:** In all, responses from 1319 men (mean age 54.2 ± 10.2 years) are analysed. Of these, 267 report LUTS: 58.4% (156) report moderate to severe LUTS and 51.7% (138) are yet to seek medical care. As regards seeking medical care, all the men reporting LUTS of 3 months, 35.7% of 126 men reporting moderate LUTS, and 20.0% of 30 men reporting severe LUTS are yet to seek medical care. LUTS being non-bothersome (not financial constraint) is the most prevalent reason for not seeking medical care early. Delay is encouraged by limited access to health information (OR 3.10; $p < 0.001$), but discouraged by literacy (OR 0.86; $p < 0.001$) and aging (OR 0.93; $p = 0.002$).

**Conclusion:** From the community perspective, the prevalent challenge to seeking medical care for LUTS early is absence of bother. Empowering men through formal education and researched health information will influence positively the time that LUTS in men is appreciated as bothersome.

**Keywords:** LUTS, Men, Medical-care, Challenges, Delay

## Background

Lower urinary tract symptoms (LUTS) are a set of symptoms that usually indicate that there is dysfunction in the storage and controlled evacuation of urine from the urinary bladder [1]. These symptoms can occur in any age group, but the reasons for the symptoms vary from age to age and from one gender to the other [2]. Irrespective of the primary diagnosis, it is suspected that LUTS could have a common pathway [3]. The occurrence of any or some of these symptoms is an indication that there is altered bladder compliance, altered infravesical resistance, increased flow of urine into the bladder, or a combination of these in varying proportions [4]. LUTS may vary from sudden onset transient LUTS, to insidious onset progressive LUTS [5]. In men who are 40 years of age and older, common disease conditions associated with insidious onset progressive LUTS include enlarging benign and malignant prostates, chronic prostatitis, urethral stricture disorders, neoplastic diseases of the urinary bladder,

* Correspondence: ikenna.nnabugwu@unn.edu.ng
[1]Department of Surgery, College of Medicine, University of Nigeria Ituku-Ozalla, Enugu PMB 01129, Nigeria

neurogenic bladder disorders, diuresis-causing disorders and many more [6–8]. Some of these disease conditions have attendant grave consequences if not promptly and appropriately addressed medically [9].

Men experiencing LUTS seek medical care at varying points in symptom progression [10]. A number of individual constitutional, social and economic factors, interacting with each other, have been documented to influence the intention to seek medical care: some of them are cultural belief and practice, self-perceived aging [11], literacy level [12], poor finances and accessibility of medical care especially in the absence of robust health insurance [13], and exposure to health information [14].

Left unattended, most of the disease conditions resulting in progressive LUTS and worsening bladder outlet obstruction have increasing risk of life-threatening complications such as obstructive nephropathy, septicaemia, acute urinary retention, and so on [15]. In fact, some of these disease conditions such as prostate and bladder cancers are only curable in the early stages of the diseases, when LUTS alone may be the pointer to the possibility of the diagnosis. Yet allegedly, many men express challenges to appropriate medical care at this early phase of disease evolution [16].

In a typical low-income country with poor health insurance coverage, hospital-based studies report that men diagnosed of benign prostate enlargement (BPE), prostate cancer, bladder cancer, and other disease conditions whose early clinical features are LUTS predominantly present to appropriate hospitals late with complications beyond LUTS [17]. On the other hand, in other climes it has been documented that there is more to seeking medical care for LUTS by men than providing free healthcare services [18]. LUTS of varying severity and duration are considered non-bothersome by men. In addition, men feel embarrassed discussing their LUTS with someone else including medical care providers [19]. The prevalent challenge to early presentation with LUTS in low-income setting may not be financial constraints. The aim of this study therefore is to identify, from the community perspective, the challenges to early presentation to appropriate medical care for LUTS in men. This knowledge will help focus on the right strategies towards improving on early presentation for medical care.

## Methods

This interviewer-assisted, questionnaire-based cross-sectional survey was conducted from March 5th to May 25th, 2018 in Enugu, southeast Nigeria. From the 2006 population figures, Enugu has an estimated population of 983,000 persons, 22.0% of which are men who are 40 years and above [20].

The survey questionnaire which was administered by pre-tutored trainee Urologists and intern doctors, captured respondent's age and presence or not of LUTS. Where LUTS were reported, the duration of the reported LUTS was ascertained. In addition, the questionnaire assessed respondent's attitude to seeking medical care early using a 4-point Likert scale on 5 question stems as adapted from Davis et al. [21] The severity of LUTS and the quality of life (QoL) due to the reported LUTS were assessed using validated International Prostate Symptom Score (IPSS) chart [22]. For respondents that had sought medical care for the reported LUTS, the duration of LUTS before medical care was sought as well as the reason for seeking medical care was determined. The nature of medical care sought in the first instance was noted.

Access to possible health information on LUTS was captured in terms of discussions on LUTS with family and peers as well as exposure to conventional media and internet health broadcasts and write ups.

Finally, household living conditions and durable assets adapted from Nigeria-General Household Survey, Panel 2015–2016, Wave 3 [23], were assessed for the purpose of creating respondent's wealth index. Reliability test yielded Cronbach's $\alpha = 0.735$ for the wealth index variables.

The sample size as worked out using the formula $n = \frac{Z^2 P(1-P)}{d^2}$ is 372 subjects; where $P$ is 0.591 [24], $Z$ is 1.96 and $d$ is 0.05. As reported in Nnabugwu et al., (2019) [25] 3 of 9 settlement clusters were randomly selected in Enugu for the study. Within the clusters, the study participants were selected through a systematic random sampling technique of 1 in every 3 eligible men. To be included in the study were men 40 years and older and dwelling within the clusters. Written informed consent was obtained from each eligible participant before inclusion.

Simple frequency was used to determine prevalence of LUTS and nature of medical care sought firstly. Arithmetic mean on compute variable was used to differentiate respondents with good attitude from those with poor attitude to seeking medical care based on responses from the Likert questions focusing on attitude to seeking medical care. Principal Component Analysis (PCA) was used to create wealth indices using the data on household durable assets and living conditions. PCA was also used to create health information indices using responses on possible sources of health information on LUTS. Logistic Regression Analysis was used to evaluate factors that influence duration from onset of LUTS to seeking medical care. Significance was set at $p < 0.05$. All analyses were done with SPSS® version 20. The University of Nigeria Teaching Hospital Bioethics Committee approved of the study.

## Results

Figure 1 shows the pathway to patient recruitment in this survey. One thousand three hundred and nineteen (1319) duly completed questionnaires out of 1337 were returned for analysis. The socio-demographic characteristics of these respondents are shown in Table 1.

Majority of the respondents are between 40 and 59 years of age' acquired more than 6 years of formal education and reported no lower urinary tract symptoms.

Two hundred and sixty-seven (267) of the 1319 respondents report at least one lower urinary tract symptom which gives overall LUTS prevalence rate of 20.2%. Nocturia at a rate of 19.9% is the most prevalent lower urinary tract symptom. Within the subset of men reporting LUTS ($N = 267$) nocturia is the earliest symptom reportedly noticed (35.2%). The prevalence of LUTS increases with increasing decade of life from 10.2% in the 5th decade of life to 70.0% in the 9th decade. Similarly, the severity of LUTS determined using IPSS worsens with increasing decade of life ($\chi^2$ 152.9; df 15; $p < 0.001$).

Respondents experiencing LUTS report various durations of LUTS and those who had sought medical care report various durations from onset of symptom(s) to seeking medical care. These are shown in Table 2.

Table 2 shows that as symptoms persist or progress, increasing number of men experiencing LUTS reportedly sought medical care.

One hundred and forty-two of the 267 that reported LUTS (53.2%) demonstrate good attitude to early medical care. Eighty-seven of the 111 respondents reporting mild LUTS (78.4%) are yet to seek medical care; 45 of 126 reporting moderate LUTS (35.7%) are yet to seek medical care while 6 of 30 reporting severe LUTS (20.0%) are yet to seek medical care. Twenty-five of 94 respondents (26.6%) reporting symptoms of more than 2 years, which has progressed to moderate to severe LUTS, are yet to seek medical care. Some of the reasons for not seeking medical care yet are shown in Table 3.

From Table 3, LUTS considered non-bothersome is the most prevalent reason for not seeking medical care for LUTS of various durations.

On the other hand, of these 267 respondents reporting LUTS, 129 had sought medical care from different care providers. Figure 2 is the frequency distribution of the types of care providers sought in the first instance by these respondents. Some of the reasons for seeking medical care when medical care was sought include: worsening of symptoms (38.0%), persistence of symptoms (26.4%), fear of something worse (18.6%), pressure from family and friends (14.0%) and others including loss of erection (3.1%).

From this figure, most of the respondents that sought medical care reportedly sought the services of orthodox medical doctors firstly.

The variables that influence the decision to seek medical care at the time medical care was sought were subjected to ordinal logistic regression analysis and the result is shown in Table 4.

From Table 4, age and formal educational status of respondent, severity and duration of LUTS, as well as health information index of respondent significantly

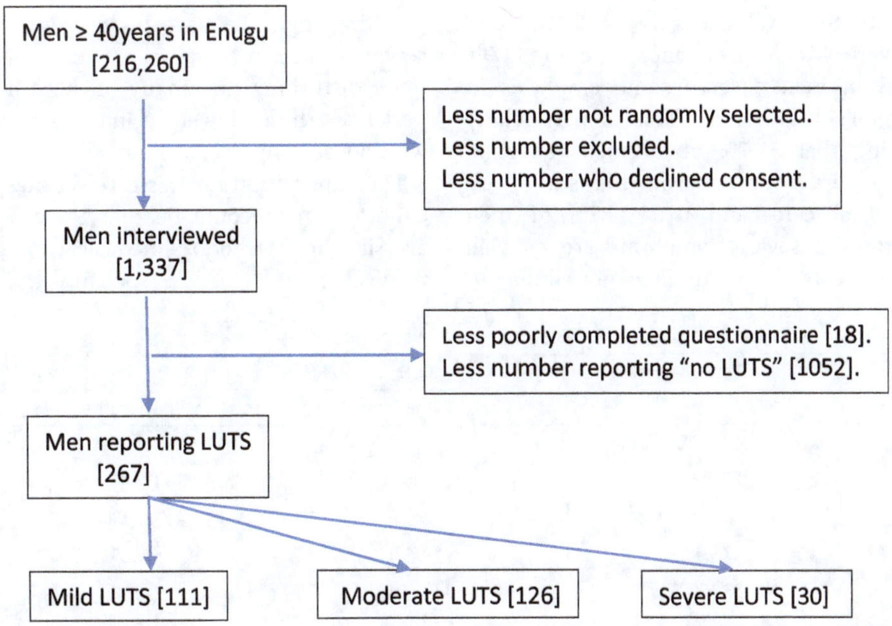


**Fig. 1** Participants' recruitment pathway

**Table 1** Socio-demographic characteristics of respondents

| Variables | | Frequency (%) |
|---|---|---|
| **Age of Respondents (years)** | **40–49** | 500 (37.9%) |
| | **50–59** | 420 (31.8%) |
| | **60–69** | 277 (21.0%) |
| | **70–79** | 110 (8.3%) |
| | **80–89** | 10 (0.8%) |
| | **90–99** | 2 (0.2%) |
| **Mean Age of Respondents (years)** | **54.2 ± 10.2** | |
| **Duration of Formal Education (years)** | **≤6** | 466 (35.3%) |
| | **>6** | 853 (64.7%) |
| **Mean Duration Formal Education (years)** | **10.5 ± 5.3** | |
| **Years in Marriage** | **Not Married** | 27 (2.1%) |
| | **≤10 years** | 350 (26.5%) |
| | **11-20 years** | 442 (33.5%) |
| | **> 20 years** | 500 (37.9%) |
| **Number of Siblings** | **None** | 14 (1.1%) |
| | **1–5** | 718 (54.4%) |
| | **> 5** | 587 (44.5%) |
| **Any LUTS** | | 267 (20.2%) |
| **Mild LUTS** | **(IPSS ≤ 7)** | 111 (8.4%) |
| **Moderate LUTS** | **(IPSS 8–19)** | 126 (9.6%) |
| **Severe LUTS** | **(IPSS ≥ 20)** | 30 (2.3%) |

[*LUTS* lower urinary tract symptoms]

influence the time in the course of LUTS that medical care is sought.

## Discussion

At an overall LUTS prevalence rate of 20.2% and moderate to severe LUTS prevalence rate of 11.9% (Table 1), LUTS in men deserve some emphasis in discussions of men's health [25]. This is particularly important realizing that 51.7% of all men reporting any lower urinary tract symptom from this survey are yet to seek medical care, and that 32.7% of men reporting moderate to severe symptoms are as well yet to seek medical care. These findings are similar to findings from other studies [24, 26, 27] and are worrisome because of the health implications of seeking medical care late in this health disorder [17]. It is obvious that some of the primary disease conditions resulting in LUTS have poor prognosis with late presentations to medical care [15, 16]. It is therefore quite disturbing that many of these men (Table 2) experience these lower urinary symptoms for years without seeking medical care.

The explanation for this care seeking behaviour in this cohort of men could be that there is some degree of aversion for orthodox medical care generally, or for medical care for LUTS specifically. However, a good

**Table 2** Duration from onset of LUTS to seeking medical care for the reported LUTS

| Duration of LUTS | Yet to seek care | Sought Medical Care | | |
|---|---|---|---|---|
| | | Within 3mths | In 4-12mths | After 12mths |
| **≤3mths (*N* = 8)** | 8 (100%) | 0 | 0 | 0 |
| **4-12mths (*N* = 51)** | 25 (49.0%) | 8 (15.7%) | 16 (31.4%) | 0 |
| **13-24mths (*N* = 40)** | 20 (50.0%) | 1 (2.5%) | 11 (27.5%) | 8 (20.0%) |
| **25-60mths (*N* = 82)** | 47 (57.3%) | 1 (1.2%) | 15 (18.3%) | 19 (23.2%) |
| **>60mths (*N* = 86)** | 38 (44.2%) | 3 (3.5%) | 13 (15.1%) | 32 (37.2%) |
| **Total (267)** | 138 (51.7%) | 13 (4.9%) | 55 (20.6%) | 59 (22.1%) |

[*mths* months]

**Table 3** Reasons for not seeking medical care across the various durations of LUTS

| Duration of LUTS | Non-Bothersome | Poor Finance | Time Constraint | Advice | Others |
|---|---|---|---|---|---|
| **≤3mths (*N* = 8)** | 4 (50.0%) | 2 (25.0%) | 2 (25.0%) | 0 | 0 |
| **4-12mths (*N* = 25)** | 20 (80.0%) | 5 (20.0%) | 0 | 0 | 0 |
| **13-24mths (*N* = 20)** | 13 (65.0%) | 5 (25.0%) | 0 | 0 | 2 (10.0%) |
| **25-60mths (*N* = 47)** | 34 (72.3%) | 8 (17.0%) | 2 (4.3%) | 2 (4.3%) | 1 (2.1%) |
| **>60mths (*N* = 38)** | 25 (65.8%) | 11 (28.9%) | 0 | 2 (5.3%) | 0 |
| **Total (138)** | 96 (69.6%) | 31 (22.5%) | 4 (2.9%) | 4 (2.9%) | 3 (2.2%) |

proportion (53.2%) of these men reportedly demonstrate good attitude towards early medical care. In addition, when they decided to seek medical care for their LUTS, most (65.9%; Fig. 2) of the respondents from this study consulted medical doctors firstly, demonstrating belief in conventional medical care. So, that these men appreciate the benefit in seeking medical care for health challenges from conventional medical care is not contestable. However, the trigger for seeking medical care for LUTS seems not to be just any lower urinary tract symptom. Curiously, this challenge to early medical care for LUTS seems not peculiar as seen from the review by Roehrborn et al. [28]

From the reasons given by respondents across all LUTS severity and symptom durations for seeking medical care belatedly, LUTS being non-bothersome ranks highest (Table 3) akin to the observation by Griffith et al. [19] So even in low-income economy with poor health insurance coverage, financial constraint does not represent the most prevalent reason for delay in seeking medical care for LUTS in men. To buttress this finding, this study also reveals that respondents' socio-economic status does not have any significant influence on when medical care is sought by men reporting LUTS (Table 4). It is only rational that one does not commit resources in terms of time and money in accessing care that is of doubtful utility. If LUTS are generally trivialized as part of aging in men, or attributed to some other factors [29], then men will fail to appreciate the utility in accessing medical care for LUTS being experienced. This stance needs to be actively corrected through enlightenment programmes since increasing level of formal education and higher exposure to health information are significantly associated with seeking medical care earlier for LUTS [30]. From this study, there is a 3.1 odd that a respondent of low health information index, due to minimal level of exposure to health information from lifestyle, will seek medical care belatedly compared to a respondent of high health information index (Table 4). Similarly, increase in level of formal education attained is associated with decrease in delay in seeking medical care for LUTS (OR 0.86; $p < 0.001$; Table 4).

As regards age of respondent, the younger the respondent, the longer the delay in seeking medical care (p 0.002). This may be because the younger respondent tends to report milder LUTS, is likely to report less bother, and to attribute higher opportunity cost to seeking medical care. On the contrary, the older respondent

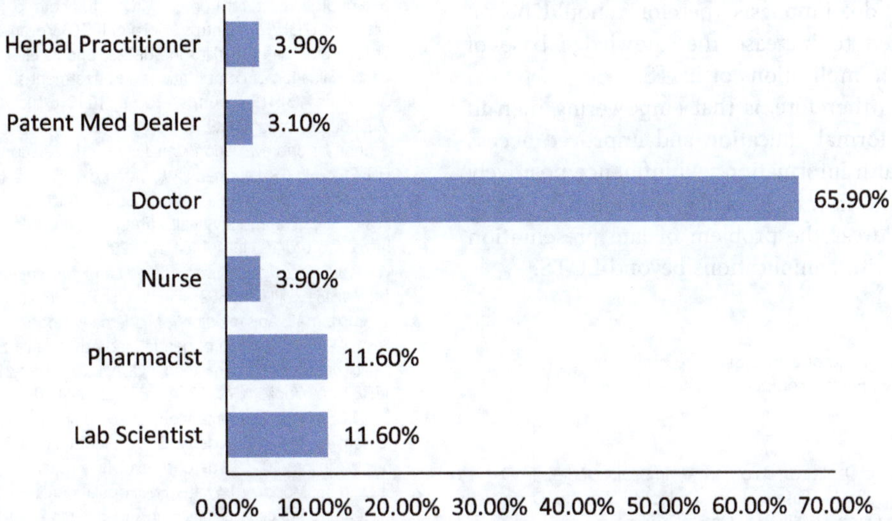


**Fig. 2** Frequency distribution of care-providers accessed firstly by respondents who had accessed medical care for reported LUTS

**Table 4** Factors that influence the decision to seek medical care for LUTS

| Variable | Odds Ratio | 95% CI | | *p*-value |
|---|---|---|---|---|
| **Age** | 0.93 | 0.90 | 0.98 | 0.002 |
| **Education** | 0.86 | 0.81 | 0.92 | < 0.001 |
| **Marriage** | 1.03 | 1.00 | 1.06 | 0.080 |
| **Siblings** | 1.00 | 0.91 | 1.09 | 0.929 |
| **Wealth Index 1** | 1.60 | 0.65 | 3.90 | 0.303 |
| **Wealth Index 2** | 1.41 | 0.61 | 3.28 | 0.425 |
| **Wealth Index 3** | 1.15 | 0.51 | 2.60 | 0.743 |
| **Wealth Index 4** | 0.87 | 0.38 | 1.98 | 0.740 |
| **Wealth Index 5** | | | | |
| **Mild LUTS** | 6.68 | 2.62 | 17.03 | < 0.001 |
| **Moderate LUTS** | 1.14 | 0.51 | 2.55 | 0.755 |
| **Severe LUTS** | | | | |
| **LUTS 4-12 months** | 0.43 | 0.22 | 0.83 | 0.012 |
| **LUTS 13-24 months** | 1.59 | 0.77 | 3.29 | 0.206 |
| **LUTS > 24 months** | | | | |
| **Low Health Information Index** | 3.10 | 1.79 | 5.38 | < 0.001 |
| **High Health Information Index** | | | | |

[*LUTS* lower urinary tract symptoms].

is, in addition, likely to be under more pressure from family and peers to seek medical care.

## Conclusion

The observed key challenge with early presentation for medical care by men experiencing LUTS is that LUTS of various severity are considered non-bothersome. Financial constraint comes into play only when LUTS become bothersome. Wealth-index does not appear to influence when LUTS become bothersome, but older age, higher formal education and higher exposure to health information significantly do. Emphasis therefore should be on strategies designed to increase the knowledge base of men on the health implications of LUTS.

The implication therefore, is that empowering men in Nigeria through formal education and improved access to researched health information will influence positively the time that LUTS in men become bothersome. This in turn will help address the problem of late presentation for medical care with complications beyond LUTS.

#### Abbreviations

LUTS: Lower urinary tract symptoms; BPE: Benign prostate enlargement; QoL: Quality of life; PCA: Principal component analysis

#### Acknowledgements

We acknowledge Dr. Louis Okolie, Dr. Solomon Anyimba, Dr. Jude Ede, Dr. Ekeoma Nwosu, Dr. Uko Uko, Dr. Casmir Nnadi, Dr. Nonso Iwenofu, Dr. Pascal Maduabuchi, Dr. Wilson Onoh, Dr. Kingsley Onyia, Dr. Njideka Oragunye, Dr. Maxwell Isiwu, Dr. Chimuanya Mogbo, Dr. Hyginus Odoh, Dr. Pamela Okafor, Dr. Princewill Osueke, Dr. Arinze Onyia, Dr. Kingsley Bassey and Dr. Nwoku Amy, Dr. Chimuanya Mogbo, Dr. Bassey K Bassey, and Dr. Chinenye Eneh for their roles during data collection.

#### Authors' contributions

IIN contributed substantially in conception, design, data acquisition, analysis and interpretation of data, and in the drafting of the manuscript. ILO contributed substantially in design, analysis and interpretation of acquired data and revision of manuscript. CAN contributed substantially in conception, design, data acquisition, analysis and interpretation of acquired data, and drafting of manuscript. All Authors read and approved of the final version being submitted and agreed to be accountable for all parts of the research work.

#### Competing interests

This manuscript is adapted from the Project work of the corresponding author in partial fulfillment of the requirements for the award of MSc degree in Health Administration and Management. No other conflicts of interest declared.

#### Author details

[1]Department of Surgery, College of Medicine, University of Nigeria Ituku-Ozalla, Enugu PMB 01129, Nigeria. [2]Department of Health Administration and Management, Faculty of Health Sciences and Technology, University of Nigeria Enugu Campus, Enugu, Nigeria.

#### References

1. Abdelmoteleb H, Jefferies ER, Drake MJ. Assessment and management of male lower urinary tract symptoms (LUTS). Int J Surg. 2016;25:164–71 https://doi.org/10.1016/j.ijsu.2015.11.043.
2. Hedlund P, Gratzke C. The endocannabinoid system – a target for treatment of LUTS. Nat Rev Urol. 2016;13(8):463–70 https://doi.org/10.1038/nrurol.2016.110.
3. Liu HT, Jiang YH, Kuo HC. Alteration of urethelial inflammation, apoptosis and junction protein in patients with various bladder conditions and storage bladder symptoms suggest common pathway involved in underlying pathophysiology. Low Urin Tract Symptoms. 2015;7(2):102–7 https://doi.org/10.1111/luts.12062.
4. Bellucci CHS, Ribeiro WO, Hemerly TS, de Bessa J Jr, Antunes AA, KRM L, Bruschini H, Srougi M, Gomes CM. Increased detrusor collagen is associated with detrusor overactivity and decreased bladder compliance in men with benign prostatic obstruction. Prostate Int. 2017;5(2):70–4 https://doi.org/10.1016/j.pmil.2017.01.008.
5. Marshall LM, Holton KF, Parsons JK, Lapidus JA, Ramsey K, Barrett-Connor E. Osteoporotic fractures in men (MrOS) study group. Prostate Cancer Prostatic Dis. 2014;17(3):265–72 https://doi.org/10.1038/pcan.2014.22.
6. Brucker BM, Kalra S. Parkinson's disease and its effect on the lower urinary tract: evaluation of complications and treatment strategies. Urol Clin North Am. 2017;44(3):415–28 https://doi.org/10.1016/j.ucl.2017.04.008.
7. Viuchoud C, Loughlin KR. Benign prostatic hyperplasia: epidemiology, economics and evaluation. Can J Urol. 2015;22(Suppl 1):1–6.
8. Hall SA, Chiu GR, Kaufman DW, Wittert GA, Link CL, McKinlay JB. Commonly used antihypertensives and lower urinary tract symptoms: results from the Boston area community health (BACH) survey. BJU Int. 2012;109(11):1676–84 https://doi.org/10.1111/j.1464-410X.2011.10593.x.
9. Weiss JP. Nocturia: focus on etiology and consequences. Rev Urol. 2012; 14(3–4):48–55 PMID: 23526404. PMCID: PMC3602727.
10. Thompson AE, Anisimowicz Y, Miedema B, Hogg W, Wodchis WP, Aubrey-Bassler K. The influence of gender and other patient characteristics on health care-seeking behaviour: a QUALICOPC study. BMC Fam Pract. 2016; 17:38 https://doi.org/10.1186/s12875-016-0440-0.
11. Sun JK, Smith J. Self-perceptions of aging and perceived barriers to care: reasons for health care delay. Gerontologist. 2017;57(suppl_2):S216–26 https://doi.org/10.1093/geront/gnx014.
12. Stewart TS, Moodley J, Walter FM. Population risk factors for late-stage presentation of cervical cancer in sub-Saharan Africa. Cancer Epidemiol. 2018;53:81–92 https://doi.org/10.1016/j.canep.2018.01.014.

13. Peng Y, Chang W, Zhou H, Hu H, Liang W. Factors associated with health-seeking behavior among migrant workers in Beijing, China. BMC Health Serv Res. 2010;10:69 https://doi.org/10.1186/1472-6963-10-69.
14. Rupert DJ, Gard Read J, Amoozegar JB, Moultrie RR, Taylor OM, O'Donoghue AC, Sullivan HW. Peer-generated health information: the role of online communities in patient and caregiver health decisions. J Health Commun. 2016;21(11):1187–97.
15. Speakman MJ, Cheng X. Management of the complications of BPH/BOO. Indian J Urol. 2014;30(2):208–13 https://doi.org/10.4103/0970-1591.127856.
16. Zargooshi J. Open prostatectomy for benign prostate hyperplasia: short-term outcome in 3000 consecutive patients. Prostate Cancer Prostatic Dis. 2007;10(4):374–7.
17. Ugwumba FO, Ozoemena OF, Okoh AD, Echetabu KN, Mbadiwe OM. Transvesical prostatectomy in the management of benign prostatic hyperplasia in a developing country. Niger J Clin Pract. 2014;17(6):797–801 https://doi.org/10.4103/1119-3077.144402.
18. Lai UC, Wun YT, Luo TC, Pang SM. In a free healthcare system, why do men not consult for lower urinary tract symptoms (LUTS)? Asia Pac Fam Med. 2011;10(1):7 https://doi.org/10.1186/1447-056X-10-7.
19. Griffith JW, Messersmith EE, Gillespie BW, Wiseman JB, Flynn KE, Kirkali Z, Kusek JW, Bavendam T, Cella D, Kreder KJ, Nero JJ, Corona ME, Bradley CS, Kenton KS, Helfand BT, Merion RM, Weinfurt KP, LURN Study Group. Reasons for seeking clinical care for lower urinary tract symptoms: a mixed methods study. J Urol. 2018;199(2):528–35 https://doi.org/10.1016/j.juro.2017.07.067.
20. Aliyu AA, Amadu L. Urbanization, cities, and health: the challenges to Nigeria –a review. Ann Afr Med. 2017;16(4):149–58 https://doi.org/10.4103/aam.aam_1_17.
21. Davis L, Ajzen I, Saunders J, Williams T. The decision of African American students to complete high school: an application of the theory of planned behaviour. Working paper 02-5, Center for Social Development, Washington University U.S.A. 2002. www.gwbweb.wustl.edu/csd. Accessed 2 Apr 2018.
22. IPSS Form. Accessed from (www.urospec.com/uro/Forms/ipss.pdf) on 4 Dec 2017.
23. Nigeria, UNDP. Human Development Report, Nigeria, 2008–2009. Abuja: United Nation Development Programme; 2009. Accessed from (www.nigerianstat.gov.ng) on 20 Feb 2018.
24. Ojewola RW, Oridota ES, Balogun OS, Ogundare EO, Alabi TO. Lower urinary tract symptoms: prevalence, perceptions, and healthcare-seeking behavior amongst Nigerian men. World J Mens Health. 2016;34(3):200–8 https://doi.org/10.5534/wjmh.2016.34.3.200.
25. Nnabugwu II, Ugwumba FO, Udeh EI, Anyimba SK, Okolie LT. The relationship between prevalence and severity of lower urinary tract symptoms (LUTS), and body mass index and mid-abdominal circumference in men in resource-poor community in Southeast Nigeria: a cross-sectional survey. BMC Urol. 2019;19(1):15 https://doi.org/10.1186/s12894-019-0444-x.
26. Lammers HA, van Wijnhoven R, Teunissen TA, Harmsen S, Lagro-Janssen AL. Why do men suffering from LUTS seek primary medical care? A qualitative study. J Eval Clin Pract. 2015;21(5):931–6 https://doi.org/10.1111/jep.12407.
27. Stothers L, Macnab AJ, Bajunirwe F, Mutabazi S, Berkowitz J. Associations between the severity of obstructive lower urinary tract symptoms and care seeking behaviour in rural Africa: a cross sectional survey from Uganda. PLoS One. 2017;12(3):e0173631 https://doi.org/10.1371/journal.pone.0173631.
28. Roehrborn CG, Miner MM, Sadovsky R. Over-the-counter medication availability could augment self-management of male lower urinary tract symptoms. Postgrad Med. 2018:1–9 https://doi.org/10.1080/00325481.2018.1487238.
29. Siu JY. Imprisoned in the cultural stereotypes of overactive bladder: cultural meanings of disease and sick role adaptation in Hong Kong. Nurs Res. 2016;65(5):352–61 https://doi.org/10.1097/NNR.0000000000000177.
30. Houle J, Meunier S, Coulome S, Mercerat C, Gaboury I, Tremblay G, de Montigny F, Cloutier L, Roy B, Auger N, Lavoie B. Peer positive social control and men's health-promoting behaviors. Am J Mens Health. 2017;11(5):1569–79 https://doi.org/10.1177/1557988317711605.

# 19

# Transverse testicular ectopia with Müllerian duct remnant in an incarcerated congenital inguinal hernia

Mostafa Kotb*, Ahmed Hassan and Mohamed Abouheba

**Abstract**

**Background:** Transverse testicular ectopia (TTE) is a rare anomaly characterized by both testes descending through a single inguinal canal. In this report, the diagnosis of TTE was discovered in the event of an incarcerated congenital inguinal hernia in a neonate.

**Case presentation:** We present a case of TTE accompanied by persistent Müllerian duct structures (PMDS) that had been discovered incidentally during inguinal exploration of a 26-day-old boy who presented with an incarcerated congenital inguinal hernia on the right side and left cryptochidism on the left side. The pathogenesis, approach and proposed management of TTE are discussed.

**Conclusion:** TTE is an extremely rare anomaly, especially in neonates, and should be suspected in patients presenting with inguinal hernia on one side and cryptorchidism on the other side.

**Keywords:** Case report, Incarcerated hernia, Müllerian duct, testicular ectopia

## Background

Transverse testicular ectopia (TTE), also named testicular pseudo-duplication or crossed testicular ectopia, is a rare anomaly characterized by both testes descending through a single inguinal canal [1]. Most of the cases (65%) are diagnosed intraoperatively during an inguinal hernia repair, while a few are diagnosed preoperatively [2]. We present a case of TTE accompanied by persistent Müllerian duct structures (PMDS) that had been discovered incidentally during inguinal exploration of a male neonate presenting with an incarcerated congenital inguinal hernia on the right side and left cryptochidism on the left side. The pathogenesis, approach and proposed management of TTE were discussed.

## Case presentation

A 26-day-old boy was referred from a peripheral hospital with a right-sided incarcerated congenital inguinal hernia. The referring pediatrician told his father that he has a palpable testis in his right inguinal canal but no palpable testis on the left side. Apart from a clinically evident right irreducible hernia and empty both hemiscrota, the rest of the examination was unremarkable. After initial resuscitation with intravenous fluids and antibiotics, an urgent operation was undertaken. On inguinal exploration, the hernia sac was found to contain a viable cecum and small bowel loops. After reduction of the contents to the peritoneal cavity, the right testis was found in the inguinal canal. However, a second testis was unexpectedly delivered through the deep inguinal ring. Both testes have independent spermatic cords, i.e. two separate sets of vas deferens and testicular vessels on either side of a T- shaped structure resembling an infantile uterus and fallopian tube (Fig. 1). Because of the shortness of the spermatic cord and the vague nature of this anomaly for the operating surgeon, only a biopsy was taken from both testes and all the structures were

* Correspondence: mostafa.rashad@alexmed.edu.eg
Pediatric Surgery, Alexandria Faculty of Medicine, Alexandria, Egypt

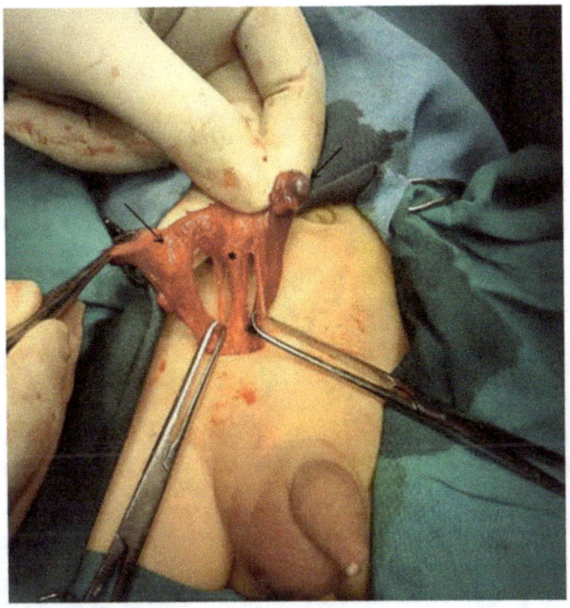

**Fig. 1** Introperative photo showing both testes (arrows) on the right side and rudimentary uterus (asterisk)

returned back to the peritoneal cavity followed by herniotomy.

Postoperative pathology showed normal testicular tissue bilaterally with absent ovarian structures. Karyotyping was done for the patient and revealed a normal 46XY male karyotype. Diagnostic laparoscopy was performed at the age of 6 months, which showed a closed left internal ring on the left side and a widely open internal ring on the right side. In addition, the left sided testis and spermatic cord were found joining their counterparts on the right side through the rudimentary uterus close to the right internal ring. The rudimentary uterus as well as the fallopian tubes were partially excised. Peritoneal dissection was made to gain extra length for both spermatic cords. Orchiopexy was done, with each testis fixed into its corresponding hemiscrotum. The patient had an uneventful recovery. Throughout the 6-month follow-up period, the size and the blood flow of both testes were normal as evaluated by Doppler ultrasound.

## Discussion and conclusions

TTE is a rare entity that usually presents in childhood, with a mean age of 4 years [3]. To our best knowledge, the present case represents the first TTE diagnosed in a neonate with irreducible inguinal hernia. The precise etiology of TTE is still unclear. Nevertheless, various anatomic factors (for instance, tearing or rupture or defective implantation of the gubernaculum, deep inguinal ring occlusion, adhesions developing between the testis and adjacent structures, late closure of the umbilical ring, etc.) are suggested to result in testicular maldescent [4].

TTE can be classified according to the presence of associated anomalies into 3 types; type 1 (associated with hernia only, 50% of the cases), type 2 (associated with PMDS, 30% of cases) and type 3 (associated with genitourinary abnormalities, 20% of cases) [5]. Our case belongs to type 2, which results from defects either in the synthesis or action of Müllerian inhibiting factor (MIF) and is characterized by the presence of uterus and fallopian tubes in otherwise phenotypically normal 46 XY males. PMDS is mostly discovered incidentally during surgery for inguinal hernia or cryptorchidism [6]. In patients with inguinal hernia and cryptorchidism, possible TTE and PMDS must be considered requiring radiologic evaluation of the genitourinary system and karyotyping [7].

Unfortunately, the overall occurrence of malignant transformation is 18%, which is nearly equal to that of abdominal testes in otherwise normal men [8]. Among the tumors which were reported with PMDS are seminoma, embryonal carcinoma, yolk sac tumor and teratoma. Moreover; these testes are subjected to a higher risk of malignant transformations arising from Müllerian remnants to squamous cell carcinoma, adenocarcinoma and papillary cystadenocarcinoma. Hence, long term follow-up for tumors is required [9].

The optimal surgical management of PMDS is still debatable. A staged procedure remains the most acceptable option as long as PMDS is usually found incidentally during surgery for inguinal hernia repair or undescended testis [10]. Testicular biopsies were taken and then replacing the testes, uterus, and fallopian tubes back through the deep inguinal ring to the abdominal cavity along with herniotomy are performed in the first stage. This is to be followed by the definitive surgery after confirming PMDS. Care should be taken as the vasa deferentia are usually found embedded in the wall of the uterus and the epididymis is contained in the mesosalpinx. Therefore, the removal of Müllerian remnants may injure these structures and interfere with the testicular blood supply as well [10]. Given the reported incidence of malignant transformation from the retained Müllerian structures along with their interference with the intrascrotal placement of the testes, as the free segment of the spermatic cord is usually short, partial removal of these structures without jeopardizing the vasa deferentia seems to be a valuable option. This was described by Guerrier et al. [11] that entails extensive dissection of the spermatic cord along with corporal hysterectomy, bilateral proximal salpingectomies while leaving fimbria and cervix attached to the epididymis to avoid vasa deferentia injury, and bilateral orchiopexy.

To sum up, TTE should be put in consideration whenever a patient presents with inguinal hernia on one side and undescended testis on the opposite side. Because of the risk of malignant transformation and interference with scrotal placement of the testis, MD remnants should be removed without jeopardizing the vas deferens, epididymis and testicular vessels in addition to herniotomy and orchiopexy. In addition, a long-term follow-up will be needed for assessment of malignant transformation and fertility in these patients.

#### Abbreviations

MIF: Müllerian inhibiting factor; PMDS: Persistent Müllerian duct structures; TTE: Transverse testicular ectopia

#### Acknowledgements

We thank Prof. Sameh Shehata, Professor of Pediatric Surgery, Alexandria Faculty of Medicine for his continuous and endless support and tips in the process of publication.

#### Authors' contributions

AH and MK has made contributions to conception and design, or acquisition of data; MA has been drafting the manuscript and revising it critically for important intellectual content. All authors read and approved the final manuscript.

#### Competing interests

The authors declare that they have no competing interests.

#### References

1. Prakash A, Jain S, Kela M, Yadav C, Lohiya R, Maheshwari T. Transverse testicular ectopia: what surgeons must know; insights in embryology and management. Arch Int Surg. 2016;6:191–4.
2. Naji H, Peristeris A, Stenman J, Svensson JF, Wester T. Transverse testicular ectopia: three additional cases and a review of the literature. Pediatr Surg Int. 2012;28:703–6.
3. Vaos G, Zavras N. Irreducible inguinal hernia due to crossed testicular ectopia in an infant. Hernia. 2004;8:397–8.
4. Ueno S, Yokoyama S, Hirakawa H. A case of transverse testicular ectopia with Müllerian duct remnant. J Pediatr Surg. 2001;36:1710–2.
5. Ozturk H, Eroglu M, Ozturk H, Uzunlar AK, Okur H. Persistent Müllerian duct syndrome associated with transverse testicular ectopia: report of two cases. FetalPediatr Pathol. 2007;26:41–6.
6. Acikalin MF, Pasaoglu O, Tokar B, Ilgici D, Ilhan H. Persistent Müllerian duct syndrome with transverse testicular ectopia: a case report with literature review. Turk J Med Sci. 2004;34:333–6.
7. Tartar T, Sarac M, Bakal U, Canpolat Ş, Kazez E. Transverse testicular ectopia: two case reports. İstanbul Med J. 2018;19:179–81.
8. Raj V, Redkar R, Krishna S, Tewari S. Rare case of transverse testicular ectopia – case report and review of literature. Int J Surg Case Rep. 2017;41:407–10.
9. Telli O, Gökçe Mİ, Haciyev P, Soygür T, Burgu B. Transverse testicular ectopia: a rare presentation with persistent Müllerian duct syndrome. J Clin Res Pediatr Endocrinol. 2014;6:180–2.
10. Naouar S, Maazoun K, Sahnoun L, et al. Transverse testicular ectopia: a three-case report and review of the literature. Pediatr Urol. 2008;71: 1070–3.
11. Guerrier D, Tran D, Vanderwinden JM, et al. The persistent Müllerian duct syndrome: a molecular approach. J Clin Endocrinol Metab. 1989;68: 46–52.

# 20

# An evidence-based self-management package for urinary incontinence in older women

Yu Fu[1*], E. Andrea Nelson[2] and Linda McGowan[3]

**Abstract**

**Background:** Urinary incontinence (UI) is a distressing condition that limits women's quality of life and places a heavy burden on health care services. Behavioural treatments are recommended as a first-line treatment. An evidence-based self-management package was developed following the Medical Research Council (MRC) framework for complex interventions. This study aimed to evaluate the feasibility and acceptability of the intervention.

**Methods:** A mixed-methods approach was undertaken, namely a randomised controlled feasibility study with nested qualitative study. Fifty women aged 55 or over living with UI, recruited from community centres were randomly assigned to either a 3-month course with the package with a support session or a control group to receive the same package only 3 months later. Principal outcome measures were: self-reported quality of life, UI severity, self-efficacy and psychological status. Analysis of covariance was undertaken to estimate within- and between- group changes for all outcomes. Acceptability was explored using individual interviews at follow-up.

**Results:** Fifty women were randomised (24 to intervention, 26 to control); mean age of 69.7 (±9.1) years and mean UI frequency 2.2 (±2.2) episodes/day at baseline. Overall, 49 women (98%) completed 3-month follow-up (24 in the intervention, 25 in the control). A positive trend was detected in the impact of UI on their personal relationships (− 3.89, $p = 0.088$), symptom severity (− 1.77, $p = 0.025$), UI symptoms scale (− 1.87, $p = 0.031$) and anxiety status (− 2.31, $p = 0.001$), respectively. Changes in quality of life and self-efficacy did not differ significantly between groups. Majority of women (71%) in the intervention group reported subjective improvement after 3 months. Spearman correlation coefficient was 0.43 ($p < 0.05$) between their subjective perception of change and self-efficacy. Women perceived the package being acceptable and described that the package had the potential to increase their knowledge and confidence to manage symptoms and improve quality of life.

**Conclusions:** The study demonstrated that the self-management package is feasible and acceptable for older women with UI. Further studies are needed with a large sample size in clinical settings to evaluate the effectiveness of this package.

**Trial registration:** ISRCTN17194896. Registered on 11th September 2019 (retrospectively registered).

**Keywords:** Urinary incontinence, Self-management, Feasibility, Randomised controlled trial, Acceptability, Mixed methods

* Correspondence: y.fu@leeds.ac.uk
[1]Leeds Institute of Health Sciences, University of Leeds, Leeds LS2 9NL, UK

## Background

Urinary incontinence (UI) is a distressing condition that limits people's quality of life and places a burden on those affected and health and social care services [1, 2]. Prevalence in women is estimated to be around about 40%, with an increase with age [3]. Women living with UI often experience functional limitations and social embarrassment, negatively impacting their mental health [4]. Although several options are available for treating and managing UI, behavioural treatments are recommended as a first-line treatment therapies for stress, urgency and mixed UI by international UI guidelines developed worldwide [5], prior to considering more intensive treatments.

Behavioural treatment programmes focusing on single elements of behavioural strategies have been extensively researched, e.g. pelvic floor muscle exercises (PFME) [6]. These programmes are sometimes challenging to deliver as they need multiple appointments, the involvement of specialised practitioners, and may lack flexibility to respond to individual needs associated with comorbidities in older women. Many women therefore choose to disengage with the service. Only a third of women with UI consult a doctor in European countries such as France, Germany, Spain and the UK, and 20 to 25% of those experiencing significant clinical symptoms seek care and less than half of them receive treatment [7]. A multifaceted intervention involving behavioural strategies may be more effective than a single component for the management of UI in older women [8, 9].

Self-management for chronic conditions is multidimensional and defined as an intervention designed to develop individuals' knowledge, skills or psychological and social resources and their ability to manage their health condition and consequences, through education, training and support [10]. Many self-management interventions have been developed to support people to cope with their health conditions and improve quality of life. Positive outcomes reported include a higher degree of self-efficacy, reduced physical interference, and improved mental health status at follow-up [11–21]. Although evidence for self-management programmes incorporating multifaceted behavioural treatments for use in UI among older women is currently limited, our systematic review concluded that multifaceted self-management interventions including PFME, bladder retraining, or combination behavioural techniques are beneficial.

Following the Medical Research Council (MRC) framework for developing and evaluating complex interventions [22], a self-management package was co-developed with older women with UI and health professionals providing treatment and care. The initial draft of the intervention was informed by synthesis of data from a systematic review and stakeholder interviews with women and health professionals. Both groups preferred an evidence-based self-management package that had the capacity to meet women's individual needs with the flexibility to modify behaviours in coping with UI without significant service provision and/or intensive interaction with health professionals. The initial draft was reviewed and discussed in detail with an expert group which consisted of four women with UI, five health professionals and two lay members. Consensus was reached on the content and format of this self-management package for older women with UI using a normal group technique [23]. However, the feasibility and acceptability of the intervention remained unknown.

## Methods

### Aim

The aim of this study was to evaluate the feasibility, acceptability, and preliminary outcomes of an evidence-based self-management package for UI in older women. Specifically, it was to 1) assess the feasibility of the intervention to evaluate the effectiveness of a self-management package; 2) assess the variation of the main outcome measures to inform sample size considerations for a full randomised controlled trial (RCT); 3) provide preliminary data on the effect of the intervention; 4) understand the benefits/limitations and acceptability of the self-management package compared to no active treatment.

### Design

A mixed-methods approach comprising a two-arm RCT feasibility study with a nested qualitative study was undertaken. The qualitative study was conducted to understand how the intervention might work and explore facilitators and barriers to acceptance of the intervention [24]. This study presented adheres to CONSORT guidelines.

### Patient and public engagement

A project advisory group comprising three older women (aged 55 plus) living with UI and one nurse working in a community continence clinic was set up prior to the commencement of this study, to ensure this study addressed issues that were important and relevant to women. The meeting was led by YF and facilitated by LMc/EAN every 6 months. Participants were provided with background information and clinical guidelines for UI management and consulted for their current experiences and expectations of managing UI. They also reviewed the findings of the systematic review and interview transcripts. All highlighted the need for evidence-based practice that has the ability to engage the wider population and indicated a willingness to use it for UI self-management. The group also supported the application of ethics approval and development of interview schedules.

### Setting

This is a single-centre, randomised controlled feasibility study of self-management package versus wait-list control with 12- week post-intervention follow up. Participants were recruited using flyers posted in community centres of a local Forum for older people in West Yorkshire, UK. A short presentation was also given by the project researcher in most centres.

### Participants

Women were eligible if they were aged 55 or over, had self-reported symptom of involuntary leakage of urine and were able to read and speak English. Individuals who self-reported their UI were caused by neurological diseases affecting the brain and spinal cord, or were cognitively impaired were excluded.

A consecutive sampling strategy was applied to recruit participants in this study. Assuming an attrition rate of 20%, a target of 25 per arm was sufficient to have 20 participants in each arm by the end of the study. This has been recommended as acceptable for a feasibility trial assuming at worst a medium effect size (Cohen's d = 0.2) for a continuous outcome and 80% power [25].

### Randomisation

All participants were recruited prior to randomisation to the intervention. Eligible women were randomised using a 1:1 ratio to either the intervention or control group. The randomisation procedure was performed by a web-based randomisation service (https://sealedenvelope.com/). Due to the nature of the intervention, this study is considered open-label and is not allocation concealed because the researcher delivering the interventions and the participants were aware of group allocation at the time of implementation.

### Intervention

The experimental intervention was the self-management package, co-developed with older women living with UI, health professionals and lay members. The aim of the package was to provide information and practical skills for women to self-manage their UI and other symptoms. Following elements were included: recognition and awareness, getting the support you need, understanding the cause, learning to manage your UI, developing a self-management plan and how can you find out more. Descriptions of self-management techniques such as PFME, bladder training and lifestyle interventions were also provided. The researcher acted as a facilitator and delivered the intervention in person immediately after the completion of baseline data collection. A self-management brochure was also distributed. The intervention group could request a single one-hour support session with the researcher if they had any difficulties in using the package.

The control group did not receive the self-management package or the support session. However they had been given a copy of the same package upon the completion of their follow-up data collection (at 3 months).

### Outcome measures

As this was a feasibility study it was appropriate to explore a range of outcome measures. Standardised self-reported measures were used to assess participants' generic and disease-specific quality of life, UI severity, self-efficacy and psychological health respectively: the EuroQol (EQ-5D-5 L) [26], King's Health Questionnaire (KHQ) [27], International Consultation on Incontinence Questionnaire – urinary incontinence short form (ICIQ-UI SF) [28, 29], Geriatric Self-Efficacy index for urinary incontinence (GSE-UI) [30], and Hospital Anxiety and Depression Scale (HADS) [31]. Data were collected at baseline and three-month follow-up. Patient Global Impression: Improvement (PGI-I) was obtained from the intervention group only at three-month follow up [32]. These measures have been commonly used in research and practice for women with UI.

### Data analysis

Descriptive analyses were undertaken to establish recruitment, drop-out rates and the distribution of baseline and follow-up characteristics and outcomes. For each of the above measures, analysis of covariance (ANCOVA) was conducted adjusting for their baseline values to take account of outcome imbalance at baseline and estimate the impact of intervention compared with control [33, 34]. T-tests and Chi-square tests were applied to compare two groups at baseline and follow-up for continuous and categorical variables, respectively. Intention-to-treat analysis was performed for this study. Data from all subjects were included in the analysis as randomised. To test the appropriateness of the analysis, complete case analysis was undertaken for each of the above outcome measures to identify the relative treatment effects using a linear (for continuous variables) and logistic (for binary outcomes) mixed model. For all analyses, a two-tailed $p$-value less than 0.05 was considered statistically significant and a p-value between 0.05 and 0.1 was interpreted as indicating a trend [35, 36].

### Nested qualitative study

Women in the intervention group were eligible to participate in this subsequent qualitative study aiming to understand the acceptability of the package. They were purposively recruited considering different types of UI, number of years living with UI, to enable wider discussions on the self-management package and their experience. The concept of data saturation guided sample size for this qualitative study [37].

Semi-structured individual interviews using open-ended questions were undertaken at follow-up. Interviews were conducted either face-to-face in the participants' homes, in a meeting room at the University, or by telephone, based on participants' preferences. Interviews were digitally recorded with permission and transcribed verbatim for analysis. Interviews focused on exploring participants' experience of managing symptoms guided by the intervention, facilitators and barriers to the use of the package, comments on the content and format, feedback on outcome measures used and suggestions on dissemination strategy.

Data analysis was commenced during the interview phase and the transcription, and continued during the analysis of the transcriptions, hence early commencement of analysis facilitated the development of subsequent interviews [38]. Data were analysed using thematic analysis [39], involving a six-step procedure: familiarising the data, generating initial codes, searching for themes, reviewing themes, defining and naming themes, and producing the report. Although they were presented as a step-by-step procedure, the analysis was an iterative and reflexive process to finalise the themes. To ensure trustworthiness and rigour of the analysis, we double coded the data as a validity check and explored alternative interpretations of the data and through discussion with members of the research team. Interview transcripts were managed and analysed using Nvivo, a qualitative software programme for organising and coding the data [40].

## Results

### Participants characteristics

Overall 50 participants ($M_{age}$ =69.7, *SD* = 9.1), were randomly allocated to either intervention ($n$ = 24, $M_{age}$ =69.5, *SD* = 8.9) or control group ($n$ = 26, $M_{age}$ =69.8, *SD* = 9.5). During the 3 months follow-up, no one in the intervention group requested the support session with the researcher. One woman in the control group dropped out due to admission to the hospital for other health conditions. A total of 49 participants with a mean age 69.6 (SD = 9.1) were included in the complete case analysis. No significant differences were found for all demographics and UI characteristics collected at baseline, indicating that randomisation was achieved between the intervention and control groups. The majority were white British (77.6%), completed secondary and higher education (91.8%), were retired (71.4%), and had delivered 2 or more children (71.5%). The number of participants was similar across different UI types. Please see participant's characteristics in Table 1.

### Outcome measures

Medians, interquartile range (IQR), mean, standard deviation (SD) and $p$-values of all baseline and follow-up outcomes are shown in Tables 2 and 3, respectively. There were no differences shown in general quality of life, UI symptoms scale and emotional health status at baseline, however groups differed with regard to KHQ severity measures (34.03 vs 48.67, $p$ = 0.028) and self-efficacy (84.96 vs 57.76, $p < 0.001$). At follow-up, differences were detected in KHQ symptom severity (6.38 vs 9.04, $p$ = 0.006), UI symptoms scale (5.38 vs 7.76, $p$ = 0.022), self-efficacy (89.13 vs 69.08, $p$ = 0.007), and anxiety (5.13 vs 7.80, $p$ = 0.049) at 3-month follow-up.

The effect of the self-management intervention on outcome measures between intervention and control groups were demonstrated in Table 4. The difference captured on each outcome measure was further shown in Figs. 1, 2, 3, 4, 5, 6, 7, 8 and 9, respectively. Participants' general quality of life were improved within both groups after the follow-up, however no significant difference was identified (see Figs. 1 and 2). Similarly, no difference was shown in UI specific quality of life (see Figs. 3 and 4), self-efficacy (see Fig. 7), or depression status (see Fig. 9) between groups. However, significant differences were detected in participants' KHQ symptom severity (− 1.77, $p$ = 0.025; also see Fig. 5), ICIQ-UI SF symptoms scale (− 1.87, $p$ = 0.031; also see Fig. 6), and their anxiety status (− 2.31, $p$ = 0.001; also see Fig. 8), respectively. A positive trend was also observed in the participants' KHQ personal relationships (− 3.89, $p$ = 0.088; also see Fig. 4).

The relationship between the participants' perceived improvement and the difference in outcomes within the intervention group was assessed using Spearman correlations (Table 5). There was a significant correlation shown between PGI-I and GSE-UI ($r_s$= 0.43, $p < 0.05$). Mean change in GSE-UI for participants who responded "better" on the PGI-I were significantly higher than those who responded "no change" or "worse".

### Qualitative findings

Individual interviews were undertaken with 15 participants from the intervention group at their homes.

**Table 1** Baseline demographics and characteristics

| Variable | Overall | | Intervention group | | Control group | | p-value |
|---|---|---|---|---|---|---|---|
| | *n* | % | *n* | % | *n* | % | |
| Total | 49 | | 24 | | 25 | | |
| Age (Mean, SD) | 69.7 | 9.1 | 69.5 | 8.9 | 69.6 | 9.6 | 0.994 |
| Ethnicity | | | | | | | 0.157 |
| White British | 38 | 77.6% | 16 | 66.7% | 22 | 88.0% | |
| Asian Indian | 9 | 18.4% | 7 | 29.2% | 2 | 8.0% | |
| Mixed White and Black African | 2 | 4.1% | 1 | 4.2% | 1 | 4.0% | |
| Education | | | | | | | 0.486 |
| Primary | 4 | 8.2% | 3 | 12.5% | 1 | 4.0% | |
| Secondary | 16 | 32.7% | 9 | 37.5% | 7 | 28.0% | |
| Further | 14 | 28.6% | 5 | 20.8% | 9 | 36.0% | |
| Higher | 15 | 30.6% | 7 | 29.2% | 8 | 32.0% | |
| Religion | | | | | | | 0.108 |
| No religion | 9 | 18.4% | 5 | 20.8% | 4 | 16.0% | |
| Christian | 31 | 63.3% | 12 | 50.0% | 19 | 76.0% | |
| Hindu | 9 | 18.4% | 7 | 29.2% | 2 | 8.0% | |
| Marital status | | | | | | | 0.365 |
| Single | 6 | 12.2% | 3 | 12.5% | 3 | 12.0% | |
| Married | 27 | 55.1% | 15 | 62.5% | 12 | 48.0% | |
| Separated | 1 | 2.0% | 0 | 0.0% | 1 | 4.0% | |
| Divorced | 3 | 6.1% | 0 | 0.0% | 3 | 12.0% | |
| Widowed | 12 | 24.5% | 6 | 25.0% | 6 | 24.0% | |
| Employment | | | | | | | 0.573 |
| Full time employed | 3 | 6.1% | 1 | 4.2% | 2 | 8.0% | |
| Part time employed | 5 | 10.2% | 3 | 12.5% | 2 | 8.0% | |
| Self employed | 1 | 2.0% | 0 | 0.0% | 1 | 4.0% | |
| Not in paid employment | 2 | 4.1% | 1 | 4.2% | 1 | 4.0% | |
| Unemployed-looking for work | 1 | 2.0% | 0 | 0.0% | 1 | 4.0% | |
| Retired | 35 | 71.4% | 19 | 79.2% | 16 | 64.0% | |
| Unable to work | 2 | 4.1% | 0 | 0.0% | 2 | 8.0% | |
| Children | | | | | | | 0.421 |
| None | 11 | 22.4% | 5 | 20.8% | 6 | 24.0% | |
| 1 | 3 | 6.1% | 1 | 4.2% | 2 | 8.0% | |
| 2 | 18 | 36.7% | 9 | 37.5% | 9 | 36.0% | |
| 3 | 11 | 22.4% | 4 | 16.7% | 7 | 28.0% | |
| UI type | | | | | | | 0.672 |
| Stress UI | 14 | 28.6% | 8 | 33.3% | 6 | 24.0% | |
| Urge UI | 17 | 34.7% | 7 | 29.2% | 10 | 40.0% | |
| Mixed UI | 18 | 36.7% | 9 | 37.5% | 9 | 36.0% | |
| Frequency of UI (average per day) | | | | | | | 0.070 |
| None | 16 | 32.7% | 12 | 50.0% | 4 | 16.0% | |
| 1 | 8 | 16.3% | 3 | 12.5% | 5 | 20.0% | |
| 2 | 5 | 10.2% | 1 | 4.2% | 4 | 16.0% | |
| 3 | 9 | 18.4% | 5 | 20.8% | 4 | 16.0% | |
| 4+ | 11 | 22.4% | 3 | 12.5% | 8 | 32.0% | |

*UI* urinary incontinence

**Table 2** Median, interquartile range (IQR), mean, standard deviation (SD) and *p*-values of outcome measurements at baseline

| Variable | Dimensions | Intervention group | | | | | | Control group | | | | | | *p*-value |
|---|---|---|---|---|---|---|---|---|---|---|---|---|---|---|
| | | *n* | % | Median | IQR | Mean | SD | *n* | % | Median | IQR | Mean | SD | |
| EQ-5D-5L | Mobility | | | | | | | | | | | | | 0.675 |
| | No/slight problem | 18 | 75.0% | | | | | 20 | 80.0% | | | | | |
| | Moderate/Severe/extreme problem | 6 | 25.0% | | | | | 5 | 20.0% | | | | | |
| | Selfcare | | | | | | | | | | | | | 0.527 |
| | No/slight problem | 22 | 91.7% | | | | | 24 | 96.0% | | | | | |
| | Moderate/Severe/extreme problem | 2 | 8.3% | | | | | 1 | 4.0% | | | | | |
| | Usual activities | | | | | | | | | | | | | 0.662 |
| | No/slight problem | 19 | 79.2% | | | | | 21 | 84.0% | | | | | |
| | Moderate/Severe/extreme problem | 5 | 20.8% | | | | | 4 | 16.0% | | | | | |
| | Pain & discomfort | | | | | | | | | | | | | 0.315 |
| | No/slight problem | 14 | 58.3% | | | | | 18 | 72.0% | | | | | |
| | Moderate/Severe/extreme problem | 10 | 41.7% | | | | | 7 | 28.0% | | | | | |
| | Anxiety & depression | | | | | | | | | | | | | 0.524 |
| | No/slight problem | 20 | 83.3% | | | | | 19 | 76.0% | | | | | |
| | Moderate/Severe/extreme problem | 4 | 16.7% | | | | | 6 | 24.0% | | | | | |
| | Index | 24 | | 0.90 | 0.23 | 0.82 | 0.17 | 25 | | 0.83 | 0.14 | 0.79 | 0.19 | 0.643 |
| | VAS | 24 | | 77.50 | 27.50 | 71.67 | 18.04 | 25 | | 70.00 | 25.00 | 64.40 | 25.59 | 0.258 |
| KHQ | Part I | | | | | | | | | | | | | |
| | General health perception (0-100) | 24 | | 25.00 | 25.00 | 33.33 | 21.70 | 25 | | 25.00 | 25.00 | 32.00 | 15.34 | 0.804 |
| | Incontinence impact (0-100) | 24 | | 33.33 | 33.33 | 45.83 | 23.70 | 24 | | 66.67 | 33.33 | 56.94 | 20.80 | 0.091 |
| | Part II | | | | | | | | | | | | | |
| | Role limitations (0-100) | 24 | | 16.67 | 33.33 | 20.14 | 22.51 | 25 | | 33.33 | 33.33 | 33.33 | 24.06 | 0.054 |
| | Physical limitations (0-100) | 24 | | 16.67 | 41.67 | 22.92 | 22.42 | 25 | | 33.33 | 33.33 | 30.67 | 20.79 | 0.216 |
| | Social limitations (0-100) | 24 | | 0.00 | 13.89 | 9.03 | 13.19 | 25 | | 0.00 | 22.22 | 16.44 | 24.40 | 0.195 |
| | Personal relationships (0-100) | 15 | | 0.00 | 0.00 | 5.56 | 12.06 | 14 | | 0.00 | 0.00 | 11.90 | 25.68 | 0.396 |
| | Emotions (0-100) | 24 | | 11.11 | 22.22 | 16.67 | 19.93 | 24 | | 11.11 | 11.11 | 17.59 | 14.98 | 0.856 |
| | Sleep/energy (0-100) | 24 | | 33.33 | 41.67 | 37.50 | 28.34 | 25 | | 50.00 | 50.00 | 47.33 | 32.16 | 0.263 |
| | Severity measures (0-100) | 24 | | 33.33 | 29.17 | 34.03 | 22.10 | 25 | | 41.67 | 33.33 | 48.67 | 22.91 | **0.028** |
| | Part III | | | | | | | | | | | | | |
| | Symptom severity scale (0-30) | 24 | | 7.50 | 5.50 | 8.00 | 4.39 | 25 | | 10.00 | 3.00 | 9.92 | 4.06 | 0.119 |
| ICIQ-UI SF | Scale (0-21) | 24 | | 8.00 | 6.50 | 8.63 | 4.03 | 25 | | 9.00 | 6.00 | 9.68 | 4.19 | 0.374 |
| GSE-UI | Scale (0-120) | 24 | | 84.50 | 33.50 | 84.96 | 18.89 | 25 | | 55.00 | 23.00 | 57.76 | 23.55 | **0.000** |
| HADS | Anxiety scale (0-21) | 24 | | 6.50 | 6.50 | 7.13 | 5.12 | 25 | | 7.00 | 5.00 | 7.56 | 4.56 | 0.755 |
| | Normal | 13 | 54.2% | | | | | 13 | 52.0% | | | | | 0.868 |
| | Mild | 7 | 29.2% | | | | | 6 | 24.0% | | | | | |
| | Moderate | 2 | 8.3% | | | | | 4 | 16.0% | | | | | |
| | Severe | 2 | 8.3% | | | | | 2 | 8.0% | | | | | |
| | Depression scale (0-21) | 24 | | 3.00 | 3.50 | 3.67 | 3.29 | 25 | | 3.00 | 4.00 | 3.88 | 4.02 | 0.840 |
| | Normal | 20 | 83.3% | | | | | 23 | 92.0% | | | | | 0.318 |
| | Mild | 2 | 8.3% | | | | | 0 | 0.0% | | | | | |
| | Moderate | 2 | 8.3% | | | | | 1 | 4.0% | | | | | |
| | Severe | 0 | | | | | | 0 | | | | | | |

T-tests for continuous variables and chi-square tests for categorical variables*VAS* Visual Analogue Scale, *KHQ* King's Health Questionnaire, *ICIQ-UI SF* International Consultation on Incontinence Questionnaire – urinary incontinence short form, *GSE-UI* Geriatric Self-Efficacy index for urinary incontinence, *HADS* Hospital Anxiety and Depression Scale

**Table 3** Median, interquartile range (IQR), mean, standard deviation (SD) and p-values of outcome measurements at 12-week follow up

| Variable | Dimensions | Intervention group | | | | | | Control group | | | | | | *p*-value |
|---|---|---|---|---|---|---|---|---|---|---|---|---|---|---|
| | | *n* | % | Median | IQR | Mean | SD | *n* | % | Median | IQR | Mean | SD | |
| EQ-5D-5L | Mobility | | | | | | | | | | | | | 0.478 |
| | No/slight problem | 21 | 87.5% | | | | | 20 | 80.0% | | | | | |
| | Moderate/Severe/extreme problem | 3 | 12.5% | | | | | 5 | 20.0% | | | | | |
| | Selfcare | | | | | | | | | | | | | 0.322 |
| | No/slight problem | 24 | 100.0% | | | | | 24 | 96.0% | | | | | |
| | Moderate/Severe/extreme problem | 0 | 0.0% | | | | | 1 | 4.0% | | | | | |
| | Usual activities | | | | | | | | | | | | | 0.950 |
| | No/slight problem | 20 | 83.3% | | | | | 21 | 84.0% | | | | | |
| | Moderate/Severe/extreme problem | 4 | 16.7% | | | | | 4 | 16.0% | | | | | |
| | Pain & discomfort | | | | | | | | | | | | | 0.682 |
| | No/slight problem | 17 | 70.8% | | | | | 19 | 76.0% | | | | | |
| | Moderate/Severe/extreme problem | 7 | 29.2% | | | | | 6 | 24.0% | | | | | |
| | Anxiety & depression | | | | | | | | | | | | | 0.957 |
| | No/slight problem | 21 | 87.5% | | | | | 22 | 88.0% | | | | | |
| | Moderate/Severe/extreme problem | 3 | 12.5% | | | | | 3 | 12.0% | | | | | |
| | Index | 24 | | 0.92 | 0.26 | 0.86 | 0.16 | 25 | | 0.88 | 0.16 | 0.83 | 0.19 | 0.471 |
| | VAS | 24 | | 80.00 | 20.00 | 78.54 | 17.60 | 25 | | 75.00 | 15.00 | 73.00 | 14.93 | 0.240 |
| KHQ | Part I | | | | | | | | | | | | | |
| | General health perception (0-100) | 24 | | 25.00 | 12.50 | 30.21 | 23.29 | 25 | | 25.00 | 25.00 | 31.00 | 20.77 | 0.900 |
| | Incontinence impact (0-100) | 24 | | 33.33 | 33.33 | 45.83 | 21.56 | 25 | | 33.33 | 33.33 | 49.33 | 25.68 | 0.609 |
| | Part II | | | | | | | | | | | | | |
| | Role limitations (0-100) | 24 | | 16.67 | 33.33 | 20.14 | 23.04 | 25 | | 33.33 | 33.33 | 30.67 | 23.90 | 0.123 |
| | Physical limitations (0-100) | 24 | | 16.67 | 33.33 | 22.92 | 22.42 | 25 | | 33.33 | 33.33 | 32.67 | 24.76 | 0.156 |
| | Social limitations (0-100) | 24 | | 0.00 | 5.56 | 5.56 | 10.87 | 25 | | 0.00 | 11.11 | 8.22 | 20.98 | 0.581 |
| | Personal relationships (0-100) | 16 | | 0.00 | 0.00 | 0.00 | 0.00 | 16 | | 0.00 | 0.00 | 5.21 | 11.74 | **0.086** |
| | Emotions (0-100) | 24 | | 11.11 | 22.22 | 12.50 | 14.40 | 25 | | 11.11 | 22.22 | 16.44 | 20.06 | 0.435 |
| | Sleep/energy (0-100) | 24 | | 16.67 | 33.33 | 27.08 | 31.01 | 25 | | 33.33 | 33.33 | 37.33 | 31.28 | 0.255 |
| | Severity measures (0-100) | 24 | | 25.00 | 16.67 | 26.39 | 17.66 | 25 | | 33.33 | 25.00 | 37.33 | 20.99 | **0.055** |
| | Part III | | | | | | | | | | | | | |
| | Symptom severity scale (0-30) | 24 | | 6.00 | 4.00 | 6.38 | 2.93 | 25 | | 10.00 | 4.00 | 9.04 | 3.51 | **0.006** |
| ICIQ-UI SF | Scale (0-21) | 24 | | 4.50 | 4.00 | 5.38 | 2.83 | 25 | | 9.00 | 5.00 | 7.76 | 4.08 | **0.022** |
| GSE-UI | Scale (0-120) | 24 | | 94.50 | 31.00 | 89.13 | 23.86 | 25 | | 67.00 | 34.00 | 69.08 | 25.46 | **0.007** |
| HADS | Anxiety scale (0-21) | 24 | | 5.00 | 6.00 | 5.13 | 4.59 | 25 | | 7.00 | 5.00 | 7.80 | 4.65 | **0.049** |
| | Normal | 19 | 79.2% | | | | | 16 | 64.0% | | | | | 0.593 |
| | Mild | 2 | 8.3% | | | | | 4 | 16.0% | | | | | |
| | Moderate | 2 | 8.3% | | | | | 2 | 8.0% | | | | | |
| | Severe | 1 | 4.2% | | | | | 3 | 12.0% | | | | | |
| | Depression scale (0-21) | 24 | | 2.00 | 3.50 | 3.08 | 3.28 | 25 | | 3.00 | 3.00 | 3.44 | 3.92 | 0.732 |
| | Normal | 21 | 87.5% | | | | | 22 | 88.0% | | | | | 0.720 |
| | Mild | 2 | 8.3% | | | | | 1 | 4.0% | | | | | |
| | Moderate | 1 | 4.2% | | | | | 1 | 4.0% | | | | | |
| | Severe | 0 | 0.0% | | | | | 0 | | | | | | |

T-tests for continuous variables and chi-square tests for categorical variables *VAS* Visual Analogue Scale, *KHQ* King's Health Questionnaire, *ICIQ-UI SF* International Consultation on Incontinence Questionnaire – urinary incontinence short form, *GSE-UI* Geriatric Self-Efficacy index for urinary incontinence, *HADS* Hospital Anxiety and Depression Scale

**Table 4** Mean, standard error (SE) and p-values of pre-post intervention differences and treatment effect

| Variable | Dimensions | Baseline difference[a] | | | Follow-up difference[a] | | | Treatment effect[c] | | |
|---|---|---|---|---|---|---|---|---|---|---|
| | | OR[b]/Coef. | SE | *p*-value | OR[b]/Coef. | SE | *p*-value | OR[b]/Coef. | SE | *p*-value |
| EQ-5D-5L | Mobility | | | | | | | | | |
| | No/slight problem | | | | | | | | | |
| | Moderate/Severe/extreme problem | 1.33 | 0.92 | 0.675 | 0.57 | 0.45 | 0.481 | 0.32 | 0.33 | 0.267 |
| | Selfcare | | | | | | | | | |
| | No/slight problem | | | | | | | | | |
| | Moderate/Severe/extreme problem | | | | | | | | | |
| | Usual activities | | | | | | | | | |
| | No/slight problem | | | | | | | | | |
| | Moderate/Severe/extreme problem | 1.38 | 1.02 | 0.663 | 1.05 | 0.81 | 0.950 | 0.74 | 0.77 | 0.774 |
| | Pain & discomfort | | | | | | | | | |
| | No/slight problem | | | | | | | | | |
| | Moderate/Severe/extreme problem | 1.84 | 1.12 | 0.317 | 1.30 | 0.85 | 0.683 | 0.63 | 0.62 | 0.637 |
| | Anxiety & depression | | | | | | | | | |
| | No/slight problem | | | | | | | | | |
| | Moderate/Severe/extreme problem | 0.63 | 0.46 | 0.526 | 1.05 | 0.91 | 0.957 | 1.24 | 1.14 | 0.811 |
| | Index | 0.02 | 0.05 | 0.643 | 0.04 | 0.05 | 0.471 | 0.02 | 0.03 | 0.540 |
| | VAS | 7.27 | 6.35 | 0.258 | 5.54 | 4.66 | 0.240 | 3.82 | 4.51 | 0.402 |
| KHQ | Part I | | | | | | | | | |
| | General health perception (0-100) | 1.33 | 5.35 | 0.804 | -0.79 | 6.30 | 0.900 | -1.63 | 5.38 | 0.763 |
| | Incontinence impact (0-100) | -11.11 | 6.44 | **0.091** | -3.50 | 6.79 | 0.609 | 3.07 | 6.26 | 0.626 |
| | Part II | | | | | | | | | |
| | Role limitations (0-100) | -13.19 | 6.66 | **0.054** | -10.53 | 6.71 | 0.123 | -1.06 | 4.96 | 0.831 |
| | Physical limitations (0-100) | -7.75 | 6.17 | 0.216 | -9.75 | 6.76 | 0.156 | -3.82 | 4.96 | 0.446 |
| | Social limitations (0-100) | -7.42 | 5.64 | 0.195 | -2.67 | 4.80 | 0.581 | 1.66 | 3.61 | 0.648 |
| | Personal relationships (0-100) | -6.35 | 7.37 | 0.396 | -5.21 | 2.93 | **0.086** | -3.89 | 2.19 | **0.088** |
| | Emotions (0-100) | -0.93 | 5.09 | 0.856 | -3.94 | 5.01 | 0.435 | -3.44 | 3.24 | 0.294 |
| | Sleep/energy (0-100) | -9.83 | 8.67 | 0.263 | -10.25 | 8.90 | 0.255 | -3.68 | 6.92 | 0.598 |
| | Severity measures (0-100) | -14.64 | 6.44 | **0.028** | -10.94 | 5.55 | **0.055** | -1.36 | 3.86 | 0.725 |
| | Part III | | | | | | | | | |
| | Symptom severity scale (0-30) | -1.92 | 1.21 | 0.119 | -2.67 | 0.93 | **0.006** | -1.77 | 0.76 | **0.025** |
| ICIQ-UI SF | Scale (0-21) | -1.06 | 1.18 | 0.374 | -2.39 | 1.01 | **0.022** | -1.87 | 0.84 | **0.031** |
| GSE-UI | Scale (0-120) | 27.20 | 6.11 | **0.000** | 20.05 | 7.05 | **0.007** | -4.90 | 5.16 | 0.348 |
| HADS | Anxiety scale (0-21) | -0.44 | 1.38 | 0.755 | -2.68 | 1.32 | **0.049** | -2.31 | 0.66 | **0.001** |
| | Normal | | | | | | | | | |
| | Ill | 0.92 | 0.53 | 0.879 | 0.47 | 0.31 | 0.245 | 0.34 | 0.28 | 0.188 |
| | Depression scale (0-21) | -0.21 | 1.05 | 0.840 | -0.36 | 1.03 | 0.732 | -0.17 | 0.46 | 0.715 |
| | Normal | | | | | | | | | |
| | Ill | 2.30 | 2.11 | 0.364 | 1.05 | 0.91 | 0.957 | 0.44 | 0.54 | 0.505 |

*VAS* Visual Analogue Scale, *KHQ* King's Health Questionnaire, *ICIQ-UI SF* International Consultation on Incontinence Questionnaire – urinary incontinence short form, *GSE-UI* Geriatric Self-Efficacy index for urinary incontinence, *HADS* Hospital Anxiety and Depression Scale[a]Difference=intervention-control; [b]OR: odds ratio; [c]For each outcome, analysis of covariance (ANCOVA) model with the baseline outcome was used to estimate the treatment effect

Participants ranged in age from 55 to 86 years. The majority were retired (11; 73%) and had suffered from UI for more than 5 years (11; 73%), but had received no support (13; 87%) from health services.

Each interview lasted between 15 and 48 min. A total of four themes were generated. Facilitators and barriers to the use of the self-management package followed by suggestions were also explored under each theme.

#### *Raising awareness and gaining/refreshing knowledge*

All participants found that this package had raised their attention to UI management as well as the

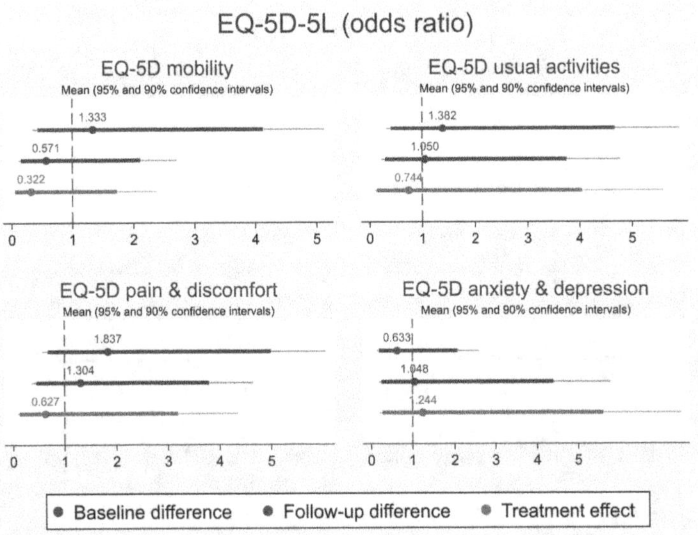


**Fig. 1** Mean (95 and 90% confidence intervals) of pre-post intervention differences and treatment effect for EQ-5D

resources and support available. Some participants learned new knowledge and management skills, while others found it useful to help refresh their memory. Positive comments were received on the fact that this package gathered both information and practical skills in a systematic and structured manner, accompanied by tips shared by women and health professionals.

> *"Yeah, I found the information on how to do the pelvic floor muscle exercises really good, it describes exactly what you should do and how much you should do.." (W5)*

A few participants also expressed the need for more detailed information and tips to meet their needs. For instance, information and explanation were desired for biofeedback, vaginal cones, pads and how certain lifestyles impacted on UI symptoms and severity. In addition, some participants shared strategies and experiences of managing UI, including yoga, weight management programmes, and using reminders to practice PFME.

Half of the participants also identified the bladder diary as a potential barrier to the use of this book. For people who were in employment or regularly involved in outdoor activities, they felt that it was

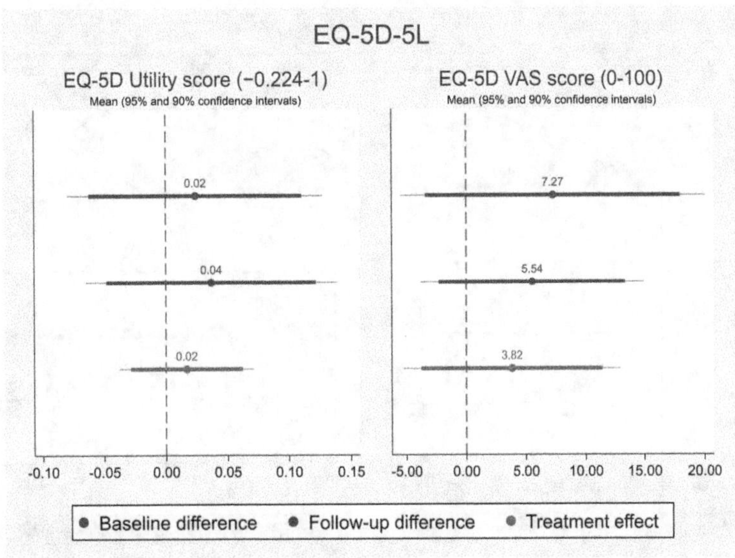


**Fig. 2** Mean (95 and 90% confidence intervals) of pre-post intervention differences and treatment effect for EQ-5D utility and VAS scores

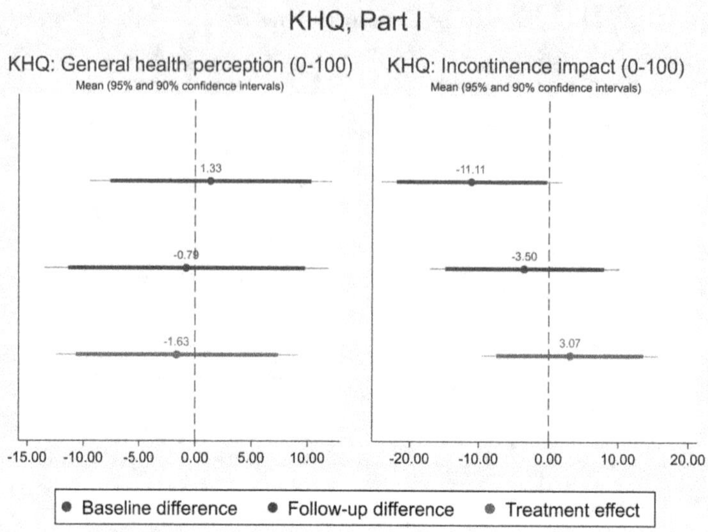


**Fig. 3** Mean (95 and 90% confidence intervals) of pre-post intervention differences and treatment effect for KHQ, Part I

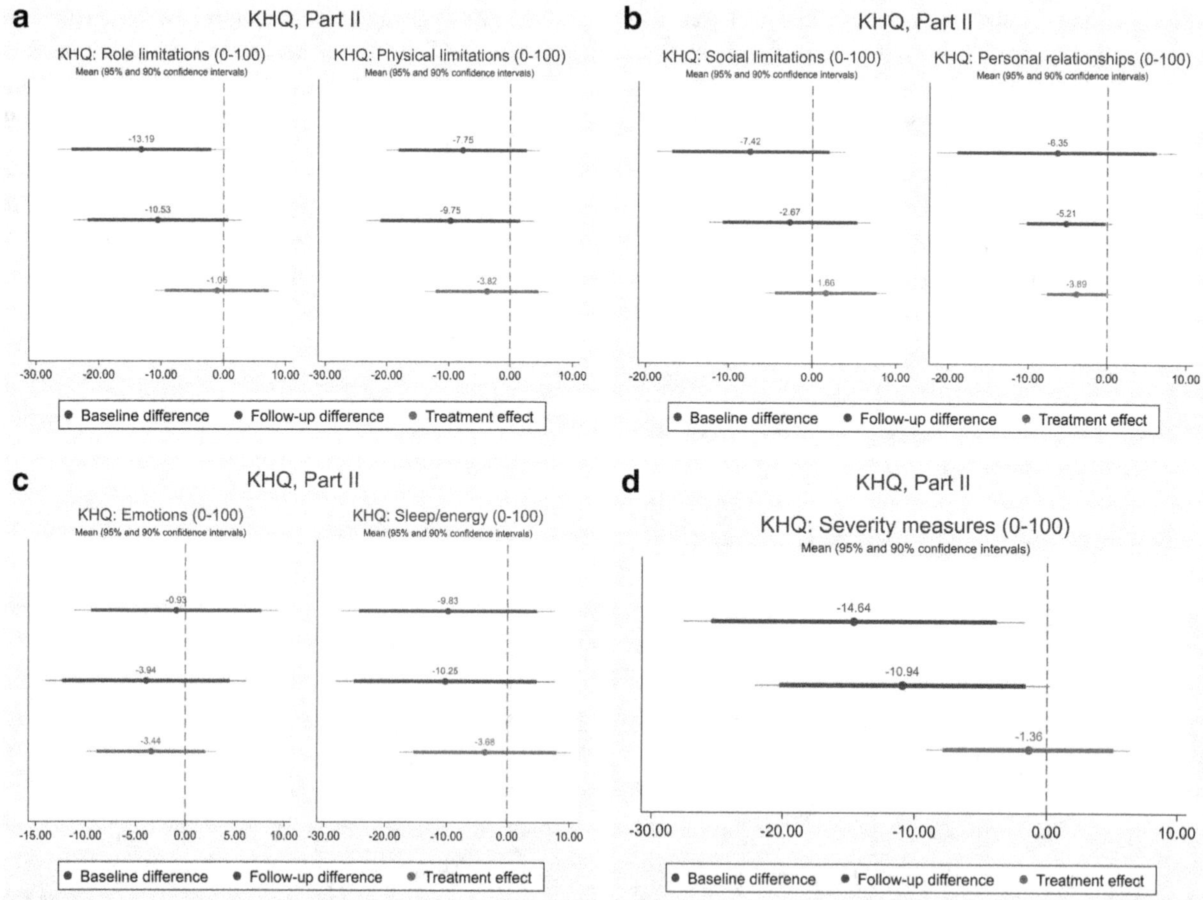


**Fig. 4** Mean (95 and 90% confidence intervals) of pre-post intervention differences and treatment effect for KHQ, Part II

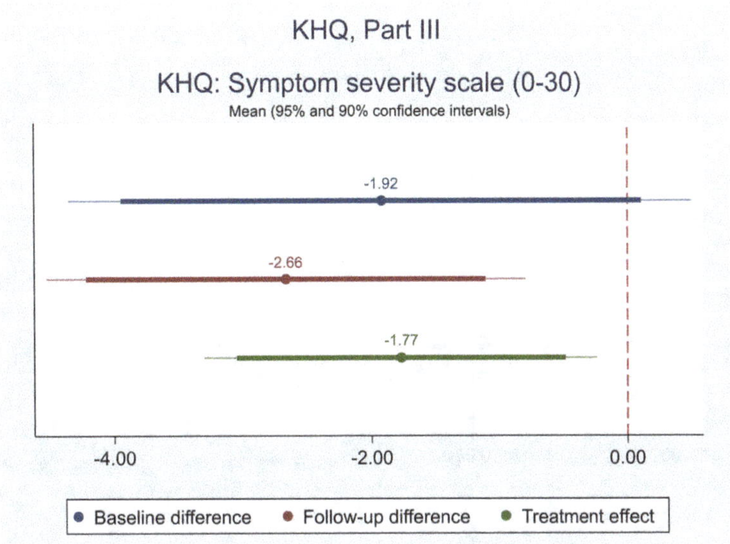


**Fig. 5** Mean (95 and 90% confidence intervals) of pre-post intervention differences and treatment effect for KHQ, Part III

difficult and infeasible to measure intake of fluids and volume voided.

#### *Feeling more confident and motivated to management UI*

Participants generally felt more equipped and confident in managing their UI with resources and support supplied in the package.

> *"...we can do this, at least we know where to contact, we can tell the doctors also but if it happens to somebody you can tell them and they can do this."(W24)*

Participants also expressed their desire to motivate for self-management, however many of them did not practice as much as they would like to due to other commitments. Hence they suggested the inclusion of information and strategies on how to stay motivated and develop adherence.

> *"I suspect a lot of people would read the book, and think, oh yeah, that's a really good idea, I ought to be doing that, and then never, ever actually do it."(W46)*

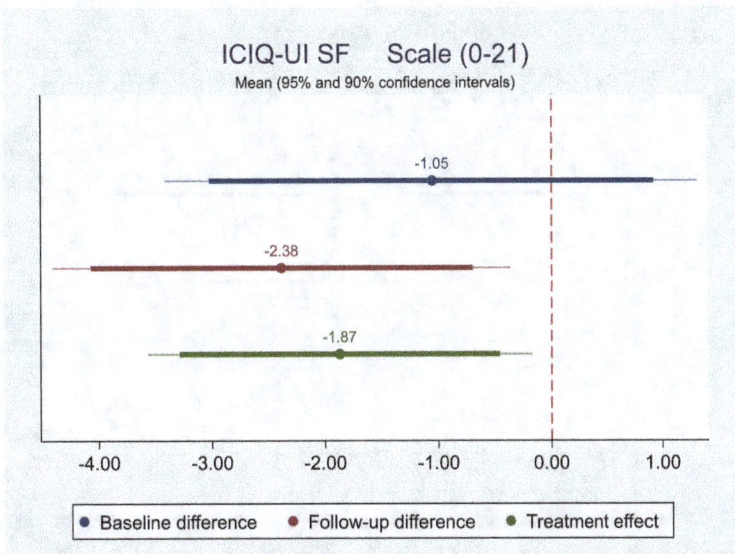


**Fig. 6** Mean (95 and 90% confidence intervals) of pre-post intervention differences and treatment effect for ICIQ-UI SF

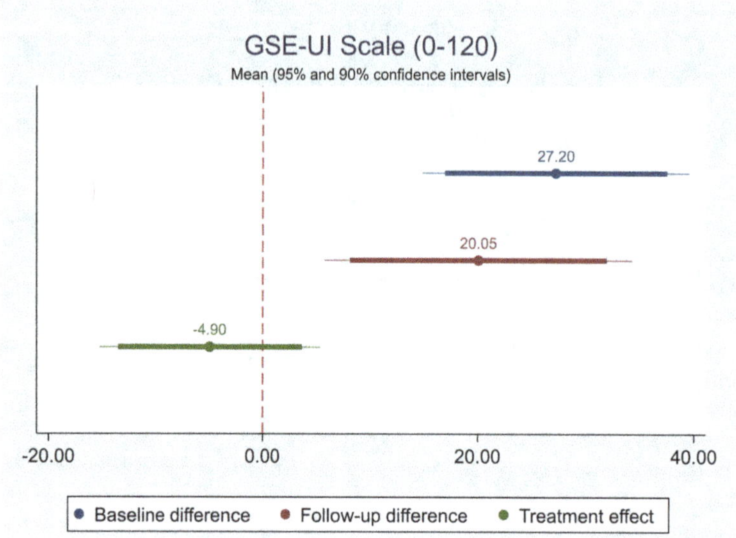


**Fig. 7** Mean (95 and 90% confidence intervals) of pre-post intervention differences and treatment effect for GSE-UI

***Being a useful and user-friendly package***

All participants preferred the fact that this package was colour coded, making it easy to read and follow. They found the texts being easy to read and understand and the illustrations being appropriate, indicating that there was no need to book the support session. Some participants described benefit gained as a result of using this package.

> *"The book was very well put together, and very clear, very easy to read, and it was very informative." (W6)*

> *"I'm still having the occasional accident, but now I'm sort of going oh well, I will get there. It's not a major setback. But it's not affecting my life like it used to." (W5)*

Some of them preferred a smaller size of the package so they could carry in their handbags, whereas some believed that people tended to put it away if it was a small book. A few concerned about the phrase "older women" used in the title of the package and suggested to remove it or simply indicate "women over 55".

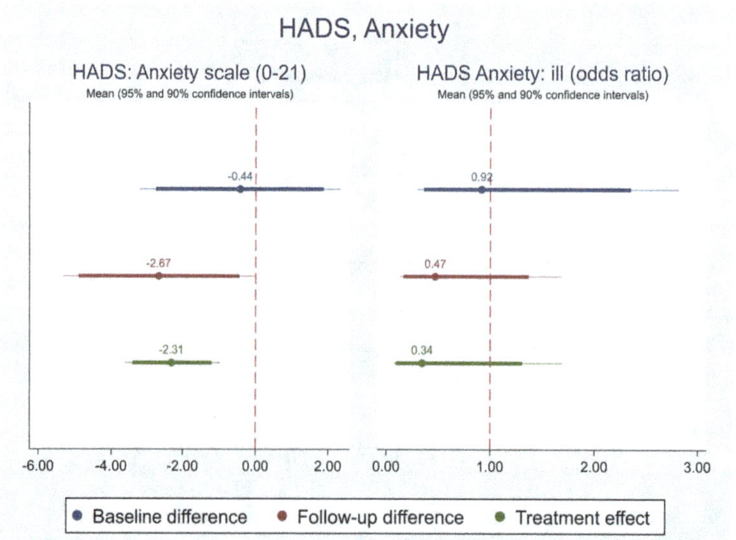


**Fig. 8** Mean (95 and 90% confidence intervals) of pre-post intervention differences and treatment effect for HADS, Anxiety

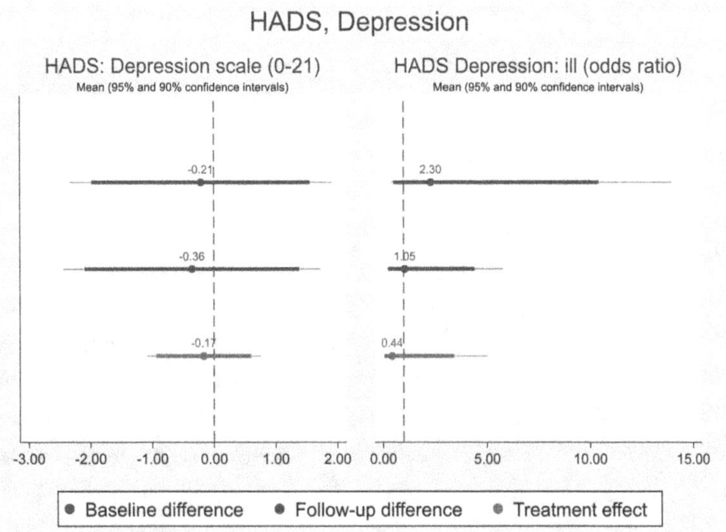


**Fig. 9** Mean (95 and 90% confidence intervals) of pre-post intervention differences and treatment effect for HADS, Anxiety

***Exploring dissemination strategies***

All participants found the self-reported questionnaires in the feasibility study acceptable and considered them being necessary. Some appreciated being involved in this study. All participants recommended places where appropriate to distribute the package, including doctor's surgeries, hospitals, pharmacies, workplaces, public libraries, local leisure centres, and other meeting places for women.

Some participants also expressed the need to design the package in multiple languages groups who may have limited access to support and resources. In addition to delivering the package to individuals, a couple of participants expressed their preference for a group to enable peer support.

## Discussion

This results of this study provide supporting evidence for the feasibility and acceptability of the self-management package as a complementary strategy for the management of UI in older women. This results of the feasibility RCT have confirmed that recruitment of women with UI from local community centres who were not actively engaged with health services is feasible and the drop-out rate is low. Completion and follow up of the questionnaires were successful. The findings of the acceptability study have suggested that the package may be a useful resource in improving women's knowledge and practical skills for the management of UI. Women also expressed the need for such intervention for this condition and commented that questionnaires used to capture information were acceptable.

The feasibility RCT showed that women's UI severity, symptoms and anxiety status were improved after the intervention for 3 months. This provides initial evidence that this self-management package has the capacity to reduce both physical and emotional impact of UI on women. There is an increasing interest in the self-management of UI consisting in both research and practice, however many interventions only focused on one particular skill or technique [6]. The UK Continence Society has recommended a support package for patients with UI as a minimum standard for continence care [41]. With no evidence-based package being available, this study developed the intervention consisting of multiple components and also demonstrated the acceptability of the intervention and potential benefit on women's physical and psychological health. Therefore, future studies are needed to evaluate the intervention in other settings in a larger multicentre trial in order to gain robust evidence.

Although the difference in women's quality of life or self-efficacy was not detected, women described that they felt more confident and motivated to self-manage their condition and some of them gained improvement after using the package. Qualitative interviews further supported these findings and participants reported that the package was informative and useful in raising their awareness. A significant correlation was observed between women's self-efficacy and their subjective perception of improvement. This suggests that women who gained a higher level of self-efficacy were likely to experience an improved subjective perception of their UI condition. Therefore, individual's self-efficacy level needs to be assessed as a way to stratify participants before randomisation process. For those with extremely low

**Table 5** Correlation between PGI-I and changes in outcomes within intervention group

| Mean change (SD) | PGI-I | | | | | | | Spearman's correlation |
|---|---|---|---|---|---|---|---|---|
| | Very much worse | Much worse | A little worse | No change | A little better | Much better | Very much better | |
| | 0 (0%) | 0 (0%) | 4 (16.7) | 3 (12.5) | 9 (37.5) | 7 (29.2) | 1 (4.2) | |
| EQ-5D-5L | | | | | | | | |
| Index | NA | NA | 0.03 (0.10) | 0.08 (0.01) | 0.05 (0.09) | 0.05 (0.14) | 0.00 (.) | -0.05 |
| VAS | NA | NA | 2.50 (16.58) | 8.33 (23.63) | 13.89 (18.33) | 2.86 (14.39) | -15.00 (.) | -0.04 |
| KHQ | | | | | | | | |
| Part I | | | | | | | | |
| General health perception (0-100) | NA | NA | 12.50 (43.30) | 8.33 (14.43) | -8.33 (17.68) | -14.29 (13.36) | 25.00 (.) | -0.25 |
| Incontinence impact (0-100) | NA | NA | -8.33 (16.67) | 0.00 (33.33) | 7.41 (27.78) | -4.76 (12.60) | 0.00 (.) | 0.05 |
| Part II | | | | | | | | |
| Role limitations (0-100) | NA | NA | -8.33 (9.62) | 5.56 (9.62) | -0.00 (18.63) | 2.38 (17.82) | 0.00 (.) | 0.15 |
| Physical limitations (0-100) | NA | NA | 8.33 (28.87) | 0.00 (16.67) | 1.85 (15.47) | -4.76 (8.13) | -16.67 (.) | -0.19 |
| Social limitations (0-100) | NA | NA | -5.56 (6.42) | 0.00 (0.00) | -0.62 (14.28) | -7.94 (12.36) | 0.00 (.) | -0.05 |
| Personal relationships (0-100) | NA | NA | -16.67 (16.67) | 0.00 (.) | 0.00 (0.00) | -6.67 (14.91) | 0.00 (.) | 0.29 |
| Emotions (0-100) | NA | NA | -11.11 (20.29) | 0.00 (0.00) | -3.70 (9.62) | -6.35 (8.74) | 22.22 (.) | 0.08 |
| Sleep/energy (0-100) | NA | NA | -4.17 (20.97) | -22.22 (9.62) | -7.41 (23.73) | -21.43 (20.89) | 50.00 (.) | -0.02 |
| Severity measures (0-100) | NA | NA | -12.50 (4.81) | -22.22 (17.35) | -3.70 (10.30) | -4.76 (13.49) | 0.00 (.) | 0.38* |
| Part III | | | | | | | | |
| Symptom severity scale (0-30) | NA | NA | -1.25 (6.50) | 0.00 (4.36) | -1.89 (3.92) | -2.43 (3.78) | 0.00 (.) | -0.13 |
| ICIQ-UI SF | | | | | | | | |
| Scale (0-21) | NA | NA | -2.75 (2.22) | -1.33 (4.51) | -3.89 (3.66) | -3.86 (4.34) | -1.00 (.) | -0.02 |
| GSE-UI | | | | | | | | |
| Scale (0-120) | NA | NA | -15.00 (17.03) | 0.67 (11.02) | 8.78 (9.87) | 10.71 (15.64) | 4.00 (.) | 0.43** |
| HADS | | | | | | | | |
| Anxiety scale (0-21) | NA | NA | -1.75 (0.96) | -0.67 (1.53) | -1.11 (1.96) | -4.14 (3.34) | 0.00 (.) | -0.22 |
| Depression scale (0-21) | NA | NA | -1.00 (1.63) | 0.33 (0.58) | -0.56 (1.88) | -0.86 (2.12) | 0.00 (.) | -0.02 |

*PGI-I* Patient Global Impression: Improvement, *VAS* Visual Analogue Scale, *KHQ* King's Health Questionnaire, *ICIQ-UI SF* International Consultation on Incontinence Questionnaire – urinary incontinence short form, *GSE-UI* Geriatric Self-Efficacy index for urinary incontinence, *HADS* Hospital Anxiety and Depression Scale**$p < 0.05$; *$p < 0.1$

self-efficacy, interventions with a purpose to build their confidence may be needed before providing self-management package.

Existing literature has shown modest benefit of self-management interventions in older women with UI. Compared to pharmacological therapies alone, nonpharmacological interventions, such as behavioural therapy either alone or combined with other intervention, are more effective in achieving cure or improvement both stress and urge UI [42]. Clinical effectiveness of self-management of UI has also been with respect to symptoms, UI severity, quality of life and perceptions of improvement when being delivered in group format with effects maintained (12 months [43]. Similarly, this study has observed improvement in symptoms and severity with the self-management package, and effects on psychological health. This package appears feasible to modify women's quality of life living with UI. Further studies may be needed to investigate the effectiveness of self-management interventions on both physical and psychosocial outcomes in women with UI, at both short and long term.

### Strengths and limitations

The intervention was co-developed with key stakeholders including women with UI and health professionals. The feasibility and acceptability of the intervention were evaluated with women who were not actively engaged with clinical services for UI. Potential positive effects were observed in women's UI symptoms and their psychological status, which were further supported by the women's experiences. However, careful interpretation is needed. The study was not allocation concealed and the sample size was not sufficiently powered to make robust inferences about the effectiveness of the intervention. Further studies are needed with a large sample size in multiple clinical settings to evaluate the effectiveness of this package. There is a possibility of bias associated with the self-reported measures. Objective information such as pad test or measure of PFM strength may be needed. It is worth noting that pad tests are not recommended in the routine assessment of women with UI by the NICE [44]. Also, women may be less in favour of the invasiveness of the measures such as vaginal dynamometer.

## Conclusions

The self-management package consisting of multifaceted behavioural techniques appears feasible to improve UI symptoms, severity and anxiety status in older women living with UI. Women also found it useful for increasing their awareness, motivation and knowledge of UI management. This study suggested that this package has the potential to be implemented in routine practice with further evaluation of effectiveness in clinical settings.

### Abbreviations

MRC: Medical Research Council; PFME: Pelvic floor muscle exercises; RCT: Randomised controlled trial; UI: Urinary incontinence

### Acknowledgements

We thank women and health professionals' involvement and their contribution to this study.

### Authors' contributions

All authors have read the manuscript, discussed the results and commented on the manuscript. All authors have met the criteria for authorship and approved the final. YF: study design, data collection and analysis, drafting and revising the manuscript. EAN: study design and analysis, revising the manuscript. LM: study design and analysis, revising the manuscript.

### Competing interests

The authors declare that they have no competing interests.

### Author details

[1]Leeds Institute of Health Sciences, University of Leeds, Leeds LS2 9NL, UK. [2]School of Health and Life Sciences, Glasgow Caledonian University, Glasgow, UK. [3]School of Healthcare, University of Leeds, Leeds, UK.

### References

1. Abrams P, Andersson KE, Apostolidis A, Birder L, Bliss D, Brubaker L, Cardozo L, Castro-Diaz D, O'Connell PR, Cottenden A, et al. 6th international consultation on incontinence. Recommendations of the international scientific committee: evaluation and treatment of urinary incontinence, pelvic organ prolapse and faecal incontinence. Neurourol Urodyn. 2018; 37(7):2271–2.
2. Rubilotta E, Balzarro M, D'Amico A, Cerruto MA, Bassi S, Bovo C, Iacovelli V, Bianchi D, Artibani W, Finazzi Agrò E. Pure stress urinary incontinence: analysis of prevalence, estimation of costs, and financial impact. BMC Urol. 2019;19(1):44.
3. Cooper J, Annappa M, Quigley A, Dracocardos D, Bondili A, Mallen C. Prevalence of female urinary incontinence and its impact on quality of life in a cluster population in the United Kingdom (UK): a community survey. Primary Health Care Res Dev. 2015;16(4):377–82.
4. Abrams P, Smith AP, Cotterill N. The impact of urinary incontinence on health-related quality of life (HRQoL) in a real-world population of women aged 45–60 years: results from a survey in F rance, G ermany, the UK and the USA. BJU Int. 2015;115(1):143–52.
5. Syan R, Brucker BM. Guideline of guidelines: urinary incontinence. BJU Int. 2016;117(1):20–33.
6. Dumoulin C, Hay-Smith J, Habée-Séguin GM, Mercier J. Pelvic floor muscle training versus no treatment, or inactive control treatments, for urinary incontinence in women: a short version Cochrane systematic review with meta-analysis. Neurourol Urodyn. 2015;34(4):300–8.
7. O'Donnell M, Lose G, Sykes D, Voss S, Hunskaar S. Help-seeking behaviour and associated factors among women with urinary incontinence in France, Germany, Spain and the United Kingdom. Eur Urol. 2005;47(3):385–92.
8. Tannenbaum C, Agnew R, Benedetti A, Thomas D, van den Heuvel E. Effectiveness of continence promotion for older women via community organisations: a cluster randomised trial. BMJ Open. 2013;3(12):e004135.
9. Tannenbaum C, Fritel X, Halme A, van den Heuvel E, Jutai J, Wagg A. Long-term effect of community-based continence promotion on urinary symptoms, falls and healthy active life expectancy among older women: cluster randomised trial. J Age Ageing. 2019;48(4):526–32. https://doi.org/10.1093/ageing/afz038.
10. Taylor SJ, Pinnock H, Epiphaniou E, Pearce G, Parke HL, Schwappach A, Purushotham N, Jacob S, Griffiths CJ, Greenhalgh T. A rapid synthesis of the evidence on interventions supporting self-management for people with long-term conditions: PRISMS–practical systematic review of self-management support for long-term conditions; 2014.
11. Gurden M, Morelli M, Sharp G, Baker K, Betts N, Bolton J. Evaluation of a general practitioner referral service for manual treatment of back and neck pain. Primary Health Care Res Dev. 2012;13(3):204.
12. Lorig K. Self-management of chronic illness: a model for the future. Generations. 1993;17(3):11–4.
13. Lorig K. Self-management education: more than a nice extra. Med Care. 2003;41(6): 699–701.
14. Lorig K, González VM, Laurent DD, Morgan L, Laris B. Arthritis self management program variations: three studies. Arthritis Rheumatism. 1998;11(6):448–54.
15. Lorig K, Holman H. Arthritis self-management studies: a twelve-year review. Health Educ Q. 1993;20(1):17–28.
16. Barlow J, Wright C, Sheasby J, Turner A, Hainsworth J. Self-management approaches for people with chronic conditions: a review. Patient Educ Couns. 2002;48(2):177–87.
17. Barlow JH, Turner AP, Wright CC. A randomized controlled study of the arthritis self-management Programme in the UK. Health Educ Res. 2000;15(6):665–80.
18. Bourbeau J, Van Der Palen J. Promoting effective self-management programmes to improve COPD. Eur Respir J. 2009;33(3):461–3.
19. Effing TW, Bourbeau J, Vercoulen J, Apter AJ, Coultas D, Meek P, van der Valk P, Partridge MR, van der Palen J. Self-management programmes for COPD moving forward. Chronic Respiratory Dis. 2012;9(1):27–35.
20. Lennon S, McKenna S, Jones F. Self-management programmes for people post stroke: a systematic review. Clin Rehabil. 2013; 0269215513481045.
21. Smith-Turchyn J, Morgan A, Richardson J. The effectiveness of group-based self-management Programmes to improve physical and psychological outcomes in patients with Cancer: a systematic review and meta-analysis of randomised controlled trials. Clin Oncol. 2015;28(5):292–305.
22. Craig P, Dieppe P, Macintyre S, Michie S, Nazareth I, Petticrew M. Developing and evaluating complex interventions: the new Medical Research Council guidance. Int J Nurs Stud. 2013;50(5):587–92.
23. Lennon R, Glasper A, Carpenter D: Nominal Group Technique: its utilisation to explore the rewards and challenges of becoming a mental health nurse, prior to the introduction of the all graduate nursing curriculum in England. In.: Working Papers in Health Sciences 1: 2 ISSN 2051–6266/20120000; 2012.
24. Campbell M, Fitzpatrick R, Haines A, Kinmonth AL, Sandercock P, Spiegelhalter D, Tyrer P. Framework for design and evaluation of complex interventions to improve health. Bmj. 2000;321(7262):694–6.
25. Whitehead AL, Julious SA, Cooper CL, Campbell MJ. Estimating the sample size for a pilot randomised trial to minimise the overall trial sample size for the external pilot and main trial for a continuous outcome variable. Stat Methods Med Res. 2016;25(3):1057–73.
26. Herdman M, Gudex C, Lloyd A, Janssen M, Kind P, Parkin D, Bonsel G, Badia X. Development and preliminary testing of the new five-level version of EQ-5D (EQ-5D-5L). Qual Life Res. 2011;20(10):1727–36.
27. Kelleher C, Cardozo L, Khullar V, Salvatore S. A new questionnaire to assess the quality of life of urinary incontinent women. BJOG Int J Obstet Gynaecol. 1997;104(12):1374–9.
28. Avery K, Donovan J, Peters TJ, Shaw C, Gotoh M, Abrams P. ICIQ: a brief and robust measure for evaluating the symptoms and impact of urinary incontinence. Neurourol Urodynamics. 2004;23(4):322–30.

29. Klovning A, Avery K, Sandvik H, Hunskaar S. Comparison of two questionnaires for assessing the severity of urinary incontinence: the ICIQ-UI SF versus the incontinence severity index. Neurourol Urodynamics. 2009; 28(5):411–5.
30. Tannenbaum C, Brouillette J, Korner-Bitensky N, Dumoulin C, Corcos J, Tu LM, Lemieux MC, Ouellet S, Valiquette L. Creation and testing of the geriatric self-efficacy index for urinary incontinence. J Am Geriatr Soc. 2008; 56(3):542–7.
31. Zigmond AS, Snaith RP. The hospital anxiety and depression scale. Acta Psychiatr Scand. 1983;67(6):361–70.
32. Yalcin I, Bump RC. Validation of two global impression questionnaires for incontinence. Am J Obstet Gynecol. 2003;189(1):98–101.
33. Vickers AJ, Altman DG. Analysing controlled trials with baseline and follow up measurements. Bmj. 2001;323(7321):1123–4.
34. Senn SS: Statistical issues in drug development, vol. 69. United States: Wiley; 2008.
35. Drummond GB, Tom BD. Statistics, probability, significance, likelihood: words mean what we define them to mean. Adv Physiol Educ. 2011;35(4): 361–4.
36. Halsey LG, Curran-Everett D, Vowler SL, Drummond GB. The fickle P value generates irreproducible results. Nat Methods. 2015;12(3):179.
37. Guest G, Bunce A, Johnson L. How many interviews are enough? An experiment with data saturation and variability. Field Methods. 2006;18(1): 59–82.
38. Morse JM, Field PA. Principles of data analysis. In: Nursing Research edn. United States: Springer; 1996. p. 103–23.
39. Braun V, Clarke V. Using thematic analysis in psychology. Qual Res Psychol. 2006;3(2):77–101.
40. QSR International: NVivo qualitative data analysis software: QSR international Pty ltd; 2018.
41. Minimum Standards for Continence Care in the United Kingdom. http://www.ukcs.uk.net/wp-content/uploads/2016/04/15091716_Revised_Min_Standards_for_CC_in_UK.pdf. Accessed 16 Nov 2019.
42. Balk EM, Rofeberg VN, Adam GP, et al. Pharmacologic and nonpharmacologic treatments for urinary incontinence in women: a systematic review and network meta-analysis of clinical outcomes. Ann Intern Med. 2019;170:465–79. [Epub ahead of print 19 March 2019]. https://doi.org/10.7326/M18-3227.
43. Diokno AC, Newman DK, Low LK, Griebling TL, Maddens ME, Goode PS, Raghunathan TE, Subak LL, Sampselle CM, Boura JA, et al. Effect of group-administered behavioral treatment on urinary incontinence in older women: a randomized clinical TrialEffect of group-administered behavioral treatment on urinary incontinence in older WomenEffect of group-administered behavioral treatment on urinary incontinence in older women. JAMA Intern Med. 2018;178(10):1333–41.
44. NICE. Urinary incontinence in women: management. In. Edited by National Institute for health and care excellence. London: NICE; 2013.

# 21

# Clinical characteristics and endoscopic treatment of hematospermia with postcoital hematuria

Zao-Ming Huang[1], Yan-Feng Li[1*], Qi Wang[2], Yong Zhang[1], Yong Luo[1], Zhi-Lin Nie[1], Ke Li[1], Qing-Xing Feng[1] and Xu-Dong Liu[1]

**Abstract**

**Background:** Recurrent hematospermia accompanied by postejaculatory hematuria is a very rare phenomenon, has not been well understood in the clinical setting, and usually leads to misdiagnosis and mistreatment. The aim of this study was to summarize the clinical characteristics, etiologic diagnosis, and endoscopic treatment of hematospermia with postcoital hematuria.

**Methods:** We collected the clinical data from 39 patients of hematospermia with postcoital hematuria, who were admitted to our hospital from May 2014 to October 2019. The etiologic diagnostic process and endoscopic surgery were analyzed retrospectively, and we observed and evaluated the efficacy and any complications during follow-up.

**Results:** The average age of the 39 patients was 44.1 years (range, 18–61 years), and the disease history ranged from 1 month to 20 years, with a median duration of 24 months. All of the patients were observed by urethrocystoscopy, which showed 38 cases of posterior urethral hemangioma (PUH) or abnormal varicose vessels, and 1 case of anterior urethral hemangioma. Of these, 18 patients underwent transurethral resection of urethral hemangioma, and 21 patients underwent transurethral electrocauterization. Postoperative follow-up ranged from 1 to 56 months, with a median of 16 months. The symptoms disappeared in 37 patients and recurred in 2 patients two to 3 months after the operation. The two recurrent patients were treated again by transurethral electrocauterization, and their symptoms then disappeared.

**Conclusions:** PUH is the most common cause of hematospermia with postejaculatory hematuria. Herein, we demonstrated that transurethral resection or electrocauterization provides a safe, effective, and minimally invasive method for the treatment of PUH.

**Keywords:** Posterior urethral hemangioma (PUH), Hematuria, Hematospermia, Urethrocystoscopy, Electroresection

## Background

Hematospermia accompanied by postejaculatory or posterection hematuria is a very rare clinical symptom in male patients. Although studies in recent years have shown that this phenomenon is primarily caused by posterior urethral hemangioma (PUH) [1–5], it is still easy to misdiagnose and mistreat due to its atypical clinical manifestations and an overall lack of relevant knowledge in this area [6]. According to our knowledge, until the end of 2019, the total number of reported male urethral hemangiomas in the MEDLINE database was less than 70 since the first case report in 1895 [1–21]. The clinical features, diagnosis, and treatment of this disease is still not well understood. From May 2014 to October

* Correspondence: 1738401063@qq.com
[1]Department of Urology, Daping Hospital, Army Medical University, No.10, Daping Changjiangzhilu, Yuzhong District, Chongqing 400042, China

2019, 39 patients with intractable hematospermia accompanied by postejaculatory hematuria were treated at our hospital, and we herein summarize the clinical characteristics, etiologic diagnosis, and endoscopic treatment effects.

## Methods

Thirty-nine patients of intractable hematospermia with postcoital hematuria were treated at our hospital from May 2014 to October 2019. The clinical data were collected and retrospectively analyzed, including age, course of disease, principal symptoms, routine urine test results, coagulation function, imaging features, endoscopic findings, causes of bleeding, location and size of lesions, surgical operative skills, postoperative pathologic results, complications, and follow-up results.

All patients received conservative treatment for more than 1 month prior to admission, but no improvement was observed. After admission, all of the patients were excluded from hematuric conditions caused by urinary tumors, urinary calculi, infections, trauma, and abnormal coagulation function by relevant laboratory, or imaging examinations. All the patients were also further diagnosed and treated by urethrocystoscopy. Bladder mucosae, bilateral ureteral openings, posterior urethra, and anterior urethra were observed carefully, and we paid special attention to any suspicious abnormal indications such as bleeding, neoplasms, or abnormal protuberances. We also performed transrectal seminal vesicle massage to observe the color of the seminal vesicle fluid seeping from the bilateral ejaculatory orifices. Most of the patients had obvious hemangioma-like protuberances at the 6:00 position between the verumontanum and the external urethral sphincter in lithotomy position, which was significantly different from the surrounding normal urethral mucosa. A few patients had a circular, abnormal vascular protuberance in this area, and some individuals had localized abnormal hemangioma-like protuberances in the anterior urethral area. Electroresection either alone or along with electrocautery (using an SM10 bipolar plasma system at 100 W of output power for electroresection and 80 W for electrocautery) to the abnormal blood vessels or hemangioma-like protuberances were performed carefully and precisely. The range of resection was slightly more than the edge of the lesion by approximately 2 mm, and the depth was usually 4–5 mm (equivalent to the depth of an electric cutting loop). The bottom was usually fulgurated at the same time to destroy the abnormal blood vessels at the edge of the lesion. Foley urethral catheters were routinely retained for 1 or 2 days after the operation.

We used SPSS 18.0 statistical software for all of the statistical analyses. Measurement data that conformed to a normal distribution are expressed by $x \pm s$, whereas non-normally distributed measurement data are expressed by medians and range.

## Results

The age range of the patients was 18–61 years (mean age was 44.1 ± 10.2 years). The duration of symptoms ranged from 1 month to 20 years, and the median symptom duration was 24 months. Of these, 15 cases had a history of less than 1 year, 24 cases of more than 1 year, and 9 cases of more than 5 years. According to the age at onset, there were 5 patients aged less than 30 years, 13 patients aged 30–39 years, 12 patients aged 40–49, and 9 patients aged 50–59 years.

All of the patients showed typical recurrent or persistent hematospermia accompanied by hematuria on the first urination after sexual intercourse or even presented a large amount of fresh blood or blood clots from the urethral orifice after sexual intercourse or masturbation. The amount of blood in the urine was usually significantly more than that in the semen, and the hematuria then disappeared on the second and later urinations after sexual intercourse. The overall characteristic symptoms of the 39 patients are shown in Table 1.

All of the patients underwent ultrasonography of the urinary system (and CT examination if necessary), and we excluded the lesions caused by tumors, stones, or other common causes of urinary system bleeding. Pelvic magnetic resonance imaging (MRI) was usually performed before surgery, and the results showed that the size and shape of the seminal vesicles were normal and without signs of bleeding. Via urethrocystoscopy, we initially excluded hematuria from the bladder and ureters, and then transrectal seminal vesicle massage further confirmed that there was no bleeding in the seminal vesicles. The typical manifestation we found was a 0.5–0.8 cm × 1.0 cm dark red hemangioma-like mass located at 6:00 in lithotomy position between the verumontanum and the external urethral sphincter, approximately 0.5–1 cm from the distal part of the verumontanum, which was significantly different from the surrounding normal urethral mucosa and prone to bleeding (34/39) (Figs. 1, 2). We observed that some patients had obviously active episodes of hemorrhaging. Lesion localization and patterns in the 39 patients are summarized in Table 2.

We treated all the lesions with electrocautery alone or along with electroresection. Twenty-one cases underwent direct fulguration at the lesion site because of the small size of the hemangioma or the presence of only varicose blood vessels, and no pathologic specimens were obtained. Eighteen patients underwent electrosurgical excision of abnormal hemangioma-like tissue at the lesion site, and postoperative pathologic findings were cavernous hemangiomas in 15 cases, racemose

**Table 1** Symptoms of 39 patients with hematospermia and postcoital hematuria

| Symptoms | Number of patients (%) |
|---|---|
| Hematuria after sexual intercourse | 39 (100) |
| Hematuria with blood clots after sexual intercourse | 31 (79.5) |
| Hematuria after sexual excitement or erection without ejaculation | 19 (48.7) |
| Dysuria with repeated urinary retention and massive hematuria after sexual intercourse | 1 (2.6) |
| Blood dripping from urethra with hematuria after sexual intercourse | 2 (5.1) |

hemangioma in 1 case, and unclassified hemangiomas in 2 cases.

Each patient was followed up from 3 to 56 months, with a median follow-up period of 16 months. Early postoperative hematuria or urethral bleeding usually disappeared within 2–6 weeks. Except for one case of unilateral acute epididymitis in the early stages after the operation, we uncovered no other related complications—including urethral stricture, dysuria, incontinence, or change in sexual function—in any other patient. The symptoms of hematospermia and hematuria completely disappeared in 37 of the 39 patients during the entire follow-up period, whereas 2 out of the 39 had a recurrence of hematospermia with hematuria 2–3 months after the operation. When re-observed by urethrocystoscopy, the original hemangioma at the 6:00 position disappeared. One patient showed a newly formed circumferential varicosity or hemangioma-like change outside the 6:00 position, whereas the other had hemangioma-like changes in the distal area of the original lesion at the 6:00 position. These patients' symptoms, however, disappeared after re-electrocautery.

## Discussion

Patients with recurrent or intractable hematospermia accompanied by postejaculatory hematuria are seen very rarely in the clinic, and it is usually easy to misdiagnose or mistreat them due to its atypical clinical manifestations [6]. In an etiologic study of hematospermia, Leary and Aguilo in 1974 found that 4.6% of the 174 cases

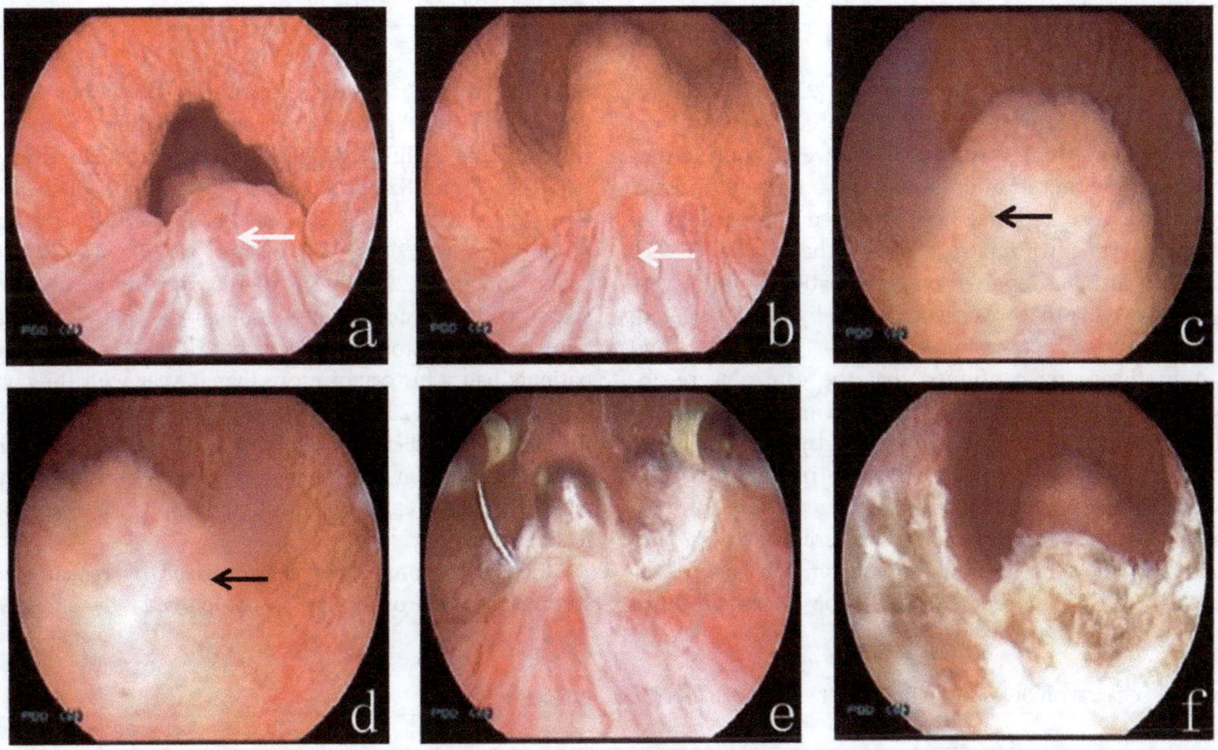


**Fig. 1** Typical case 1. Endoscopic observation and management of PUH. **a**, **b** There is a dark red hemangioma-like mass located at 6:00 in the lithotomy position, between the verumontanum and the external urethral sphincter, and 0.5–1 cm from the distal part of the verumontanum (white arrow). **c**, **d** There is seepage of milky white, jelly-like seminal vesicle fluid from the orifices of the bilateral ejaculatory ducts upon transrectal seminal vesicle massage, but there was no bleeding in the seminal tract (black arrow). **e**, **f** The PUH was treated by electroscission either alone or electrocautery

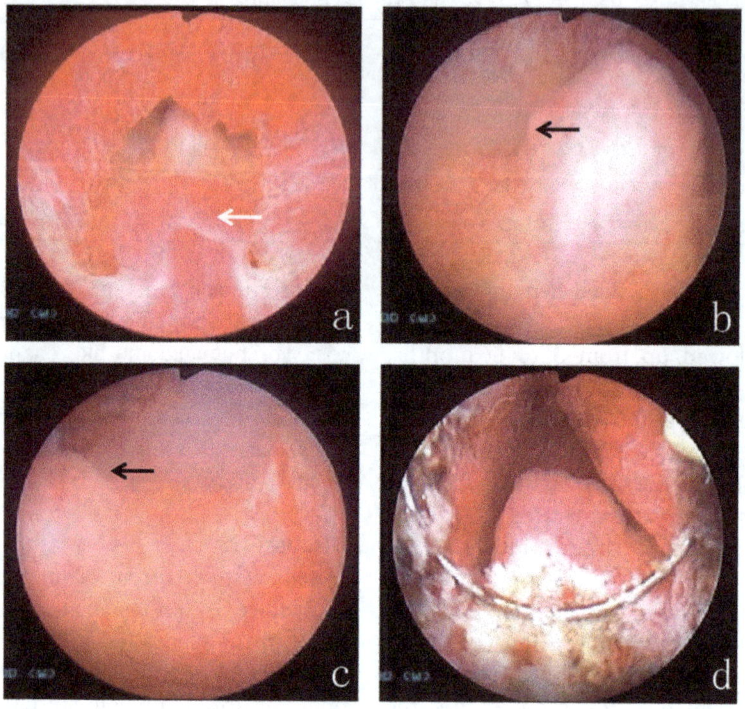

**Fig. 2** Typical case 2. Endoscopic observation and management of PUH. **a** Typical dark red, hemangioma-like bulge observed 0.5–1 cm from the distal part of the verumontanum, between the verumontanum and the external urethral sphincter (white arrow). **b**, **c** There is seepage of milky white, jelly-like seminal vesicle fluid from the orifices of the bilateral ejaculatory ducts upon transrectal seminal vesicle massage but no bleeding in the seminal tract (black arrow). **d** The PUH was treated by electroscission either alone or along with electrocautery

surveyed were due to urethral varices [22], and more recently, Papp reported that 4–7% of 122 cases were caused by urethral varices [23]. However, only a few studies in the literature during the past 30 years (most of which are case reports) have reported the etiology of hematospermia with postejaculatory hematuria [1–21]. Cattolica in 1982 reported on three patients with severe hematospermia that was accompanied by hematuria, clot formation, and occasional urinary retention, and cystourethroscopy confirmed that the causes were abnormal non-variceal blood vessels in the posterior urethra [24]. In 1997, Hayashi and Furuya reported that the lesions in their patients (characterized by hematospermia and massive hematuria after ejaculation) were located close to the distal end of the verumontanum, and these proved to be urethral hemangiomas by histopathology [25, 26]. Our report featured the largest group of patients studied thus far. Previous reports have suggested that most patients presented in their second or third decade of life [27, 28]. Saito reported 20 patients between 38 and 82 years (mean, 63) with 90% of the patients older than 50 [1]. Our results showed that the age of onset in 64.1% (25/39) of the patients was 30–49 years, and in 87.2% (34/39) of the patients was 30–59 years—certainly an elevated incidence. Analysis of patient medical histories showed that 61.5% (24/39) of the patients had a history of more than 1 year with the condition, of which, 23.1% (9/39) had a history of more than 5 years. This indicated that most of these patients were still affected after repeated treatments, and they had failed to obtain early diagnosis and appropriate and effective treatment.

Patient symptoms were characterized by repeated or stubborn hematospermia accompanied by massive

**Table 2** Localization of lesions in the 39 patients as confirmed by urethrocystoscopy

| Lesion location | Number of patients (%) |
|---|---|
| Hemangioma-like mass between the verumontanum and the external urethral sphincter in the 6:00 lithotomy position | 34 (87.2) |
| Abnormal blood vessels with obvious varicosities around the prostatic urethra and verumontanum | 3 (7.7) |
| Circumferential abnormal varicose blood vessels in the plane of the external urethral sphincter | 1 (2.6) |
| Hemangioma-like changes in the bulbourethral area | 1 (2.6) |

hematuria, and the amount of hemorrhage can be much greater than in simple hematospermia. Blood clots are common in hematuria, and individual patients may also have recurrent urinary retention. At the same time, a few patients may manifest obvious hematuria or urethral bleeding, even if they do not ejaculate after erection or from other sexual stimulation, and this may lead to a fear of sexual intercourse. One patient refused to have sex for as long as 1–2 years for fear of bleeding, which caused stress in this individual's marriage.

We noted that a previous report suggested that transrectal power Doppler ultrasonography was helpful in the diagnosis of hemangioma, as it revealed a strong blood flow site in the urethra near the apex of the prostate [1]. Unfortunately, we did not perform ultrasonographic examination via Doppler of the entire urethral tract in every patient. However, in order to clarify the etiology, patients in this group were carefully examined by urethrocystoscopy, and our observations were focused on the posterior urethral prostatic region, the verumontanum region, and the distal 1–2 cm region of the verumontanum. The possibility of hematospermia originating from the seminal ducts was completely excluded by our MRI examination before the operation and seminal vesicle massage during the operation. Under the pressure of the endoscopy sheath, abnormal blood vessels are sometimes difficult to observe clearly. Cattolica suggested that cystoscopy during penile flaccidity may miss these lesions that enlarge and become more visible during an erection [24]. Saito proposed that endoscopy with reduced irrigation flow immediately after ejaculation will increase the probability of diagnosing these lesions [1]. Our experience is that it is necessary to constantly adjust the angle of the front end of the endoscope, repeatedly moving it forward and backward, and to reduce the flushing pressure to carefully observe the integrity and smoothness of the urethral mucosa in the aforementioned areas. We usually found that there were isolated smooth pink or dark red, vein-like mass protrusions with clear boundaries at the 6:00 position between the distal part of the verumontanum and the external urethral sphincter. A few patients also showed a circular protrusion in this area. In addition to the above typical manifestations, we also had three patients with widespread and abnormal varicose blood vessels around the prostatic urethra, and verumontanum; one patient showed a circular abnormal enlargement of blood vessels on the plane of the external urethral sphincter; and one patient manifested localized hemangioma-like changes in the anterior urethra (bulbar urethra). Because urethral lesions in this type of patients occur in different areas and are of different extent and size, it is necessary to observe the abnormal changes carefully throughout the entire urethra so as to deliver an appropriate diagnosis and treatment.

Usual methods for the endoscopic resection of PUH are electroresection/electrocautery and Holmium laser resection [3, 5, 19, 20]. The former is a simple and effective method with fewer complications and less recurrence. It has also been reported that endoscopic injection of a sclerosing agent, pingyangmycin, is an alternative therapy for the treatment of hemangiomas [6, 29]. In addition, De León and others believe that Holmium laser treatment of prostatic urethral hemangiomas is effective, without complications, and should become one of the preferred methods for the treatment of prostatic urethral hemangiomas [19]. Regardless of the treatment method used, the objective is to improve the therapeutic effect and reduce the recurrence rate and complications. Thirty-nine patients in our group were treated with transurethral electroscission either alone or along with electrocautery, and we observed no complications during the operation. Only one patient developed acute epididymitis early after the operation, and he was successfully treated with active anti-infection therapy. No other complications such as urethral stricture, dysuria, incontinence, or change in sexual function occurred. Only two cases showed recurrence within 2–3 months postoperatively, and all recovered well after a second use of the same method.

It is reported that depending upon the pattern, hemangioma of the urinary tract is classified as cavernous, capillary, venous, or racemose—with cavernous being the most common [21]. In our study, 18 patients received a histopathologic diagnosis—with cavernous hemangioma in 15 cases, racemose hemangioma in one case, and unclassified hemangioma in two cases. The pathologic types of the cases in our group were obviously consistent with a previous report [21].

The etiology and pathogenesis of PUH—which often occurs between the verumontanum and the external urethral sphincter—remain unclear. Some scholars believe that vascular endothelial growth factor is an important influencing factor, whereas others believe that urethral hemangioma is a congenital disease. The latter may originate from residual embryonic angioblasts—which cannot successfully differentiate into normal blood vessels—leading to the formation of hemangiomas [25]. This possibility cannot be ruled out as it may be due to a degenerative process associated with chronic stimuli and atrophy. A few cases may also be associated with some congenital diseases, including Sturge Weber or Klippel-Trenaunay syndrome [17, 30, 31]. Saito suggested that there was a high intraluminal urethral pressure around the external urethral sphincter, and high venous pressure led to the formation of hemangiomas [1]. From our cases and previously reported data [1, 2, 5], we believe that PUH is more common than reported in the published literature. The possibility of urethral hemangiomas should be considered when patients present with hematospermia accompanied by postejaculatory or posterection hematuria.

This study has several limitations: We did not evaluate the imaging pattern of hemangiomas by Doppler ultrasonography, and we included only a limited number of patients because of low disease prevalence. Only one bipolar plasma system for electroresection either alone or along with electrocautery was used, and we did not compare it with any other methods for the treatment of PUH.

## Conclusion

In summary, as an exceedingly rare and easily misdiagnosed clinical symptom, hematospermia accompanied by postejaculatory or posterection hematuria can be diagnosed by its characteristic manifestations. PUH and abnormal blood vessels in the prostate (as confirmed by cystourethroscopy) were common causes of hematospermia and postejaculatory hematuria. We showed that transurethral resection or fulguration of urethral hemangioma or abnormal blood vessels constitutes a minimally invasive, simple, safe, and effective treatment method.

### Abbreviations

PUH: Posterior urethral hemangioma; MRI: Magnetic resonance imaging; CT: Computerized tomography

### Acknowledgements

Not applicable.

### Authors' contributions

YFL designed the study, performed the operation. ZMH participated in the operation and drafted the manuscript. QW participated in the analysis and interpretation of the data. YZ, YL, ZLN, KL, QXF and XDL participated in the operation and clinical follow-up. All authors read and approved the final manuscript.

### Competing interests

The authors declare that they have no competing interests.

### Author details

[1]Department of Urology, Daping Hospital, Army Medical University, No.10, Daping Changjiangzhilu, Yuzhong District, Chongqing 400042, China. [2]Department of Urology, Chongqing Renji Hospital, University of Chinese Academy of Sciences, Chongqing 400062, China.

### References

1. Saito S. Posterior urethral hemangioma: one of the unknown causes of hematuria and/or hematospermia. Urology. 2008;71(1):168 e11–4.
2. Tian L, Han H, Lei HE, Zhang XD. Clinical features of haematospermia associated with seminal vesicle calculi versus posterior urethral haemangioma. Andrologia. 2018;50(8):e13072.
3. Han H, Zhou XG, Fan DD, Tian L, Zhang XD. An unusual etiology for hematospermia and treatments that were successful. Urology. 2015;86(4): 740–3.
4. Kang DH, Lee JY, Jung DC, Oh YT, Cho ES, Park SY, Lee KS, Cho KS. Tertiary referral hospital experiences of men presenting with painless postcoital gross hematuria and a suggestion for the management algorithm. Urology. 2018;115:112 8.
5. Soleimani MJ, Shadpour P, Mehravaran K, Kashi AH. Laser treatment for urethral hemangiomas: report of three cases. Urol J. 2017;14(3):3094–9.
6. Yong F, Juan L, Jinhuan W, Haohua Y, Wei C, Jiacong M, Junhang L, Wenwei W. Urethral cavernous hemangioma: a highly misdiagnosed disease (a case report of two patients and literature review). BMC Urol. 2019;19(1):13.
7. Mandal S, Nayak P, Purkait S, Das M, Mahalingam R. Rare images of urethral hemangioma and its management. Urology. 2019;124:e9–e11.
8. Varea-Malo R, Campos-Juanatey F, Portillo Martín JA, Castillo CL. Multiple urethral hemangiomas associated with urethral stricture: an uncommon aetiology for urethral bleeding. Case Rep Urol. 2019;2019:9071327.
9. Itesako T, Eura R, Okamoto Y, Tatarano S, Yoshino H, Nishimura H, Yamada Y, Enokida H, Nakagawa M. Oral propranolol in a child with infantile hemangioma of the urethra. Urology. 2018;122:165–8.
10. Hamada A, Hattahara K, Oyama R, Hirayama K, Masui K, Shichiri Y. Urethral hemangioma with repeated urinary retention by posterection hematuria. Hinyokika Kiyo. 2017;63(12):533–5.
11. Parshad S, Yadav SP, Arora B. Urethral hemangioma. An unusual cause of hematuria. Urol Int. 2001;66(1):43–5.
12. Lauvetz RW, Malek RS, Husmann DA. Treatment of extensive urethral hemangioma with KTP/532 laser. Lasers Surg Med. 1996;18(1):92–5.
13. Singh DV, Mandal AK. Unusual cause of urethral bleeding in an adolescent: a case in dilemma. Int J Adolesc Med Health. 2014;26(1):149–51.
14. Abbinante M, Crivellaro S, Guaitoli P, Mastrocinque G, Ammirati E, Frea B. Cavernous hemangioma of the spongious body of the urethra: a case report. Urologia. 2012;79(3):211–3.
15. Serizawa RR, Nørgaard N, Horn T, Vibits H. Hemangioma of the prostate--an unusual cause of lower urinary tract symptoms: case report. BMC Urol. 2011;11:4.
16. Noviello C, Cobellis G, Romano M, Amici G, Martino A. Posterior urethral polyp causing haematuria in children. Pediatr Med Chir. 2011;33(3):134–6.
17. Tepeler A, Yeşilolva Y, Kılınç A, Aktoz T, Onen A. A mild and rare form of Klippel-Trenaunay syndrome presenting with urethral bleeding due to penile hemangioma. Urology. 2011;77(2):463–5.
18. Efthimiou I, Kavouras D, Vasilakis P, Katsanis S. Hemangioma of penile urethra-treatment with simple transurethral excision: a case report. Cases J. 2009;2:6199.
19. de León JP, Arce J, Gausa L, Villavicencio H. Hemangioma of the prostatic urethra: holmium laser treatment. Urol Int. 2008;80(1):108–10.
20. Khaitan A, Hemal AK. Urethral hemangioma: laser treatment. Int Urol Nephrol. 2000;32(2):285–6.
21. Jahn H, Nissen HM. Haemangioma of the urinary tract: review of the literature. Br J Urol. 1991;68(2):113–7.
22. Leary FJ, Aguilo JJ. Clinical significance of hematospermia. Mayo Clin Proc. 1974;49(11):815–7.
23. Papp GK, Kopa Z, Szabo F, et al. Aetiology of haemospermia. Andrologia. 2003;35(5):317–20.
24. Cattolica EV. Massive hemospermia: a new etiology and simplified treatment. J Urol. 1982;128(1):151–2.
25. Hayashi T, Igarashi K, Sekine H. Urethral hemangioma: case report. J Urol. 1997;158(2):539–40.
26. Furuya S, Ogura H, Tanaka Y, et al. Hemangioma of the prostatic urethra: hematospermia and massive postejaculation hematuria with clot formation. Int J Urol. 1997;4(5):524–6.
27. Manuel ES, Seery WH, Cole AT. Capillary hemangioma of the male urethra: case report with literature review. J Urol. 1977;117(6):804.
28. Roberts JW, Devine CJ Jr. Urethral hemangioma: treatment by total excision and grafting. J Urol. 1983;129(5):1053–4.
29. Bissada NK, Frangos DN, Ferentzi C. Management of extensive urethral hemangiomas with endoscopic sclerotherapy:case report. J Urol. 1994; 151(4):1015–6.
30. Klein TW, Kaplan GW. Klippel- Trenaunay syndrome associated with urinary tract hemangiomas. J Urol. 1975;114(4):596–600.
31. Lei H, Guan X, Han H, et al. Painless urethral bleeding during penile erection in an adult man with Klippel-Trenaunay syndrome: a case report. Sex Med. 2018;6(2):180–3.

# 22

# Efficacy of dapoxetine treatment in Chinese patients with premature ejaculation and possible factors affecting efficacy in the real-world practice

Jing Peng[1†], Dong Fang[1†], Huixi Li[1†], Yuan Tang[1], Yiming Yuan[1], Wanshou Cui[1], Bing Gao[1], Hongjun Li[2*] and Zhichao Zhang[1*]

**Abstract**

**Background:** The treatment effect of dapoxetine in real-world practice is not well established. This study was to investigate the factors influencing efficacy of dapoxetine for the treatment of Premature ejaculation (PE) in the real-world setting.

**Methods:** Altogether 154 patients were followed up between Jan 2015 and Dec 2015. The clinical global impression of change (CGIC), premature ejaculation profile (PEP), the estimated intravaginal ejaculation latency time (eIELT) and estimated number of intravaginal thrusts before ejaculation (NITBE) were collected. The clinical characteristics of patients with CGIC = 0 and CGIC≥1 were compared.

**Results:** After 4 weeks treatment, an obvious improvement compared with the baseline was found regarding mean eIELT (2.4 ± 1.6 min vs 1.0 ± 0.7 min, $P < 0.001$) and mean NITBE (85.9 ± 61.9 times vs 37.4 ± 28.6 times, $P < 0.001$). The proportion of patients with a self-evaluation of at least "slightly better" and were categorized into "CGIC≥1" group was 70.1%. There were significant differences between patients in the "CGIC = 0" and "CGIC≥1" groups regarding mean NITBE ($P = 0.010$) and PEDT ($P = 0.009$) score at baseline. The adverse effects were acceptable.

**Conclusion:** Dapoxetine was well-tolerated and improved the sexual satisfaction of patients with PE. The severity of PE based on PEDT and NITBE suggest that there could be an effectiveness change with dapoxetine use in real-world practice.

**Keywords:** Premature ejaculation, Dapoxetine, Sexual dysfunction, Efficacy

## Background

Premature ejaculation (PE) is one of the most of prevalent male sexual disorders, with a reported incidence of 21–33% in some populations [1, 2]. Dapoxetine hydrochloride, a short-acting selective serotonin reuptake inhibitors (SSRIs), is the currently the only on-label oral treatment [3]. This on-demand agent has been proved to increase the quality of life for the patient and their sexual partner by a pooled analysis of five randomized, placebo-controlled, phase 3 clinical trials ($N = 6081$) [4] and by a critical review [5].

Most data on the efficacy of dapoxetine are derived from clinical trials involving Western participants, and results from clinical trials may not be consistent with the results observed in the real-world practice. Clinical trials follow strict protocols involving patients with pre-defined inclusion criteria and results are obtained under ideal conditions. In contrast, clinical practice has several associated challenges including low rates of compliance, economic considerations, and a lack of awareness of the condition by the spouse, and these factors may influence the real-world utility of treatments for PE. In real-world

* Correspondence: lihongjun@pumch.cn; zhangzhichao@bjmu.edu.cn
[†]Jing Peng, Dong Fang and Huixi Li contributed equally to this work.
[2]Department of Urology, Peking Union Medical College Hospital, Peking Union Medical College, Chinese Academy of Medical Sciences, No. 1 Shuaifuyuan, Dongcheng District, Beijing 100730, China
[1]Andrology Center, Department of Urology, Peking University First Hospital, Institute of Urology, Peking University, No. 59A, Di'anmen West St., Xicheng District, Beijing 100034, China

setting dapoxetine treatment discontinuation was high. Mondaini et al. [6] reported that 68.7% of patients would discontinue dapoxetine treatment in a short time. The main reason was effect below expectations. It is important to achieve a reasonable effect in a short term.

Furthermore, stopwatch-determined intravaginal ejaculation latency time (IELT) is the most common measure to diagnose and evaluate treatment efficacy in clinical trials, which is not appropriate in real world practice. In the clinical setting, stopwatch-determined IELT is substituted by self-estimated IELT, which is often overestimated by patients [7].

In this study, we sought to evaluate the treatment effect of dapoxetine on Chinese patients with PE in the real-world practice, and to investigate factors influencing treatment efficacy of dapoxetine.

## Methods

### Patients inclusion

This open-label, retrospective and observational study included patients with PE who accepted dapoxetine treatment in real-world practice. All patients reported short intravaginal latency, and at least 'moderate' distress or interpersonal difficulty relating to their PE at baseline. To be included in the study, patients had to be over 18 years, and were required to be in a heterosexual, stable, and monogamous sexual relationship with the same partner for at least 6 months. The Premature Ejaculation Diagnostic Tool (PEDT) was used to diagnose PE [8] and subjects with a PEDT score ≥ 11 were included. The linguistic validation of PEDT questionnaire has been performed and the Chinese version was used [9, 10]. Patients were excluded from the study if they experienced primary erectile dysfunctions, engaged in sexual intercourse less than once per week, abused alcohol or illicit substances, had a history of medical or psychiatric illness, or if their partner experienced any sexual dysfunction. The study received the ethics approval by committee of Peking University First Hospital. All patients agreed and signed the informed consent, that their information (including clinical information and surveillance) would be collected for scientific study and by published in professional medical journals.

### Patients treatment and outcome measures

After a 4-week run-in period, patients were asked to take dapoxetine 30 mg 1–3 h before planned sexual intercourse. No other PE therapies were provided during the study period. Patients were assessed after 4 weeks of treatment, and were required to engage in sexual intercourse at least 6 times during the 4-week study period.

All measures including eIELT and estimated number of intravaginal thrusts before ejaculation (NITBE) were evaluated at baseline and at week 4. The definition of NITBE was the frequency of penile moving forward and backward in female vaginal. The patients were demanded using the similar frequency and depth of insertion as before and recorded the average NITBE.

Patient were required to answer the question from CGIC "Compared to the start of the study, would you describe your premature ejaculation problem as much worse, worse, slightly worse, no change, slightly better, better, or much better?" and the answers were scored from 0 to 3 (0: no change, 1: Slightly better, 2: better, 3: much better) respectively. Patients were also assessed based on the Premature Ejaculation Profile (PEP) [11]; a validated tool that includes measures of perceived control over ejaculation, satisfaction with sexual intercourse, ejaculation-related personal distress, and ejaculation-related interpersonal difficulty. Part of the database is attached in Additional file 1.

Patient Health Questionnaire (PHQ-9) and General Anxiety Disorder-7 (GAD-7) questionnaire were used to evaluate patients' depression and anxiety [12, 13]. The linguistic validation of PHQ-9 and GAD-7 questionnaires have also been performed and the Chinese versions were used [14, 15].

### Statistical analysis

Statistical analysis was carried by using SPSS 20.0 (IBM Corp, Armonk, NY, USA). Continuous variables normally distributed were expressed as mean ± SD, otherwise median and range (min, max) were used. For categorical variables, frequency and percentile were used to describe the data. Patients were categorized into two groups based on their answer to CGIC after 4 weeks treatment: "CGIC = 0" group vs "CGIC≥1".

Clinical characteristics between the two groups were compared using Chi-square or Mann-Whitney test. The comparison of IELT and NITBE before and after treatment was performed using paired T test. All statistical tests were two-tailed and a $P$ value of less than 0.05 was considered as statistically significant. The receiver-operating curve for treatment effect was also analyzed.

## Results

One hundred seventy-two patients with PE received dapoxetine therapy (30 mg on-demand) for 4 weeks were included in this study. One hundred fifty-four patients were followed up and their data were analyzed and compared at baseline and after dapoxetine treatment. The mean age was 32.5 ± 6.8 (range: 21–61) years. After 4 weeks treatment, there was an obvious improvement compared with the baseline regarding mean eIELT (2.4 ± 1.6 min vs 1.0 ± 0.7 min, $P < 0.001$) and mean NITBE (85.9 ± 61.9 times vs 37.4 ± 28.6 times, $P < 0.001$) (Fig. 1).

Substantial improvements were found in all PEP measures (Fig. 2). At baseline, 9.7 and 0% of patients reported fair or good control over ejaculation which increased to 31.2 and 38.3% at week 4, respectively ($P < 0.001$). At

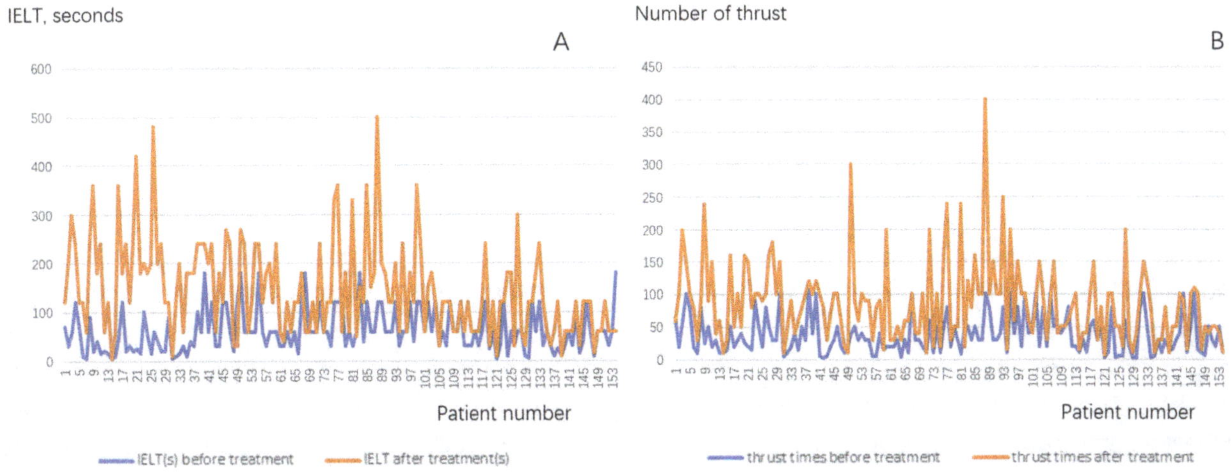


**Fig. 1** IELT distribution (**a**) and thrust times distribution (**b**). IELT: intravaginal ejaculation latency time

baseline, 20.1 and 0% of patients reported fair or good satisfaction with sexual intercourse which increased to 35.1 and 35.7% at week 4, respectively ($P < 0.001$). At baseline, 30.5 and 41.6% of patients reported moderate or quite a bit of ejaculation-related personal distress which decreased to 19.5 and 7.8% at week 4, respectively ($P < 0.001$). At baseline, 35.7 and 15.6% of patients reported moderate or quite a bit of interpersonal difficulty which decreased to 16.9 and 4.6% at week 4, respectively ($P < 0.001$).

Overall, 108 patients (70.1%) answered the CGIC question with "slightly better", "better" or "much better", and were categorized into "CGIC≥1" group (Table 1). Regarding the clinical characteristics between the two groups, the mean NITBE at baseline was 28.0 ± 22.0 and 41.5 ± 30.1 times ($P = 0.010$) and mean PE severity at baseline measured by the PEDT was 15.7 ± 2.7 and 14.5 ± 2.6, respectively ($P = 0.009$), which indicated that the severity of PE and reduced NITBE prior to treatment may be associated with reduced treatment effect. A ROC curve was made to illustrate the relationship between PEDT scores and treatment effect (Fig. 3). Based on Youden index, the best cut-off value was 14.5, with sensitivity 65.2% and specificity 57.4%. A PEDT score of lower than 14.5 points would indicate a possibly better treatment effect. Notably, no significant difference in terms of baseline eIELT was found between the two groups (56.3 ± 44.4 vs 63.0 ± 42.5, $p = 0.262$). Baseline characteristics were also similar, including age, PE duration, previous treatment, and intercourse frequency (all $p > 0.05$).

Regarding adverse effects, 21 patients (13.6%) eventually discontinued dapoxetine treatment, and the reasons included lack of efficacy ($n = 13$), side effects ($n = 5$), and low frequency of sexual intercourse ($n = 3$). Of the patients who completed the 4-week treatment regimen, 72.2%

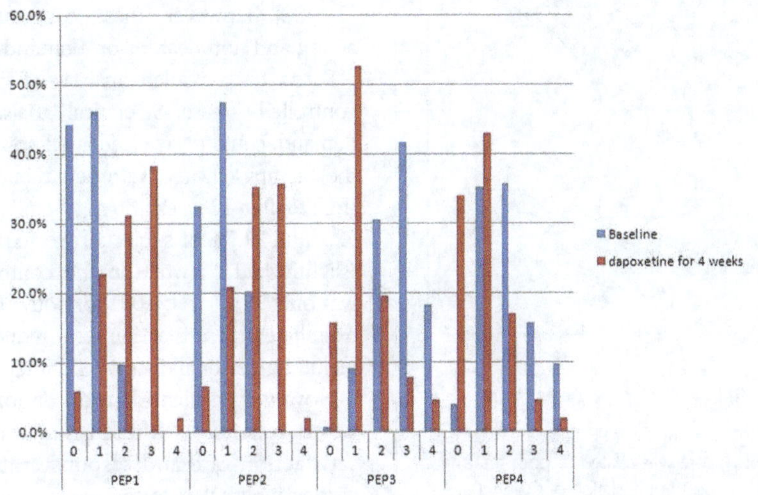


**Fig. 2** Comparison of PEP before and after dapoxetine treatment. All PEP measures showed significant improvements with dapoxetine treatment at week 4 vs. baseline. PEP: premature ejaculation profile

**Table 1** Possible factors affecting the efficacy of dapoxetine 30 mg treatment for 4 weeks

| Parameters | CGIC-C | | P |
|---|---|---|---|
| | 0 (n = 46) | ≥1 (n = 108) | |
| Age (yeas, mean ± SD) | 33.8 ± 8.1 | 31.9 ± 6.1 | 0.213 |
| Marital Status: Married | 88.6% | 84.5% | 0.508 |
| PE duration (years, mean ± SD) | 6.4 ± 5.7 | 8.2 ± 6.8 | 0.058 |
| Type of PE (% of primary PE) | 84.8% | 70.4% | 0.060 |
| Percentage of Intercourse frequency ≥ 2 times | 43.4% | 53.7% | 0.245 |
| Percentage of CP | 41.3% | 41.7% | 0.967 |
| Percentage of previous SSRI use | 10.9% | 18.5% | 0.239 |
| Percentage of previous Effective SSRI use | 10.0% | 28.6% | 0.097 |
| Percentage of history of Circumcision or penile dorsal nerve transection | 28.3% | 34.3% | 0.467 |
| PHQ-9(median [min, max]) | 6.0 [0, 27] | 6.0 [0, 26] | 0.835 |
| GAD-7(median [min, max]) | 4.0 [0, 25] | 3.5 [0, 21] | 0.253 |
| IELT (Seconds, mean ± SD) | 56.3 ± 44.4 | 63.0 ± 42.5 | 0.262 |
| NITBE (times, mean ± SD) | 28.0 ± 22.0 | 41.5 ± 30.1 | 0.010* |
| PEDT (mean ± SD) | 15.7 ± 2.7 | 14.5 ± 2.6 | 0.009* |

*CGIC* Clinical Global Impression of Change, *CP* chronic prostatitis, *ED* erectile dysfunction, *GAD-7* General Anxiety Disorder Questionnaire, *IELT* intravaginal ejaculatory latency time, *NITBE* number of intravaginal thrusts before ejaculation, *PE* premature ejaculation, *PEDT* Premature Ejaculation Diagnostic Tool, *PHQ-9* Patient Health Questionnaire-9 items, *SD* standard deviation, *SSRI* selective serotonin reuptake inhibitors
*statistical significance

would like to continue dapoxetine therapy. Treatment emergent adverse events (TEAEs) were reported in 32 patients (20.8%), that mainly included headache (7.1%), dizziness (7.1%), nausea (4.5%), somnolence (1.9%) and nasal congestion (1.9%). Most TEAEs were mild or moderate in severity and resolved without treatment.

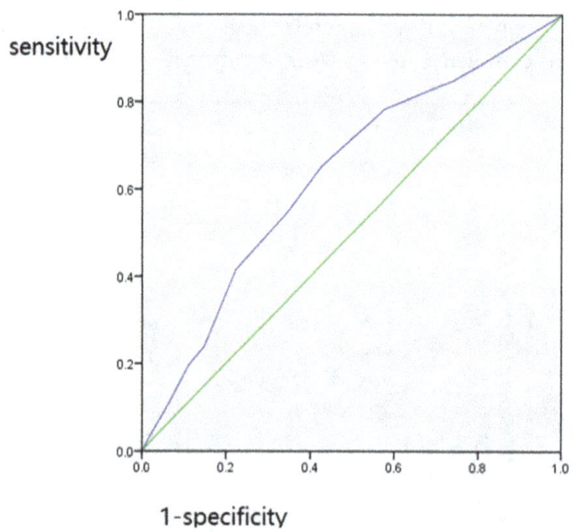


**Fig. 3** The receiver-operating curve (ROC) of PEDT for treatment effect. Note: since higher PEDT score was related to poor treatment effect, the ROC curves are showing the prediction of CGIC = 0, NOT CGIC≥1 (better results). PEDT: Premature Ejaculation Diagnostic Tool; CGIC: clinical global impression of change

## Discussion

PE can interfere with sexual satisfaction, leading to decreased quality of life for the patients and their partners [16–18]. The mechanism for developing PE has not been fully elucidated, especially considering the role of physiological components. SSRIs had been introduced to the treatment of PE following the psychopharmacological studies regarding pathways that control ejaculation [19, 20]. SSRIs could inhibit neuronal re-uptake of serotonin and subsequent potentiation of serotonin activity, and since the serotonergic neurotransmission is related to the pathways which control ejaculation, the delayed ejaculation is a commonly reported side effect [21, 22]. However, these compounds are off-label, long-acting and not ideal for on-demand use.

Based on a pooled analysis of five randomized, placebo-controlled, phase 3 clinical trials, dapoxetine, given on-demand, could delay ejaculation approximately 2.5–3 fold and the therapy efficacy were better in those with lower baseline IELT. After 12 weeks 30 mg or 60 mg dapoxetine treatment, 62.1 and 71.7% of subjects reported that their PE was at least "slightly better", while in the control group this proportion was only 36.0% ($P < 0.001$ for both). Dapoxetine also improved overall sexual satisfaction, and reduced mental consequences including personal distress and interpersonal difficulty [4].

However, clinical data on dapoxetine treatment in real world practice is limited. Jiann et al. [23] reported the satisfaction rate and response rate were 45.0 and 74.6%, respectively. We found dapoxetine treatment was well-accepted by patients with PE and 70.1% of patients reportedly responded to dapoxetine treatment on demand.

In this study, a total of 70.1% of patients reported that their PE was at least “slightly better” with dapoxetine treatment, and 40% of patients evaluated their treatment effect as “better”. Yang et al. [24] reported similar results in Chinese men with PE. The rate of improvement and excellence with dapoxetine 30 mg was 63.5 and 36.5%, respectively. This reflects what was reported in five combined phase 3 trials of 6081 patients, whereby 62.1% of subjects taking dapoxetine 30 mg reported that their PE was at least “slightly better” and 30.7% reported “better” compared with 13.9% in the placebo arm ($P < 0.001$) [4]. Only those who reported that their PE was “better” were satisfied with sexual intercourse.

Dapoxetine was well-tolerated with 72.2% of patients stating that they would continue dapoxetine therapy. In our study, 64.4% of patients who discontinued dapoxetine treatment complained of lack of efficacy which was consistent with the main reasons for discontinuation of dapoxetine or SSRIs in phase 3 clinical trials [6, 25].

In the reported phase 3 trials, 64.9% of the study population were primarily categorized as patients with lifelong PE [4]. In our study, alongside primary PE incidence, we investigated other factors including, marital status, chronic prostatitis, intercourse frequency, prior use and reported efficacy of SSRIs, circumcision or penile dorsal nerve transection, ED and PE severity. While no correlation between efficacy of dapoxetine and the clinical factors listed above were identified, the severity of PE prior to treatment was found to be associated with the efficacy of dapoxetine.

Several factors may impact IELT and thus causing strong interpersonal differences which are reflected in the distribution of IELT values [26], including the performance of foreplay, the interval from last sexual experience, the gesture for sexual intercourse, the depth and force of thrusting, and the partner's vaginal lubrication [27]. We compared patient clinical characteristics and found that most factors would not affect CGI-C, including PE category, effective SSRI use, and estimated IELT. McMahon et al. [28] reported PE category ($P = 0.5$) and estimated baseline IELT ($P = 0.16$) did not affect CGIC rating of “slightly better” in 285 Asia-Pacific men with PE. Patients with a lower PEDT score and a higher NITBE at baseline responded better to dapoxetine.

Interestingly, eIELT was not significantly different between” CGIC = 0″ and” CGIC≥1″ groups, suggesting that eIELT might be poorly estimated in the real-world setting. Lee et al. [7] compared stopwatch-determined IELT and eIELT in healthy men and found that eIELT was overestimated by approximately 1 min.

The stopwatch-determined IELT measured by female partner might not be suitable in real world practice, although it is considered the most objective measure for PE evaluation in clinical trials. Therefore, there is a need for a simple, relative and reliable tool for PE evaluation in real world practice. In this study, we have introduced NITBE as a measure for PE evaluation. We found that baseline NITBE could predict dapoxetine treatment efficacy, and therefore, might be a useful measure for PE evaluation and might be more accurate than eIELT.

Waldinger et al. [29] proposed NITBE in 1994 and found that NITBE between patient assessment and partner assessment was consistent. However, NITBE was not used in subsequent studies. As a very convenient method, it would be possible to evaluate the IELT in daily life and might be a useful tool for PE diagnosis and treatment evaluation in real word practice; however, further validation is required.

Our study has several strengths, including the analysis of co-existing clinical factors that potentially impact PE, and we firstly used NITBE to evaluate PE and found better role of NITBE on PE evaluation than eIELT. In further studies, we will compare NITBE with stopwatch-determined IELT in healthy men and patients with PE. Despite its novel findings, the present study does have some limitations. This was a retrospective, open-label study and the sample size was small relative to clinical trials; there might be some inevitable bias due to the retrospective nature. A further prospective study would be required to reduce bias and increase the strength. A further limitation of the study was that objective stopwatch-determined IELT is difficult to obtain accurately in real world practice, thus clinical trials are required to testify the impact of frequency of penile movement on NITBE. Therefore, patients were included in the study based on the PEDT score, and patient-reported measures included PEP, CGIC and NITBE. Besides although PEP questionnaire has been used in previous studies focusing on Chinese patients [30], the linguistic validation has not been performed.

## Conclusions

Dapoxetine treatment increased CGIC, eIELT and NITBE and was well-tolerated with an acceptable safety profile. Patients with less severe PE based on PEDT and higher NITBE seemed to have better efficacy with dapoxetine.

### Abbreviations

CGIC: Clinical global impression of change; eIELT: Intravaginal ejaculation latency time; NITBE: Number of intravaginal thrusts before ejaculation; PE: Premature ejaculation; PEDT: Premature Ejaculation Diagnostic Tool; PEP: Premature ejaculation profile

### Acknowledgements

We thank Sainan Zhu for the help of critical analysis of data.

### Authors' contributions

JP, HongjunL, ZZ: Protocol/project development; JP, DF, HuixiL, YT, YY, WC, BG: Data collection or management; DF, HuixiL: Data analysis; JP, DF, HuixiL: Manuscript writing/editing; HongjunL, ZZ: Critical revision of the manuscript. All authors read and approved the final manuscript.

**Competing interests**

The authors declare that they have no competing interests.

**References**


1. Porst H, Montorsi F, Rosen RC, Gaynor L, Grupe S, Alexander J. The premature ejaculation prevalence and attitudes (PEPA) survey: prevalence, comorbidities, and professional help-seeking. Eur Urol. 2007;51(3):816–23.
2. Laumann EO, Paik A, Rosen RC. Sexual dysfunction in the United States: prevalence and predictors. JAMA. 1999;281(6):537–44.
3. Modi NB, Dresser MJ, Simon M, Lin D, Desai D, Gupta S. Single- and multiple-dose pharmacokinetics of dapoxetine hydrochloride, a novel agent for the treatment of premature ejaculation. J Clin Pharmacol. 2006;46(3):301–9.
4. McMahon CG, Althof SE, Kaufman JM, Buvat J, Levine SB, Aquilina JW, Tesfaye F, Rothman M, Rivas DA, Porst H. Efficacy and safety of dapoxetine for the treatment of premature ejaculation: integrated analysis of results from five phase 3 trials. J Sex Med. 2011;8(2):524–39.
5. Russo A, Capogrosso P, Ventimiglia E, La Croce G, Boeri L, Montorsi F, Salonia A. Efficacy and safety of dapoxetine in treatment of premature ejaculation: an evidence-based review. Int J Clin Pract. 2016;70(9):723–33.
6. Mondaini N, Fusco F, Cai T, Benemei S, Mirone V, Bartoletti R. Dapoxetine treatment in patients with lifelong premature ejaculation: the reasons of a "Waterloo". Urology. 2013;82(3):620–4.
7. Lee WK, Cho ST, Lee YS, Lee YG, Oh CY, Yoo C, Cho JS, Shin TY, Lee SK, Lee SH, Ko K, Yang DY. Can estimated intravaginal ejaculatory latency time be used interchangeably with stopwatch-measured intravaginal ejaculatory latency time for the diagnosis of lifelong premature ejaculation? Urology. 2015;85(2):375–80.
8. Kam SC, Han DH, Lee SW. The diagnostic value of the premature ejaculation diagnostic tool and its association with intravaginal ejaculatory latency time. J Sex Med. 2011;8(3):865–71.
9. Huang YP, Chen B, Ping P, Wang HX, Hu K, Zhang T, Yang H, Jin Y, Yang Q, Huang YR. The premature ejaculation diagnostic tool (PEDT): linguistic validity of the Chinese version. J Sex Med. 2014;11(9):2232–8.
10. Jiang H, Liu D, Deng C, Shang X, Hong K, Deng J, Wang Z, Yang H, Shi Y, Huang Y, Wang P, Zhang Y, Liang J, Shen B, Li F, Zhang C. Reliability and validity of the Chinese version of the premature ejaculation diagnostic tool. Natl J Androl. 2015;21(7):598–603.
11. Patrick DL, Giuliano F, Ho KF, Gagnon DD, McNulty P, Rothman M. The premature ejaculation profile: validation of self-reported outcome measures for research and practice. BJU Int. 2009;103(3):358–64.
12. Kroenke K, Spitzer RL, Williams JB. The PHQ-9: validity of a brief depression severity measure. J Gen Intern Med. 2001;16(9):606–13.
13. Ruiz MA, Zamorano E, García-Campayo J, Pardo A, Freire O, Rejas J. Validity of the GAD-7 scale as an outcome measure of disability in patients with generalized anxiety disorders in primary care. J Affect Disord. 2011;128(3):277–86.
14. Wang W, Bian Q, Zhao Y, Li X, Wang W, Du J, Zhang G, Zhou Q, Zhao M. Reliability and validity of the Chinese version of the patient health questionnaire (PHQ-9) in the general population. Gen Hosp Psychiatry. 2014; 36(5):539–44.
15. Zeng QZ, He YL, Liu H, Miao JM, Chen JX, Xu HN, Wang JY. Reliability and validity of Chinese version of the Generalized Anxiety Disorder 7-item (GAD-7) scale in screening anxiety disorders in outpatients from traditional Chinese internal department. Chin Mental Health J. 2013;27(3):163–8 [Article in Chinese].
16. Symonds T, Roblin D, Hart K, Althof S. How does premature ejaculation impact a man s life? J Sex Marital Ther. 2003;29(5):361–70.
17. Montague DK, Jarow J, Broderick GA, Dmochowski RR, Heaton JP, Lue TF, Nehra A, Sharlip ID. AUA erectile dysfunction guideline update panel. AUA guideline on the pharmacologic management of premature ejaculation. J Urol. 2004;172(1):290–4.
18. Byers ES, Grenier G. Premature or rapid ejaculation: heterosexual couples' perceptions of men's ejaculatory behavior. Arch Sex Behav. 2003;32(3):261–70.
19. Waldinger MD, Berendsen HH, Blok BF, Olivier B, Holstege G. Premature ejaculation and serotonergic antidepressants-induced delayed ejaculation: the involvement of the serotonergic system. Behav Brain Res. 1998;92(2):111–8.
20. Waldinger MD. The neurobiological approach to premature ejaculation. J Urol. 2002;168(6):2359–67.
21. McMahon CG, Touma K. Treatment of premature ejaculation with paroxetine hydrochloride as needed: 2 single-blind placebo controlled crossover studies. J Urol. 1999;161(6):1826–30.
22. Waldinger MD, Hengeveld MW, Zwinderman AH, Olivier B. Effect of SSRI antidepressants on ejaculation: a double-blind, randomized, placebo-controlled study with fluoxetine, fluvoxamine, paroxetine, and sertraline. J Clin Psychopharmacol. 1998;18(4):274–81.
23. Jiann BP, Huang YJ. Assessing satisfaction in men with premature ejaculation after dapoxetine treatment in real-world practice. Int J Clin Pract. 2015;69(11):1326–33.
24. Yang L, Luo L, Chen XF, Fan JH, Liu RM, Wang XN, Nan XY, Zhang Y, Lin XF, Wang MZ, Xing JP, Yang ZS, Jian BL, He H, Wu DP, He DL. Efficacy and tolerability of dapoxetine in the treatment of premature ejaculation. Zhonghua Nan Ke Xue. 2015;21(10):892–5 [Article in Chinese].
25. Salonia A, Rocchini L, Sacca' A, Pellucchi F, Ferrari M, Carro UD, Ribotto P, Gallina A, Zanni G, Deho' F, Rigatti P, Montorsi F. Acceptance of and discontinuation rate from paroxetine treatment in patients with lifelong premature ejaculation. J Sex Med. 2009;6(10):2868–77.
26. Waldinger MD, Zwinderman AH, Olivier B, Schweitzer DH. Geometric mean IELT and premature ejaculation: appropriate statistics to avoid overestimation of treatment efficacy. J Sex Med. 2008;5(2):492–9.
27. McMahon CG, Althof SE, Waldinger MD, Porst H, Dean J, Sharlip ID, Adaikan PG, Becher E, Broderick GA, Buvat J, Dabees K, Giraldi A, Giuliano F, Hellstrom WJ, Incrocci L, Laan E, Meuleman E, Perelman MA, Rosen RC, Rowland DL, Segraves R. An evidence-based definition of lifelong premature ejaculation: report of the International Society for Sexual Medicine (ISSM) ad hoc committee for the definition of premature ejaculation. J Sex Med. 2008;5(7):1590–606.
28. McMahon C, Lee SW, Kim SW, Moon du G, Kongkanand A, Tantiwongse K. The Asia-Pacific flexible dose study of dapoxetine and patient satisfaction in premature ejaculation therapy: the PASSION study. Sex Med. 2016;4(1):e18–27.
29. Waldinger MD, Hengeveld MW, Zwinderman AH. Paroxetine treatment of premature ejaculation: a double-blind, randomized, placebo-controlled study. Am J Psychiatry. 1994;151(9):1377–9.
30. Ya Z, Zhang X, Shen L, Peng D, Tang D, Huang Z, Cheng P, Dou X, Mao J, Gao J, Liang C. Efficacy and discontinuation reasons of dapoxetine in the treatment of lifelong premature ejaculation. Chin J Androl. 2018;32(3):12–6.

23

# Case report on secondary testicular necrosis due to fulminant epididymitis: Ultrasonographic evaluation and diagnosis

Wout Devlies[1,2*], Mattias Seghers[3] and Kurt Dilen[2]

**Abstract**

**Background:** Scrotal pain is a common complaint in the clinical practice, with many underlying causes. Infectious causes, like epididymitis, are frequently encountered in the work-up of scrotal pain. The presentation of epididymitis is mostly mild, yet major complications can occur.

**Case presentation:** We present a 35-year-old male presenting with scrotal pain and swelling of the testicle. Epididymitis with testicular necrosis was diagnosed using repeated doppler ultrasonography measurements. An orchiectomy was performed which showed a hemorrhagic process with affected spermatic cord. Funiculitis together with epididymal swelling can impede testicular blood flow, with testicular necrosis possibly resulting in orchiectomy. This is the first case that proved funiculitis to co-exist in loss of colour doppler on pathological evaluation.

**Conclusions:** In order to reduce major complications, medical therapy should be promptly initiated when there is a suspicion of epididymitis.

**Keywords:** Testicular necrosis, Epididymitis, UTI, Complication

## Background

Acute scrotal pain is frequently encountered at the emergency department. The differential diagnosis is broad, with sometimes difficult differentiation [1]. Different causes consist of acute epididymitis, testicular torsion, Fournier's gangrene, torsion of appendix testis, trauma, post-vasectomy pain, inguinal hernia, mumps orchitis, testicular cancer, immunoglobulin A (IgA) vasculitis, and acute idiopathic scrotal edema. Due to the extensive list of diagnosis the standard of care is to identify causes that need immediate action. Testicular torsion and Fournier's gangrene [2] are examples needing urgent surgical intervention. In acute epididymitis/ epididymo-orchitis medical treatment should start promptly, ultrasonography can help to prove the diagnosis and help with the prognosis of this infection [3].

Testicular torsion and major epididymo-orchitis can be difficult to distinguish. This distinction is made on blood results with infectious episodes resulting in higher C-reactive protein levels. One rare complication in epididymitis is testicular necrosis, with an incidence of 1–2% of epididymitis cases. In case of post-infectious necrosis, the presentation to surgery-time was significantly longer than in testicular torsion [4].

On ultrasonography epididymo-orchitis necrosis can be recognized by a juxta-epididymal string-of-bead sign, contrasting the whirlpool/knot sign, seen in testicular torsion [4]. Reduction of color doppler signalling with high intratesticular resistive indices and negative diastolic flow increase the likelihood of testicular necrosis associated with epididymo-orchitis [5, 6]. Further

* Correspondence: wout.devlies@outlook.com
[1]Faculty of Medicine, KU Leuven, Leuven, Belgium
[2]Department of Urology, Regional hospital St. Franciskus, Heusden-Zolder, Belgium

assessment of suspected testicular necrosis and its vascularity can be performed using ultrasound microbubble contrast [7].

Surgical management in necrosed testis is an orchiectomy. Fasciotomy in early hypoperfusion has been suggested in the past, but no clinical outcomes have been reported [8]. This is therefore not routinely done. Partial hypoperfusion and necrosis of the testis can be treated conservatively with close follow-up.

A Medline search was initiated to discuss similar cases and their treatment approaches using MeSH terms: testis, orchitis, epididymitis, necrosis and infection. There is currently a lack of data and clinical guidance in patients presenting with these complications. Together with the available literature, this case report can support clinicians in their daily practise.

## Case presentation

A 35-year old male, with no relevant past medical history, presented to the emergency room with local swelling, fever of 39.4 °C (103 °F) and pain in the right hemiscrotum. It started mildly a week earlier and he was started on ciprofloxacin 500 mg since 4 days. There was no history of trauma and no recent disease signs. A scrotal ultrasound was performed on admission showing an enlargement of the epididymis on the right side with septal hydrocoele (Fig. 1a). By using scrotal color doppler ultrasound scanning an increased signal was seen in the right testis (Fig. 1b). Blood results initially showed C-reactive protein (CRP) of 69 mg/L with a leucocytosis of 20,000/mm$^3$ and left shift.

The diagnosis of epidymo-orchitis was made with a prompt start of IV antibiotics (ceftriaxone 2 g 1x/day with amikacin 1 g/day). On repeated bloods the next day, the CRP rose to 230 and 320 mg/L one and 2 days after presentation respectively with remaining leucocytosis of 29,000/mm$^3$ and 22,000/mm$^3$. Initial urine culture showed the presence of an extended spectrum beta lactamase *E. coli*, sensitive to ceftriaxone and temocillin, resistant to Fluoroquinolones. After knowledge of the antibiogram, the patient was put on temocillin.

Two days after the initial presentation, the symptomatology did not improve notably. A re-assessment with ultrasonography and blood results was done. This showed a stable hypervascularisation and swelling in the epididymis. The septal hydrocele enlarged in 2 days' time with an appearance of heterogeneity in the hydrocele collection. Upon second ultrasound evaluation, no residual color Doppler signal was found in the testis (Fig. 1c).

Due to the evolving ultrasonographic findings and the loss of doppler signal an orchiectomy was performed. The testis was removed together with the epididymis and the existing pyocele. The operation field was thoroughly cleaned. Postoperative blood analysis showed a CRP level of 210 mg/L with a leucocytosis of 18,000/mm$^3$.

On anatomopathological review these structures were primarily typed of hemorrhagic substrate with mixed inflammatory cells (Fig. 2). The spermatic cord in this

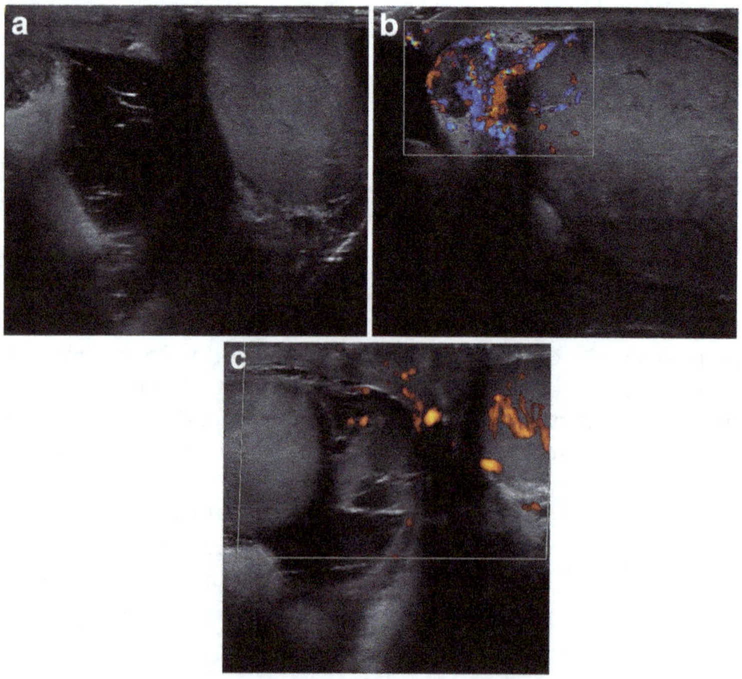

**Fig. 1 a-b**: Initial ultrasonographical images with **a**: Pyocoele, **b**: accentuated doppler of epididymo-orchitis. **c**: Images of the second ultrasonographical evaluation, with right-sided avascular necrosis with pyocoele in comparison to a normal left testis

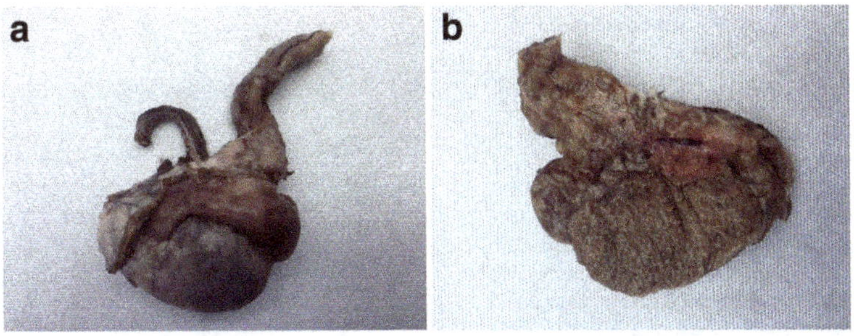

**Fig. 2** Postoperative resection specimen **a**: pathology specimen **b** cross-sectional section of the testis

resection is also taint in a similar process. No signs of malignancy are seen in the resection specimen. A microbiological examination of the orchiectomy specimen could confirm the presence of E Coli in the resection specimen, therefore providing additional evidence for an epidydimo-orchitis, yet this was not performed.

The patient went home with outpatient parenteral antimicrobial therapy of Temocillin for 7 days. The blood abnormalities gradually decreased with a reassuring clinical picture. The patient remained asymptomatic and afebrile since.

## Discussion

Testicular necrosis is a rare presentation of epididymitis in the emergency department, with an estimated incidence of 1–2% of all epididymitis cases [9, 10].

Our case highlights the benefit of ultrasonography of the testis. This case initially showed clear hyperperfusion with a rapid change to hypoperfusion. The latter being strongly associated with testicular necrosis [9].

Moreover, this paper proves to be a contemporary example of the approach in severe epididymitis and the useful ultrasonographical measures. As ultrasonography is frequently performed and relatively cheap, but on the other hand user dependent, this paper supplied us with evidence on how to diagnose similar conditions.

We preferred to surgically remove the testicle directly after loss of doppler signal, yet other authors have reported acceptable results with longer intervals between diagnosis and surgery [11]. When longer intervals are used a fistula would be formed which should then be surgically removed [12, 13].

Testicular necrosis is caused by venous occlusion from the testes [11, 14]. The mechanism of this para-infectious thrombosis is not entirely clear [11, 15]. Suggested mechanisms contributing to this testicular necrosis could be venous compression by oedema of the epididymis, swelling of the funiculus in case of funiculitis or edema at the external inguinal ring. Besides this, bacterial toxins may damage endothelial cells with induction of vascular thrombosis [15–17]. In rodents infected with E Coli, necrosis is found to be the primary cell death mechanism. This effect is primarily seen in Sertoli cells in infected testis with impaired spermatogenesis due to the lack of supporting germ cells [18]. This lowering of spermatogenesis after infectious necrosis is also seen in human testis [11].

As discussed different etiologies have been postulated with few proven cases, with few high quality evidence reported in literature. To our knowledge, this is the first case that proved funiculitis to co-exist in loss of colour doppler on pathological evaluation.

## Conclusion

Epididymitis is a common condition with possible severe complications. If epididymitis is suspected we suggest to start medical treatment promptly. In our experience, scrotal ultrasound should be performed for the diagnosis of epididymitis and orchitis and should be repeated if there is a suspicion of doubtful blood supply to the testicle. This case provides the first clinical evidence to support associated funiculitis in this disease. Also this case stresses the usefulness of ultrasonography in the diagnosis and management of testicular necrosis secondary to epididymitis/ epididymo-orchitis.

#### Abbreviations

MeSH: Medical subject headings

#### Acknowledgements

We would like to thank Michel Vanbockrijck of the Department of Pathology, Regional hospital Jessa, Hasselt, Belgium for his cooperation to this study.

#### Authors' contributions

Design and drafting of the study: WD, MS, KD. Revision of the article: WD, MS, KD. All authors have read and approved the manuscript.

#### Competing interests

The authors declare no conflict of interest.

#### Author details

Faculty of Medicine, KU Leuven, Leuven, Belgium. [2]Department of Urology, Regional hospital St. Franciskus, Heusden-Zolder, Belgium. [3]Department of Radiology, Regional hospital St. Franciskus, Heusden-Zolder, Belgium.

**References**


1. Fukuda S, Takahashi T, Kumori K, et al. Idiopathic testicular infarction in a boy initially suspected to have acute epididymo-orchitis associated with mycoplasma infection and Henoch–Schönlein purpura. J Pediatr Urol. 2009; 5(1):68–71. https://doi.org/10.1016/j.jpurol.2008.07.003.
2. Baskin LS, Carroll PR, EV C, JW M. Necrotising soft tissue infections of the perineum and genitalia: bacteriology, treatment and risk assessment. Br J Urol. 1990;65(5):524–9. https://doi.org/10.1111/j.1464-410X.1990.tb14801.x.
3. Banyra O, Shulyak A. Acute epididymo-orchitis: staging and treatment. Cent Eur J Urol. 2012;65(3):139–43. https://doi.org/10.5173/ceju.2012.03.art8.
4. Ching-di Chang JLCLYCCHYLSNSK. Acute Epididymo-orchitis–related global testicular infarction: clinical and ultrasound findings with an emphasis on the Juxta-epididymal string-of-bead sign. Ultrasound Q. 2016;32(3):283–9. https://doi.org/10.1097/ruq.0000000000000225.
5. Lefort C, Thoumas D, Badachi Y, et al. Ischemic orchiditis: review of 5 cases diagnosed by color Doppler ultrasonography. J Radiol. 2001;82(7):839–42 http://www.ncbi.nlm.nih.gov/pubmed/11507447. Accessed January 5, 2019.
6. Sue SR, Pelucio M, Gibbs M. Testicular infarction in a patient with epididymitis. Acad Emerg Med. 1998;5(11):1128–30 http://www.ncbi.nlm.nih.gov/pubmed/9835481. Accessed January 5, 2019.
7. Yusuf G, Sellars ME, Kooiman GG, Diaz-Cano S, Sidhu PS. Global testicular infarction in the presence of epididymitis. J Ultrasound Med. 2013;32(1): 175–80. https://doi.org/10.7863/jum.2013.32.1.175.
8. Vordermark JS, Favila MQ. Testicular necrosis: a preventable complication of epididymitis. J Urol. 1982;128(6):1322–4. https://doi.org/10.1016/S0022-5347(17)53482-5.
9. Pilatz A, Wagenlehner F, Bschleipfer T, et al. Acute epididymitis in ultrasound: Results of a prospective study withbaseline and follow-up investigations in 134 patients. Eur J Radiol. 2013;82(12). https://doi.org/10.1016/j.ejrad.2013.08.050.
10. Pilatz A, Hossain H, Kaiser R, et al. Acute epididymitis revisited: impact of molecular diagnostics on etiology and contemporary guideline recommendations. Eur Urol. 2015;68(3):428–35. https://doi.org/10.1016/j.eururo.2014.12.005.
11. Hourihane DO. Infected infarcts of the testis: a study of 18 cases preceded by pyogenic epididymoorchitis. J Clin Pathol. 1970;23(8):668–75 http://www.ncbi.nlm.nih.gov/pubmed/4922665. Accessed January 5, 2019.
12. PARR NJ, PRASAD BRP, HAYHURST V, McMILLAN A, LEEN CS, FOWLER JW. Suppurative Epididymo-orchitis in young "high risk" patients-a new problem? Br J Urol. 1993;72(6):949–51. https://doi.org/10.1111/j.1464-410X.1993.tb16306.x.
13. Chia D, Penkoff P, Stanowski M, Beattie K, Wang AC. Testicular infarction and rupture: an uncommon complication of epididymo-orchitis | Kopernio. J Surg Case Rep. 2016;5:1–3.
14. Eisner DJ, Goldman SM, Petronis J, Millmond SH. Bilateral testicular infarction caused by epididymitis. Am J Roentgenol. 1991;157(3):517–9. https://doi.org/10.2214/ajr.157.3.1872237.
15. Rencken RK, DJ du P, De HLS. Venous infarction of the testis - a cause of non-response to conservative therapy in epididymo-orchitis. South African Med J. 78(9):337–8 https://www.ajol.info/index.php/samj/article/view/160180/149763. Accessed January 5, 2019.
16. ERTC O, Kitson JL, Green B. Venous infarction of the testis secondary to acute epididymitis. Br J Urol. 1990;65(1):107–8. https://doi.org/10.1111/j.1464-410X.1990.tb14672.x.
17. Bird K, Rosenfield AT. Testicular infarction secondary to acute inflammatory disease: demonstration by B-scan ultrasound. Radiology. 1984;152(3):785–8. https://doi.org/10.1148/radiology.152.3.6463261.
18. Lu Y, Bhushan S, Tchatalbachev S, et al. Necrosis is the dominant cell death pathway in uropathogenic Escherichia coli elicited epididymo-orchitis and is responsible for damage of rat testis. PLoS One. 2013;8(1):e52919. https://doi.org/10.1371/journal.pone.0052919.

# 24

# A comparison of stage-specific all-cause mortality between testicular sex cord stromal tumors and germ cell tumors: Results from the National Cancer Database

Kyle B. Zuniga[1,2,3*], Samuel L. Washington III[1], Sima P. Porten[1] and Maxwell V. Meng[1]

**Abstract**

**Background:** Testicular sex cord stromal tumors (SCSTs) are managed similarly to germ cell tumors (GCTs); however, few studies have directly compared outcomes between these tumor types. Using the National Cancer Database (NCDB), we sought to compare overall and stage-specific all-cause mortality (ACM) between SCSTs versus GCTs.

**Methods:** NCDB was queried for patients diagnosed with SCSTs and GCTs between 2004 and 2013. Descriptive statistics were used to compare sociodemographic and clinical characteristics between groups. Univariable and multivariable Cox proportional hazards regression analyses were used to assess associations with ACM.

**Results:** We identified 42,192 patients diagnosed with testicular cancer between 2004 and 2013, with 280 having SCSTs and 41,912 patients having GCTs. Median age for SCSTs and GCTs was 45 (interquartile range [IQR] 34–59) and 34 (IQR 27–43), respectively ($p < 0.001$). Median follow-up was 39 and 52 months, respectively. Overall, patients with SCSTs had greater risk of ACM compared to those with GCTs (HR 1.69, 95% CI 1.14–2.50). Private insurance, greater education, and fewer comorbidities were associated with reduced risk of ACM ($p < 0.05$ for all). Among those with stage I disease, tumor type was not associated with ACM on multivariable analysis. Among those with stage II/III disease, patients with SCSTs had increased risk of ACM compared to patients with GCTs (HR 3.29, 95% CI 1.89–5.72).

**Conclusions:** Patients with advanced SCSTs had worse survival outcomes compared to those with advanced GCTs. These data suggest a need for further investigation to ascertain effective management recommendations for SCSTs.

**Keywords:** Testicular neoplasms, Leydig cell tumors, Sertoli cell tumors, Sex cord-gonadal stromal tumors, Testicular germ cell tumors

* Correspondence: kbz2102@columbia.edu
[1]Department of Urology, University of California, San Francisco, 550 16th Street, 6th Floor, San Francisco, CA 94158, USA
[2]Osher Center for Integrative Medicine, University of California, San Francisco, 1545 Divisadero Street, Suite 301, San Francisco, CA 94143, USA

## Background

Testicular cancer is a rare form of cancer, representing only 0.5% of new cancer cases in the United States (U.S.) [1]. It most commonly occurs in young adults, with 5.9 new cases per 100,000 men between 2012 and 2016 [1]. Testicular tumors can be further subclassified based on their cellular origin. Germ cell tumors (GCTs) account for roughly 95% of all testicular tumors and include seminomatous and nonseminomatous tumors (e.g., embryonal, mixed germ cell) [2]. Sex cord stromal tumors (SCSTs) make up the remaining 5% of testicular tumors and include Leydig cell tumors (LCTs) and Sertoli cell tumors (SCTs) [3].

SCSTs and GCTs differ greatly in their biological aggressiveness and survival outcomes. GCTs have an excellent prognosis, with a 99.7% 5-year disease-specific survival among those with Stage I tumors [4]. Patients with SCSTs appear to have worse survival outcomes, with the 5-year overall survival of patients with Stage I LCTs and SCTs being 91 and 77%, respectively [5]. This survival difference is multifactorial, with the inherent aggressiveness of SCSTs, differences in patient characteristics, and variable response to treatment likely contributing to this finding [6–8]. Prior studies focused on SCSTs alone, primarily small series and case studies, have demonstrated worse disease-specific and overall survival outcomes, but few studies have directly compared outcomes between SCSTs and GCTs [5, 9, 10]. These studies have been predominantly limited by the rarity of these tumors and few mortality events reported in large national cancer registries [5, 9].

Given that the American Urological Association (AUA) provides formal guidelines for the management of GCTs but none specific to SCSTs, the management of SCSTs primarily reflects that of GCTs [11]. Thus, a survival comparison between these tumor types is critical to identify whether a need for guidelines specific to SCSTs is warranted. Using a large, nationwide database of cancer patients, we sought to compare total and stage-specific all-cause mortality (ACM) outcomes between patients with GCTs and SCTSs with consideration of multiple sociodemographic and clinical characteristics.

## Methods

### Data source

The NCDB is a nationwide, facility-based cancer registry started in 1989 as a joint program between the Commission on Cancer of the American College of Surgeons and the American Cancer Society. It encompasses over 1500 institutions and contains over 70% of all cancer diagnoses in the U.S. and Puerto Rico [12, 13]. This study was approved by the Institutional Review Board at the University of California, San Francisco.

### Patient selection

Patients diagnosed between 2004 and 2013 were identified using the International Classification of Diseases for Oncology, Third Edition (ICD-O-3) codes for LCTs (8650), SCTs (8640), seminomas (9061), embryonal tumors (9070), and mixed germ cell tumors (9085). Diagnosis was determined from microscopic specimens, laboratory markers, imaging, or medical records from participating institutions. Those with unavailable staging information were excluded. Stage was defined by Clinical Stage Group or Clinical Pathological Group if the former was unavailable. Because of the low sample size of SCSTs, patients with stage II and stage III disease were collapsed into one group (stage II/III) for the survival analysis. We considered this a reasonable strategy, as both represent tumors that have spread beyond the testicle. Furthermore, this strategy has been performed in prior literature [5]. For the same reason, all forms of therapy received in addition to orchiectomy were grouped into an "adjuvant therapy" category. Of note, NCDB only reports first course treatments [14].

### Objectives and statistical analysis

The primary endpoint was ACM. Demographic, clinicopathologic, and overall survival outcome data was collected. Survival time was calculated as the time in months between diagnosis and either death or last follow-up contact. Patient characteristics were compared using Pearson's chi-squared and Fischer's exact tests for categorical variables and Wilcoxon rank-sum tests for non-parametric continuous variables. Survival curves were generated using the Kaplan-Meier plot method. Log-rank test and Cox proportional hazard regression was used to compare differences in survival among the entire cohort and on subgroup analysis by tumor stage (stage I and stage II/III). The other variables included in the multivariable models included tumor type, diagnosis year, race/ethnicity, insurance type, annual household income, percent in the patient's ZIP code without a high school diploma, residential environment (metropolitan versus urban/rural), and Charlson-Deyo comorbidity score (CDS). As the stage and adjuvant therapy variables violated the proportionality assumption, analyses were stratified on these variables (STATA 15 command: *strata*) [15]. The results are presented as hazard ratios (HR) with 95% confidence intervals (CI). HRs for patients with unknown values are not reported but were included in analyses to avoid selection bias secondary to elimination of those patients. A $p$-value $< 0.05$ was considered statistically significant. Analyses were performed using STATA 15®.

## Results

### Sociodemographic and clinical characteristics between groups

Forty-two thousand one hundred ninety-two patients diagnosed with testicular cancer between 2004 and 2013 were identified (Table 1). There were 45 patients with SCTs and 235 patients with LCTs for a total of 280 patients with SCSTs. There were 26,394 patients with seminomas, 11,358 patients with embryonal tumors, and 4160 patients with mixed germ cell tumors for a total of 41,912 patients with GCTs. Median follow-up time was 39 months (interquartile range [IQR] 20–61) for SCSTs and 52 months (IQR 28–79) for GCTs. Compared to patients with GCTs, patients with SCSTs tended to be older (45 years IQR 34–59 versus 34 years IQR 27–43, $p < 0.001$). Higher proportions of patients with SCSTs were non-Hispanic Black (17% versus 3%) and were on government insurance (25% versus 13%) (all $p < 0.001$). Higher proportions of patients with SCSTs had one or more comorbidities (10% versus 6%, $p = 0.001$) and had stage I disease at diagnosis (93% versus 77%, $p < 0.001$). A considerably lower proportion of patients with SCSTs received adjuvant therapy in addition to orchiectomy (6% versus 56%, p < 0.001). Type of adjuvant therapy received in addition to orchiectomy by tumor type can be seen in Supplementary Table 1.

The aforementioned observations remained true when broken down by stage with a few exceptions (Table 2). There was no statistically significant difference in race/ethnic distribution or insurance status among those with advanced disease. Notably, among those with advanced disease, the magnitude of difference of the proportion of those with one or more comorbidities was greater among those with SCSTs (29% versus 7%, $p < 0.001$).

### Survival analysis

On multivariable Cox proportional hazards regression of the overall group, patients with SCSTs had greater risk of ACM compared to those with GCTs (HR 1.68, 95% CI 1.13–2.49, $p = 0.010$) (Table 3) on multivariable analysis adjusting for stage and treatment via stratification. Compared to those with private insurance, those who were uninsured (HR 2.31, 95% CI 2.01–2.66, $p < 0.001$) or who had government insurance (HR 2.72, 95% CI 2.42–3.05, p < 0.001) had greater risk of ACM. Having one or more comorbidities also conferred a greater risk of ACM (HR 2.06, 95% CI 1.79–2.37, p < 0.001).

The Kaplan-Meier curves comparing overall survival outcomes between tumors types by stage can be seen in Fig. 1. At 1, 2, and 5 years, the overall survival rates for stage I SCSTs was 99% (95% CI 96–100%), 96% (95% CI 92–98%), and 94% (95% CI 89–97%), respectively and for stage I GCTs was 99% (95% CI 99–100%), 99% (95% CI 99–99%), and 97% (95% CI 97–98%), respectively

**Table 1** Overall comparison of the sociodemographic and clinical characteristics of patients with SCSTs versus GCTs

| Factor | Overall cohort | SCSTs | GCTs | *p*-value |
|---|---|---|---|---|
| N | 42,192 | 280 | 41,912 | |
| Age at diagnosis, median (IQR) | 34 (27, 43) | 45 (34, 59) | 34 (27, 43) | < 0.001 |
| Diagnosis year | | | | 0.002 |
| 2004–2005 | 8215 (20%) | 48 (17%) | 8167 (20%) | |
| 2006–2007 | 8329 (20%) | 39 (14%) | 8290 (20%) | |
| 2008–2009 | 8520 (20%) | 50 (18%) | 8470 (20%) | |
| 2010–2011 | 8561 (20%) | 81 (29%) | 8480 (20%) | |
| 2012–2013 | 8567 (20%) | 62 (22%) | 8505 (20%) | |
| Race/ethnicity | | | | < 0.001 |
| Non-Hispanic White | 32,565 (77%) | 174 (62%) | 32,391 (77%) | |
| Non-Hispanic Black | 1168 (3%) | 48 (17%) | 1120 (3%) | |
| Hispanic/Other | 7727 (18%) | 55 (20%) | 7672 (18%) | |
| Unknown | 732 (2%) | 3 (1%) | 729 (2%) | |
| Insurance | | | | < 0.001 |
| Uninsured | 4786 (11%) | 24 (9%) | 4762 (11%) | |
| Private insurance | 31,092 (74%) | 178 (64%) | 30,914 (74%) | |
| Medicaid/Medicare /other government insurance | 5487 (13%) | 70 (25%) | 5417 (13%) | |
| Unknown | 827 (2%) | 8 (3%) | 819 (2%) | |
| Income (per year) | | | | 0.42 |
| Less than $38 k | 5533 (13%) | 45 (16%) | 5488 (13%) | |
| $38 k-62,999 | 20,324 (48%) | 125 (45%) | 20,199 (48%) | |
| $63 k or greater | 15,769 (37%) | 106 (38%) | 15,663 (37%) | |
| Unknown | 566 (1%) | 4 (1%) | 562 (1%) | |
| Percent in ZIP code without a high school degree | | | | 0.81 |
| 21% or greater | 6203 (15%) | 42 (15%) | 6161 (15%) | |
| 7–20.9% | 23,172 (55%) | 159 (57%) | 23,013 (55%) | |
| Less than 7% | 12,287 (29%) | 75 (27%) | 12,212 (29%) | |
| Unknown | 530 (1%) | 4 (1%) | 526 (1%) | |
| Residence | | | | 0.48 |
| Metropolitan | 35,048 (83%) | 237 (85%) | 34,811 (83%) | |
| Urban/rural | 7144 (17%) | 43 (15%) | 7101 (17%) | |
| Charlson-Deyo comorbidity score | | | | 0.001 |
| 0 | 39,825 (94%) | 252 (90%) | 39,573 (94%) | |
| 1 or more | 2367 (6%) | 28 (10%) | 2339 (6%) | |
| Stage | | | | < 0.001 |
| Stage I | 32,463 (77%) | 259 (93%) | 32,204 (77%) | |
| Stage II | 5478 (13%) | 9 (3%) | 5469 (13%) | |
| Stage III | 4251 (10%) | 12 (4%) | 4239 (10%) | |
| Treatment received | | | | < 0.001 |
| No orchiectomy | 666 (2%) | 2 (0.7%) | 664 (2%) | |
| Orchiectomy alone | 17,885 (42%) | 260 (93%) | 17,625 (42%) | |
| Orchiectomy + adjuvant therapy | 23,585 (56%) | 18 (6%) | 23,567 (56%) | |

**Table 1** Overall comparison of the sociodemographic and clinical characteristics of patients with SCSTs versus GCTs *(Continued)*

| Factor | Overall cohort | SCSTs | GCTs | *p*-value |
|---|---|---|---|---|
| Other/unknown | 56 (0.1%) | 0 (0%) | 56 (0.1%) | |
| Last contact or death, months from diagnosis, median (IQR) | N = 37,716 | N = 249 | N = 37,467 | |
| | 52 (28, 79) | 39 (20, 61) | 52 (28, 79) | < 0.001 |
| Time from diagnosis to death in months, median (IQR) | N = 1640 | N = 27 | N = 1613 | |
| | 20 (7, 43) | 18 (7, 37) | 20 (7, 43) | 0.88 |

*GCTs* Germ cell tumors, *IQR* Interquartile range, *SCSTs* Sex cord stromal tumors

(log-rank $p < 0.001$). Among those with stage I disease, tumor type was not associated with ACM on multivariable analysis (Table 4). High income (HR 0.74 among those making >$63,000/year compared to those making <$38,000/year, 95% CI 0.56–0.98, $p = 0.032$), was associated with lower ACM.

At 1, 2, and 5 years, the overall survival rates for stage II/III SCSTs was 60% (95% CI 36–78%), 44% (95% CI 22–64%), and 25% (95% CI 8–47%), respectively and for stage II/III GCTs was 95% (95% CI 95–96%), 92% (95% CI 92–93%), and 89% (95% CI 88–90%) (log-rank $p <$ 0.001). Among those with stage II/III disease, those with SCSTs had a statistically significantly increased risk of ACM (HR 3.28, 95% CI 1.88–5.73, $p < 0.001$) on multivariable analysis adjusting for treatment via stratification (Table 4). Percent of individuals in the patient's ZIP code without a high school diploma (HR 0.67 for < 7% compared to > 21, 95% CI 0.52–0.89, $p = 0.004$) was associated with ACM.

## Discussion

Using a national registry of testicular cancer patients, we found that SCSTs conferred increased risk of ACM compared to patients with GCT. However, on multivariable subgroup analysis, this difference in overall survival was limited to those with advanced (stage II/III) disease. For these patients, the risk of ACM in the SCST group was more than three times greater than that of the GCT group. We also found that patients with SCSTs tended to be older and were more frequently of Black race.

The association between SCSTs and worse survival outcomes has been shown previously. Osbun et al. used the Surveillance, Epidemiology, and End Results (SEER) program database to estimate cancer-specific mortality (CSM) for various testicular tumor types. They found a lower overall CSM among patients with GCTs (2%) compared to those with LCTs (7%) or SCTs (32%, $p <$ 0.001) [9]. They also reported an observation of higher unadjusted CSM rates in patients with SCSTs both in stage I and stage III disease. As with our population, higher proportions of SEER patients with SCSTs were older and Black; however, in contrast to our population, a higher proportion of SEER patients with SCSTs presented with advanced disease.

The finding that there is a greater risk of ACM with SCSTs versus GCTs among patients with advanced disease regardless of receipt of adjuvant therapy use indicates that management recommendations specific to SCSTs are needed. Currently, the AUA provides guidelines for the management of seminomatous and nonseminomatous GCTs but does not specifically address SCSTs [11]. Thus, much of the management reflects that of GCTs. An initial approach of radical resection for early stage disease has been shown to be effective [6, 16]. Featherstone et al. reported that, among 36 patients with SCSTs treated with orchiectomy alone, none progressed to metastatic disease after a minimum follow-up period of 2 years [16]. These results are consistent with the high overall survival among patients with stage I disease, and perhaps translation of management of SCSTs from that of GCTs is appropriate.

Using GCTs as a reference, our data suggests that patients with disseminated SCSTs do not experience the same relatively high overall survival rates as those with localized disease. Although surgical management via retroperitoneal lymphadenectomy may have modest efficacy in those with established nodal disease, traditional chemotherapy regimens used to treat GCTs like bleomycin, etoposide, and cisplatin (BEP) or vinblastine, ifosfamide, and cisplatin (VIP) have demonstrated a transient response in SCSTs [6–8]. Radiotherapy also appears to be ineffectual for these tumors [8, 17]. This lack of effectiveness signals an opportunity to investigate the potency of newer chemotherapeutics, hormonal therapies, and immunologic agents to improve outcomes for patients with this rare tumor type. For example, it has been demonstrated that glucocorticoid treatment may inhibit a hormone-mediated cell growth mechanism in LCTs that leads to tumor regression in murine models [18]. Imatinib, a selective tyrosine kinase inhibitor, has been shown to decrease viability of Leydig tumor cell lines [19]. Furthermore, with the advent of the use of genomics and precision medicine, future therapeutic regimens could potentially be tailored for these patients and may help improve treatment outcomes in patients with advanced disease [20]. Necchi et al. performed comprehensive genome profiling on the tumors of 10 patients with metastatic SCSTs and reported that, although uncommon, several tumors expressed targetable genomic alterations indicating the potential efficacy of cell-cycle, mTOR, hedgehog, and polymerase inhibitors [20]. A case-series by Calaway et al. reported that two patients with disseminated SCSTs had tumor genetic susceptibility testing following retroperitoneal lymph

**Table 2** Stage-specific comparison of the sociodemographic and clinical characteristics of patients with SCSTs versus GCTs

| Factor | Stage I | | | Stage II/III | | |
|---|---|---|---|---|---|---|
| | SCSTs | GCTs | p-value | SCSTs | GCTs | p-value |
| N | 259 | 32,204 | | 21 | 9708 | |
| Age at diagnosis, median (IQR) | 43 (34, 57) | 34 (28, 43) | < 0.001 | 55 (42, 64) | 33 (26, 42) | < 0.001 |
| Diagnosis year | | | < 0.001 | | | 0.38 |
| 2004–2005 | 46 (18%) | 6387 (20%) | | 2 (10%) | 1780 (18%) | |
| 2006–2007 | 33 (13%) | 6416 (20%) | | 6 (29%) | 1874 (19%) | |
| 2008–2009 | 45 (17%) | 6528 (20%) | | 5 (24%) | 1942 (20%) | |
| 2010–2011 | 75 (29%) | 6487 (20%) | | 6 (29%) | 1993 (21%) | |
| 2012–2013 | 60 (23%) | 6386 (20%) | | 2 (10%) | 2119 (22%) | |
| Race/ethnicity | | | < 0.001 | | | 0.62 |
| Non-Hispanic White | 157 (61%) | 25,125 (78%) | | 17 (81%) | 7266 (75%) | |
| Non-Hispanic Black | 47 (18%) | 809 (3%) | | 1 (5%) | 311 (3%) | |
| Hispanic/Other | 52 (20%) | 5672 (18%) | | 3 (14%) | 2000 (21%) | |
| Unknown | 3 (1%) | 598 (2%) | | 0 (0%) | 131 (1%) | |
| Insurance | | | < 0.001 | | | 0.087 |
| Uninsured | 169 (65%) | 3411 (11%) | | 4 (19%) | 1351 (14%) | |
| Private insurance | 20 (8%) | 24,575 (76%) | | 9 (43%) | 6339 (65%) | |
| Medicaid/Medicare/other government insurance | 62 (24%) | 3605 (11%) | | 8 (38%) | 1812 (19%) | |
| Unknown | 8 (3%) | 613 (2%) | | 0 (0%) | 206 (2%) | |
| Income (per year) | | | 0.38 | | | 0.68 |
| Less than $38 k | 40 (15%) | 3981 (12%) | | 5 (24%) | 1507 (16%) | |
| $38 k-62,999 | 115 (44%) | 15,408 (48%) | | 10 (48%) | 4791 (49%) | |
| $63 k or greater | 100 (39%) | 12,407 (39%) | | 6 (29%) | 3256 (34%) | |
| Unknown | 4 (2%) | 408 (1%) | | 0 (0%) | 154 (2%) | |
| Percent in ZIP code without a high school degree | | | 0.69 | | | 0.75 |
| 21% or greater | 37 (14%) | 4450 (14%) | | 5 (24%) | 1711 (18%) | |
| 7–20.9% | 147 (57%) | 17,658 (55%) | | 12 (57%) | 5355 (55%) | |
| Less than 7% | 71 (27%) | 9716 (30%) | | 4 (19%) | 2496 (26%) | |
| Unknown | 4 (2%) | 380 (1%) | | 0 (0%) | 146 (2%) | |
| Residence | | | 0.42 | | | 0.51 |
| Metropolitan | 221 (85%) | 26,877 (84%) | | 16 (76%) | 7934 (82%) | |
| Urban/rural | 38 (15%) | 5327 (17%) | | 5 (24%) | 1774 (18%) | |
| Charlson-Deyo comorbidity score | | | 0.016 | | | < 0.001 |
| 0 | 237 (92%) | 30,544 (95%) | | 15 (71%) | 9029 (93%) | |
| 1 or more | 22 (9%) | 1660 (5%) | | 6 (29%) | 679 (7%) | |
| Stage | | | | | | 0.21 |
| Stage I | 259 (100%) | 32,204 (100%) | | – | – | |
| Stage II | – | – | | 9 (43%) | 5469 (56%) | |
| Stage III | – | – | | 12 (57%) | 4239 (44%) | |
| Treatment | | | < 0.001 | | | < 0.001 |
| No orchiectomy | 0 (0%) | 30 (0.1%) | | 2 (10%) | 634 (7%) | |
| Orchiectomy alone | 250 (97%) | 16,519 (51%) | | 10 (48%) | 1106 (11%) | |
| Orchiectomy + adjuvant therapy | 9 (4%) | 15,626 (49%) | | 9 (43%) | 7941 (82%) | |

**Table 2** Stage-specific comparison of the sociodemographic and clinical characteristics of patients with SCSTs versus GCTs *(Continued)*

| Factor | Stage I | | | Stage II/III | | |
|---|---|---|---|---|---|---|
| | SCSTs | GCTs | p-value | SCSTs | GCTs | p-value |
| Other/unknown | 0 (0%) | 29 (0.1%) | | 0 (0%) | 27 (0.3%) | |
| Last contact or death, months from diagnosis, median (IQR) | N = 229 | N = 28,855 | < 0.001 | N = 20 | N = 8612 | 0.002 |
| | 41 (22, 62) | 53 (29, 80) | | 19 (8, 55) | 47 (24, 75) | |
| Time from diagnosis to death, median (IQR) | N = 13 | N = 747 | | N = 14 | N = 866 | |
| | 23 (18, 43) | 31 (14, 58) | 0.78 | 11 (7, 21) | 13 (4, 28) | 0.96 |

*GCTs* Germ cell tumors, *IQR* Interquartile range, *SCSTs* Sex cord stromal tumors

**Table 3** Univariable and multivariable Cox proportional hazards regression analysis on the association between sociodemographic and clinical characteristics and mortality of the overall cohort

| | Univariable HR (95% CI) | Multivariable[a] HR (95% CI) – Overall |
|---|---|---|
| **Tumor type** | | |
| GCTs | Ref. | Ref. |
| SCSTs | 2.96 (2.03–4.33)*** | 1.68 (1.13–2.49)* |
| **Age (per 5-year increase)** | 1.21 (1.19–1.23)*** | 1.18 (1.16–1.20)*** |
| **Race/ethnicity** | | |
| Non-Hispanic White | Ref. | Ref. |
| Non-Hispanic Black | 1.80 (1.41–2.29)*** | 1.13 (0.89–1.45) |
| Hispanic/other | 1.27 (1.13–1.43)*** | 1.14 (1.01–1.30)* |
| **Insurance** | | |
| Private insurance | Ref. | Ref. |
| Uninsured | 2.63 (2.29–3.01)*** | 2.32 (2.01–2.66)*** |
| Medicaid/Medicare/other government insurance | 4.33 (3.88–4.83)*** | 2.72 (2.42–3.05)*** |
| **Income (per year)** | | |
| < $38,000 | Ref. | Ref. |
| $38,000–$62,999 | 0.71 (0.62–0.81)*** | 0.94 (0.82–1.09) |
| > $63,000 | 0.44 (0.38–0.50)*** | 0.76 (0.63–0.92)** |
| **Percent in ZIP code without a high school diploma** | | |
| > 21% | Ref. | Ref. |
| 7–20.9% | 0.63 (0.56–0.71)*** | 0.83 (0.73–0.96)* |
| < 7% | 0.43 (0.37–0.49)*** | 0.74 (0.61–0.90)** |
| **Residence** | | |
| Metropolitan | Ref. | Ref. |
| Urban/rural | 1.49 (1.33–1.67)*** | 1.13 (1.00–1.28) |
| **Charlson-Deyo comorbidity score** | | |
| 0 | Ref. | Ref. |
| ≥ 1 | 3.23 (2.82–3.70)*** | 2.06 (1.79–2.37)*** |

*CI* Confidence interval, *GCTs* Germ cell tumors, *HR* Hazard ratio, *IQR* Interquartile range, *SCSTs* Sex cord stromal tumors
*$p < 0.05$
**$p < 0.01$
***$p < 0.001$
[a]The following variables were included in the multivariable analysis: tumor type, age, diagnosis year, race/ethnicity, insurance, yearly income, percent in ZIP code without a high school diploma, residence, Charlson-Deyo comorbidity score

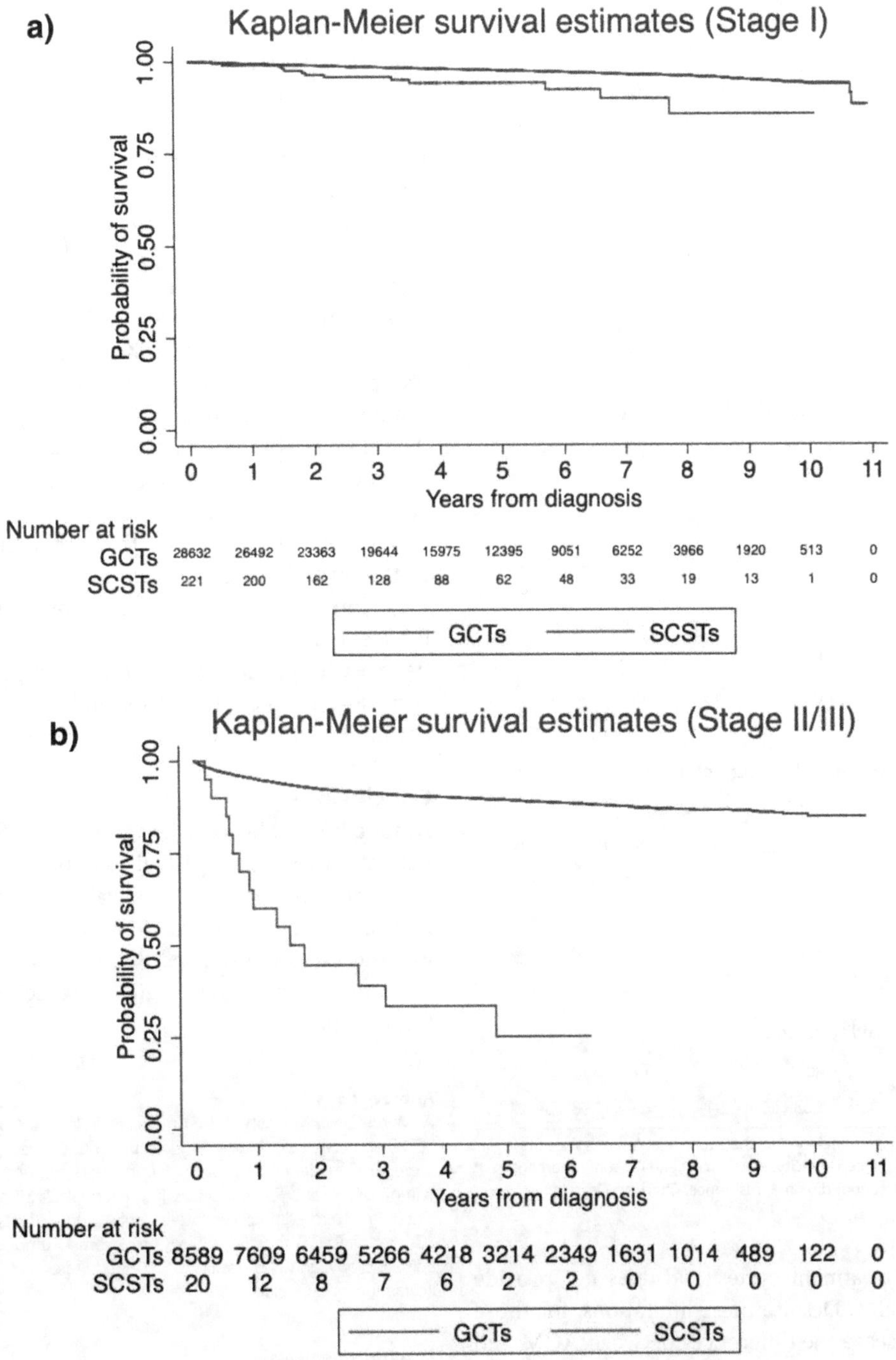


**Fig. 1** Kaplan-Meier survival estimates comparing all-cause mortality between patients with SCSTs versus GCTs among those with **a**) stage I disease and **b**) stage II/III disease

node dissection. At the time of publication, one patient was surviving on apalutamide for 4 months and another was on everolimus with slightly regressing metastatic disease for 12 months [21]. Finally, a step further would be to enhance methods for distinguishing malignant from benign LCTs for more directed adjuvant treatments.

This study is not without limitations. The inclusion of patients in this study assumes accurate designation of ICD-O-3 coding by providers and misclassification may bias the findings. This dataset also relies upon accurate reporting of histology, as there is no central pathology review. The NCDB has limited information on treatment specifics (e.g., type of chemotherapeutic agent), schedule

**Table 4** Multivariable Cox proportional hazards regression analysis on the association between sociodemographic and clinical characteristics and mortality by stage

| | Multivariable[a] HR (95% CI) – Stage I | Multivariable[a] HR (95% CI) – Stage II/III |
|---|---|---|
| **Tumor type** | | |
| GCTs | Ref. | Ref. |
| SCSTs | 1.06 (0.60–1.86) | 3.28 (1.88–5.73)*** |
| **Age (per 5-year increase)** | 1.23 (1.20–1.26)*** | 1.13 (1.10–1.16)*** |
| **Race/ethnicity** | | |
| Non-Hispanic White | Ref. | Ref. |
| Non-Hispanic Black | 1.18 (0.80–1.72) | 1.13 (0.81–1.56) |
| Hispanic/other | 1.14 (0.95–1.38) | 1.12 (0.94–1.32) |
| **Insurance** | | |
| Private insurance | Ref. | Ref. |
| Uninsured | 2.58 (2.08–3.21)*** | 2.07 (1.72–2.50)*** |
| Medicaid/Medicare/other government insurance | 3.15 (2.64–3.75)*** | 2.31 (1.97–2.70)*** |
| **Income (per year)** | | |
| < $38,000 | Ref. | Ref. |
| $38,000–$62,999 | 0.92 (0.74–1.15) | 0.96 (0.79–1.16) |
| > $63,000 | 0.74 (0.56–0.98)* | 0.77 (0.61–1.02) |
| **Percent in ZIP code without a high school diploma** | | |
| > 21% | Ref. | Ref. |
| 7–20.9% | 0.87 (0.70–1.07) | 0.80 (0.67–0.97)* |
| < 7% | 0.80 (0.61–1.06) | 0.68 (0.52–0.88)** |
| **Residence** | | |
| Metropolitan | Ref. | Ref. |
| Urban/rural | 1.18 (0.98–1.42) | 1.09 (0.91–1.29) |
| **Charlson-Deyo comorbidity score** | | |
| 0 | Ref. | Ref. |
| ≥ 1 | 2.03 (1.64–2.51)*** | 2.03 (1.68–2.45)*** |

[a]The following variables were included in the multivariable analysis: tumor type, age, diagnosis year, race/ethnicity, insurance, yearly income, percent in ZIP code without a high school diploma, residence, Charlson-Deyo comorbidity score

and sequence of treatment cycles, and does not provide information on CSM. Despite these limitations, for those with advanced disease the differences between ACM and CSM rates are reduced. Additionally, the NCDB does not contain information that may influence quality of care received (e.g., hospital quality, surgeon experience, patient healthcare access/literacy, etc.); however, many factors that contribute to this (e.g., income, insurance, education) were controlled for in our analysis. As this study is a retrospective study based on an observational dataset, there are unmeasured confounders which could impact these findings. In addition, the small sample size of SCSTs limited multivariable comparisons of ACM between SCST subtypes, and it has been proposed that LCTs and SCTs may confer different degrees of ACM risk [5]. The small sample size also precluded analysis by adjuvant treatment type, which would help provide more actionable data on the most effective management strategy for these tumors. Along those same lines, our conclusion of survival differences between patients with advanced SCSTs versus advanced GCTs is based on just 21 SCST patients. Despite its comparison to a large group of GCT patients, this may limit the accuracy of our conclusions and warrants future studies with larger populations of SCST patients. The greater proportion of stage III patients in the SCST group versus the GCT group may have had an influence on survival; however, the absolute difference between groups was quite small. Additionally, the older age and greater proportion of patients with 1 or more comorbidity among those with advanced SCSTs could have been confounders in our survival analysis; however, these differences should have been controlled for in the multivariable model. Despite these limitations, this study presents novel data comparing testicular tumors types among a large number of patients with multiple sociodemographic and clinical variables considered, and its findings may have important implications in altering management practices.

## Conclusions

Among this cohort, when comparing SCSTs to GCTs, patients with stage II/III disease but not stage I disease was associated with a statistically significantly increased risk of ACM on multivariable analysis. Increased ACM in patients with advanced SCSTs indicates an imperative for targeted treatment regimens specific to this unique tumor type.

### Abbreviations

ACM: All-Cause Mortality; AUA: American Urological Association; BEP: Bleomycin, Etoposide, and Cisplatin; CDS: Charleson-Deyo comorbidity score; CI: Confidence Interval; CSM: Cancer-Specific Mortality; GCT: Germ Cell Tumor; HR: Hazard Ratio; ICD-O-3: International Classification of Diseases for Oncology, Third Edition; IQR: Interquartile Range; LCT: Leydig Cell Tumor; SCT: Sertoli Cell Tumor; SCST: Sex Cord Stromal Tumor; SEER: Surveillance, Epidemiology, and End Results; U.S.: United States; VIP: Vinblastine, Ifosfamide, and Cisplatin

### Acknowledgements

We are grateful to Janet Cowan for assistance in preparation of this manuscript.

### Authors' contributions

KBZ, SLW, SPP, and MVM made substantial contributions to the design of this work. KBZ and SLW analysed the data. KBZ, SLW, SPP and MVM interpreted the data. KBZ drafted the work. KBZ, SLW, SPP, and MVM substantially revised the work. All authors have read and approved the manuscript.

### Competing interests

The authors declare that they have no competing interests relevant to this manuscript.

**Author details**
[1]Department of Urology, University of California, San Francisco, 550 16th Street, 6th Floor, San Francisco, CA 94158, USA. [2]Osher Center for Integrative Medicine, University of California, San Francisco, 1545 Divisadero Street, Suite 301, San Francisco, CA 94143, USA. [3]Vagelos College of Physicians and Surgeons, Columbia University Medical Center, 630 West 168th Street, New York, NY 10032, USA.

**References**

1. National Institutes of Health; National Cancer Institute; Surveillance, Epidemiology, and End Results Program: Cancer Stat Facts: Testicular Cancer. Available at https://seercancergov/statfacts/html/testis.html. Accessed 16 May 2019.
2. Bosl GJ, Motzer RJ. Testicular germ-cell Cancer. N Engl J Med. 1997;337(4): 242–54.
3. Dilworth JP, Farrow GM, Oesterling JE. Non-germ cell tumors of testis. Urology. 1991;37(5):399–417.
4. Kollmannsberger C, Tandstad T, Bedard PL, Cohn-Cedermark G, Chung PW, Jewett MA, et al. Patterns of relapse in patients with clinical stage I testicular cancer managed with active surveillance. J Clin Oncol. 2015; 33(1):51–7.
5. Banerji JS, Odem-Davis K, Wolff EM, Nichols CR, Porter CR. Patterns of care and survival outcomes for malignant sex cord stromal testicular Cancer: results from the National Cancer Data Base. J Urol. 2016;196(4):1117–22.
6. Nicolai N, Necchi A, Raggi D, Biasoni D, Catanzaro M, Piva L, et al. Clinical outcome in testicular sex cord stromal tumors: testis sparing vs. radical orchiectomy and management of advanced disease. Urology. 2015;85(2): 402–6.
7. Mosharafa AA, Foster RS, Bihrle R, Koch MO, Ulbright TM, Einhorn LH, et al. Does retroperitoneal lymph node dissection have a curative role for patients with sex cord-stromal testicular tumors? Cancer. 2003;98(4):753–7.
8. Bertram KA, Bratloff B, Hodges GF, Davidson H. Treatment of malignant leydig cell tumor. Cancer. 1991;68(10):2324–9.
9. Osbun N, Winters B, Holt SK, Schade GR, Lin DW, Wright JL. Characteristics of patients with Sertoli and Leydig cell testis neoplasms from a National Population-Based Registry. Clin Genitourin Cancer. 2017;15(2):e263–e6.
10. Kamran SC, Seisen T, Markt SC, Preston MA, Trinh QD, Frazier LA, et al. Contemporary treatment patterns and outcomes for clinical stage IS testicular Cancer. Eur Urol. 2018;73(2):262–70.
11. Stephenson A, Eggener SE, Bass EB, Chelnick DM, Daneshmand S, Feldman D, et al. Diagnosis And Treatment Of Early Stage Testicular Cancer: Aua Guideline. J Urol. 2019;202(2):272–81. https://doi.org/10.1097/JU.0000000000000318..
12. Raval MV, Bilimoria KY, Stewart AK, Bentrem DJ, Ko CY. Using the NCDB for cancer care improvement: an introduction to available quality assessment tools. J Surg Oncol. 2009;99(8):488–90.
13. American College of Surgeons; National Cancer Database: About the National Cancer Database Avalable at https://www.facs.org/quality-programs/cancer/ncdb/about Accessed 15 May 2019.
14. American College of Surgeons; National Cancer Database: National Cancer Data Base Participant User File (PUF) Data Dictionary Version: PUF 2016 Available at https://www.facs.org/~/media/files/quality%20programs/cancer/ncdb/puf_data_dictionary.ashx Accessed 20 May 2019.
15. Pitblado J. Survey data analysis in Stata. 2009. https://www.stata.com/meeting/canada09/ca09_pitblado_handout.pdf.
16. Featherstone JM, Fernando HS, Theaker JM, Simmonds PD, Hayes MC, Mead GM. Sex cord stromal testicular tumors: a clinical series--uniformly stage I disease. J Urol. 2009;181(5):2090–6 discussion 6.
17. Sawin PD, VanGilder JC. Spinal cord compression from metastatic Leydig's cell tumor of the testis: case report. Neurosurgery. 1996;38(2):407–11.
18. Panza S, Malivindi R, Chemi F, Rago V, Giordano C, Barone I, et al. Glucocorticoid receptor as a potential target to decrease aromatase expression and inhibit Leydig tumor growth. Am J Pathol. 2016;186(5):1328–39.
19. Basciani S, Brama M, Mariani S, De Luca G, Arizzi M, Vesci L, et al. Imatinib mesylate inhibits Leydig cell tumor growth: evidence for in vitro and in vivo activity. Cancer Res. 2005;65(5):1897–903.
20. Necchi A, Bratslavsky G, Shapiro O, Elvin JA, Vergilio JA, Killian JK, et al. Genomic Features of Metastatic Testicular Sex Cord Stromal Tumors. Eur Urol Focus. 2019;5(5):748–55.
21. Calaway AC, Tachibana I, Masterson TA, Foster RS, Einhorn LH, Cary C. Oncologic outcomes following surgical Management of Clinical Stage II sex cord stromal tumors. Urology. 2019;127:74–9.

# 25

# Renal pelvis and ureteropelvic junction incarceration in a Grynfeltt-Lesshaft hernia

Saadat Mehrabi, Mohammad Javad Yavari Barhaghtalab* and Mehdi Babapour

**Abstract**

**Background:** Grynfeltt–Lesshaft hernia is a kind of lumbar abdominal wall hernia in which clinical presentations may vary from an asymptomatic bulge in the lumbar area to a symptomatic lumbar mass with back pain. It has been accepted to be a rare entity, and incarceration of the kidney through this hernia is shown to be very rare, and very few previous cases have been reported in this regard.

We present a case of renal pelvic and ureteropelvic junction incarceration in a Grynfeltt-Lesshaft hernia and provide an overview of the existing literature on it.

**Case presentation:** A 76-year-old lady presented to the outpatient clinic with the chief complaint of right flank pain and swelling. Computed tomography (CT) scan of the abdomen was revealed a large herniated sac (60*30 mm) in the upper lumbar triangle with protrusion of retroperitoneal and omental fat, right renal pelvis, ureteropelvic junction and proximal ureter with consecutive hydronephrosis. Herniated retroperitoneal and omental fat was reduced, and closure of the abdominal wall defect was done using retro-muscular Mesh and was fixed to the fascia. The patient was discharged 24 h after the surgery without any complications.

**Conclusion:** Kidney herniation through the lumbar triangle is extremely rare, and the diagnosis requires careful clinical evaluation. CT scan is the modality of choice for the assessment. Management through surgery should be done in symptomatic patients.

**Keywords:** Grynfeltt–Lesshaft hernia, Renal pelvic, Ureteropelvic junction, Incarceration, Hydronephrosis, Muscular or sublay mesh

## Background

The lumbar abdominal wall hernia is uncommon. In this kind of hernia retroperitoneal (kidneys, urinary bladder, and ascending or descending colon) and intraperitoneal (small bowel, omentum, preperitoneal fat, stomach, spleen, etc) elements bulge through a defect in the dorsal posterolateral abdominal wall (upper lumbar or the Grynfeltt–Lesshaft triangle) [1–6].

The Grynfeltt-Lesshaft triangle is defined by the internal oblique muscle laterally, border of the erector spinae muscle group (quadratus lumborum) medially, the 12th rib superiorly, transversalis fascia aponeurosis on the floor, latissimus dorsi muscle on the roof [1, 7, 8]. The weakening of the transversalis fascia and the aponeurosis of the transversus abdominis is the reason for this problem [9] (Fig. 1).

It's more frequent in men between 50 and 70 years old and is more prevalent on the left side of the abdomen [10]. Risk factors are elderly, obesity, muscular atrophy, and chronic obstructive pulmonary disease (COPD) or

* Correspondence: mj.yavari.barhaghtalab@gmail.com
Department of General Surgery, Shahid Beheshti Hospital, Yasuj University of Medical Sciences, Yasuj, Iran

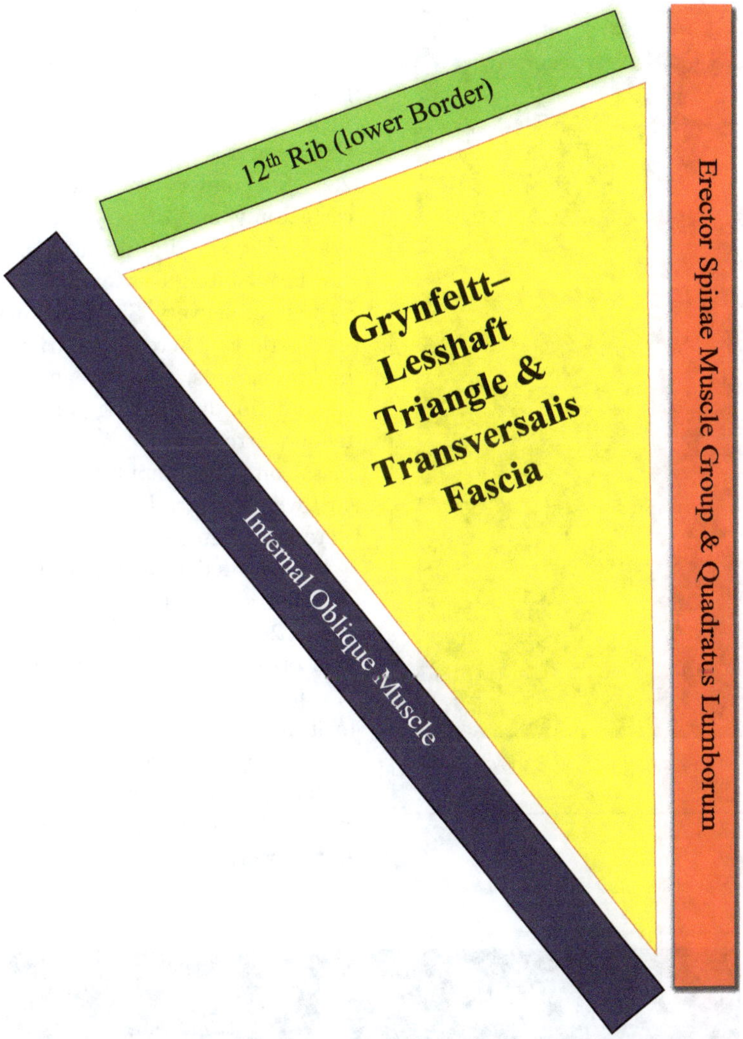


**Fig. 1** A schematic showing the parameters of the Grynfeltt–Lesshaft Hernia

any other condition that yields in increasing intra-abdominal pressure [11].

Many surgeons are unfamiliar with lumbar hernias, which may cause a delay in the diagnosis of the disease [3, 7]. Clinical presentations may vary from an asymptomatic bulge in the lumbar area to a symptomatic lumbar mass with back pain or vague abdominal symptoms and are related to the protruded contents [4]. This could have iatrogenic, congenital, and traumatic causes, while most of the patients have primary acquired hernias [1, 4]. Lumbar hernias have been misdiagnosed as lipomas [4, 7, 12–14], muscle strains, fibromas, abscesses, and kidney tumors, causing increased morbidity due to the incorrect diagnosis [3]. It is recommended to repair these hernias electively if there are no contraindications [4]. It has been said that there would be just only one case of lumbar hernia in a general surgeon's life to operate [13, 15].

A lumbar hernia is an unusual defect, and only 300 cases of primary lumbar hernias have been reported since the first case report by Garangoet in 1731 [13, 14, 16]. Their diagnosis is vital due to their substantial possible complications such as incarceration and strangulation in 25 and 8% of patients retrospectively [17]. So as this kind of hernia has been accepted to be a rare entity, incarceration of the kidney through this hernia is shown to be very rare, and very few previous cases have been reported in this regard [18–21].

We present a case of renal pelvic and ureteropelvic junction herniation in a Grynfeltt-Lesshaft hernia and provide a clear overview of the existing literature on it.

## Case presentation

A 76-year-old lady presented to the outpatient clinic with the chief complaint of right flank pain and swelling that protrudes with efforts, reduced mostly in resting

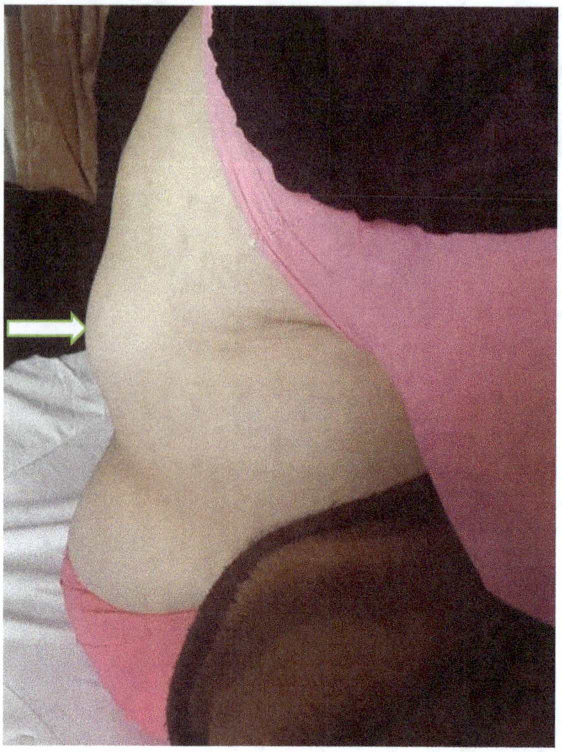

**Fig. 2** Right lumbar Hernia in a 76-year-old woman is shown with a white arrow

position and increasing in size for about 2 months before hospital admission (Fig. 2). The bulging was not associated with gastrointestinal and urinary problems. The patient's past medical history was positive for diabetes mellitus (DM), hypertension (HTN) and hyperlipidemia (HLP), and an overweight body mass index (BMI) of 28.9. She underwent hysterectomy, laparoscopic cholecystectomy, and urinary bladder prolapse repair surgery previously. She did not have any history of back trauma and heavy lifting previously. She had three children born by vaginal delivery. She used metformin and losartan for medications. There was no family history of the hernia in her parents, siblings, and children. In the physical examination in standing position, we found a soft, mildly tender, irreducible, and smooth border-right lumbar mass (on right scapular line just below the costal margin) which protruded when coughing. No bowel sounds were auscultated on the hernia.

A computed tomography (CT) scan of the abdomen revealed a large herniated sac (60*30 mm) beneath the right 12th rib in the upper lumbar triangle with protrusion of retroperitoneal fat, right renal pelvis, ureteropelvic junction and proximal ureter with consecutive hydronephrosis extended to the posterior aspect of the kidney (Figs. 3 and 4). After conducting preoperational evaluations and informed consent, the patient was operated under general anesthesia in a right lateral position. A transverse incision about 10 cm was made on the

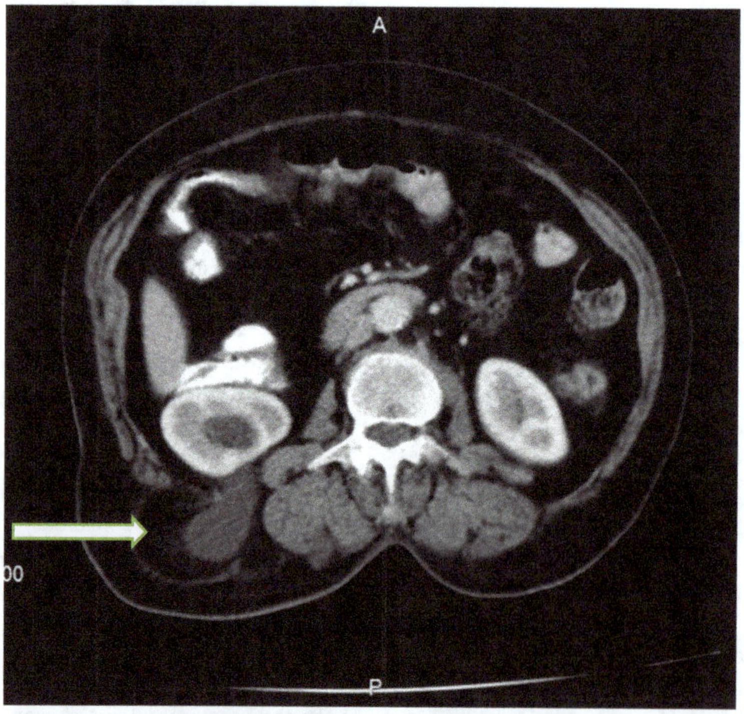


**Fig. 3** Spiral CT scan without contrast: herniated sac containing retroperitoneal and omental fat, and right renal pelvis (white arrow)

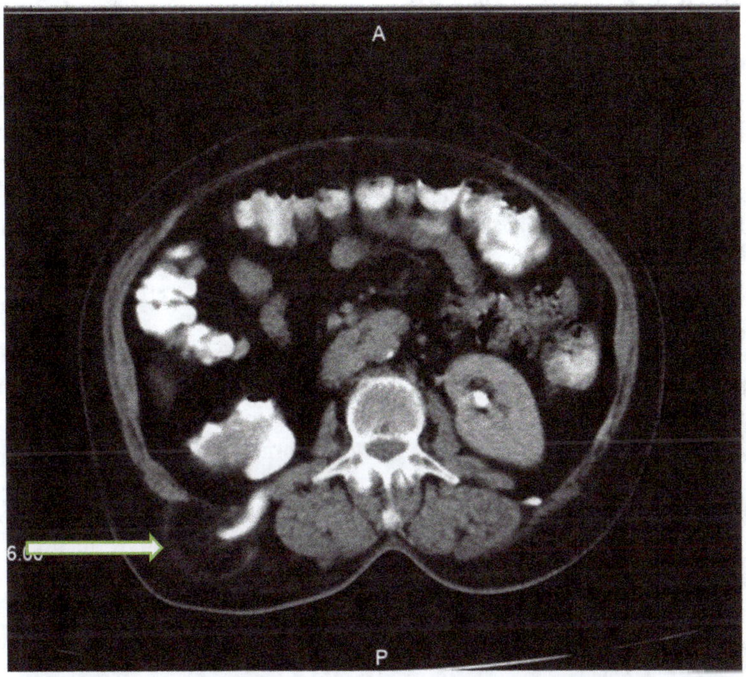


**Fig. 4** Spiral CT scan with intravenous (IV) contrast: herniated sac containing right ureter (white arrow)

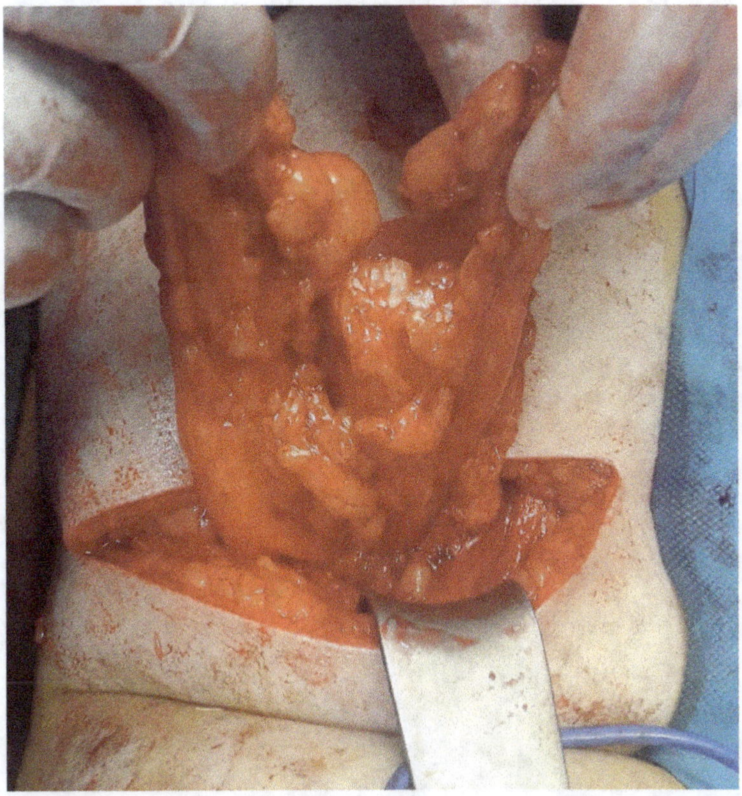

**Fig. 5** Retroperitoneal and omental fat in the herniated sac in lumbar hernia

bulging area. After dissection of skin, subcutaneous tissue, and muscle layer (latissimus dorsi), a hernia sac through a 3 cm defect was found. There was a herniated retroperitoneal and omental fat in the sac, so it was reduced back and closure of the abdominal wall defect was done using retro-muscular or sublay Monofilament Polypropylene Mesh (Paha® 8*15 cm) (Figs. 5, 6 and 7). Mesh was fixed to the fascia with non-absorbable interrupted sutures using a tension-free technique. The muscles and fascia were sutured separately with absorbable sutures, and the wound was closed. A drain catheter was not necessary to be placed. The operating time was 41 min, there were no hospital postoperative complications, and we discharged the patient 24 h after the surgery. The patient was visited and followed up on the 7th, 30th' and 60th days after discharge from the hospital, and there were good results.

## Discussion and conclusions

Lumbar hernias are rare congenital or acquired diseases (20% vs. 80% of the cases). Congenital hernias are seen in infants and children and are related to defects in the lumbar wall. Acquired hernias are divided into two groups: spontaneous (primary) hernias and secondary acquired hernias [8]. Our patient presented a primarily acquired hernia with protrusion of retroperitoneal fat, right renal pelvis, ureteropelvic junction, and proximal ureter. Reviewing the literature regarding herniation of the urinary system into the lumbar hernia has resulted in only five previous published reports. The first report presented by Presti et al. in which a 42-year-old man had a 2-week history of intermittent right flank pain and total gross hematuria. CT scan showed a right lumbar hernia with a herniated kidney in, so then the surgical repair was done [18]. Fogarty et al. presented a 76-year-old woman with right flank pain and acute renal insufficiency. CT scan revealed herniation of retroperitoneal fat, right renal pelvis, and ureteropelvic junction through a lumbar hernia [19]. Cabello et al. presented a 79-year-old woman with a tender bulging in the left lumbar area and acute ureteral colic pain, who underwent CT scan and was diagnosed to have Grynfeltt's bilateral hernia

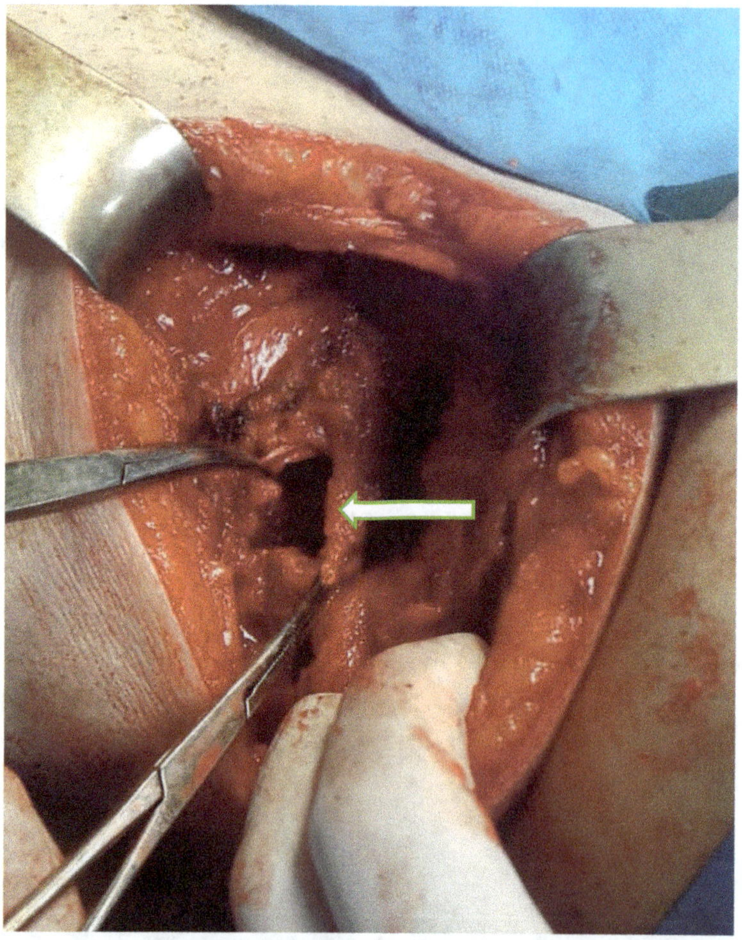

**Fig. 6** A 3 cm defect through which herniation occurred (white arrow)

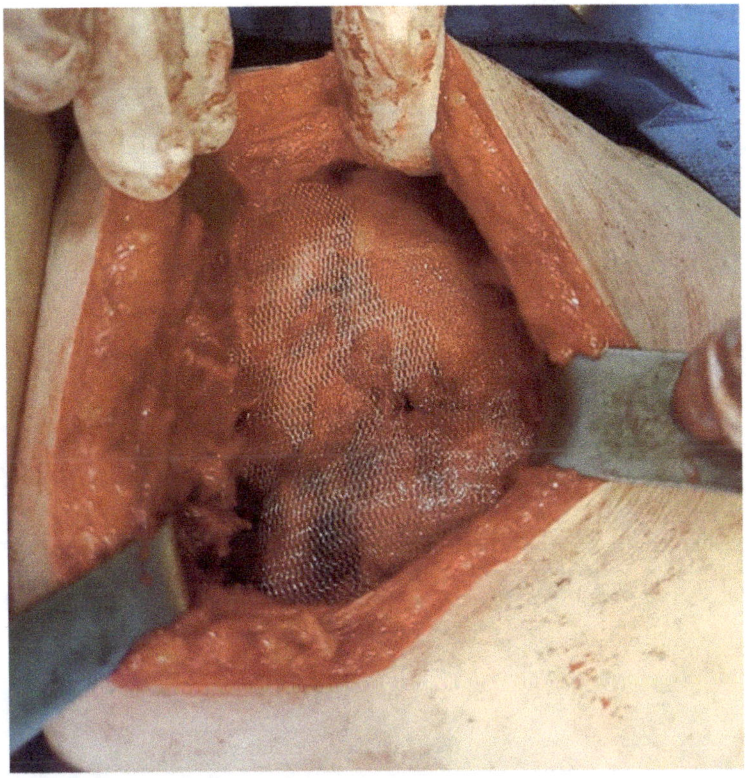

**Fig. 7** Hernioplasty with Monofilament Polypropylene Mesh

and herniation of left renal pelvis and proximal ureter [20]. Miyazato et al. reported a 59-year-old woman a known case of Cushing's syndrome who underwent laparoscopic adrenalectomy and afterward developed with lumbar herniation of the left kidney [21]. Al Hooti et al. presented a 60-year-old woman with protrusion of the right kidney lower pole through the lumbar triangle 10 years after an open right pyeloplasty. She was successfully treated conservatively in clinic and received analgesics frequently for relief of mild pain without attempting operational repair [22]. The data from the previous and our current reports are summarized in Table 1.

Therefore, the majority of patients were female patients. The mean age of the patients was $65.33 \pm 5.342$ years (with a confidence level of 95%). Pain and swelling were the dominant symptoms reported in all the patients. The pain was accompanied by gross hematuria, acute renal insufficiency, and acute renal colic pain in one patient each. The right side was more involved seen in 4 cases. Physical examination was mentioned in 4 cases, of which tenderness was found in three. Past medical history was positive for abdominal aortic aneurysm in one patient. Hypertension, diabetes, and hyperlipidemia were seen in two patients. Hypothyroidism, hyperuricemia, right adrenal Cushing's syndrome, left primary aldosteronism, right pelviureteric junction obstruction and overweight were found in one patient each retrospectively. Previous surgery history was positive in 4 cases. Laparotomy with partial right colectomy following a sharp injury, laparoscopic adrenalectomy, open right Anderson Hynes pyeloplasty and hysterectomy, laparoscopic cholecystectomy, and urinary bladder prolapse repair surgery was seen in one patient each retrospectively. CT scan was the modality used in all the cases. Intravenous urogram (IVU) was done in two patients, and an abdominal x-ray, mercaptoacetyltriglycine renal scan, and magnetic resonance imaging (MRI) were done in one patient each retrospectively. MRI was the dominant diagnostic modality used in a patient with post-laparoscopic adrenalectomy lumbar hernia. The kidney was protruded partially in all the patients. Beside, ureteropelvic junction, proximal ureter and retroperitoneal fat were seen in 2 cases each retrospectively. Urological complications were mentioned in 5 cases, of which pyelocaliectasis and hydronephrosis were seen in all the patients and ureteropelvic junction obstruction was seen in one patient.

Two patients underwent non-surgical analgesic management. Surgery was done in 4 cases, of which opened hernioplasty was done in three and was not mentioned in one. In a study done by Vagholkar et al., an open approach was implemented [23], similar to the method done in our study. They concluded that both laparoscopic and open

**Table 1** Summarized data from the previous and our current reports

| Main Author | Published Year | Country | Age (year) | Sex | Chief complaint | Physical examination | Past medical History | Past surgical History | Diagnostic modality | Herniation side and incarcerated body's part | Urological complications | Management |
|---|---|---|---|---|---|---|---|---|---|---|---|---|
| Presti [18] | 1988 | USA | 42 | Male | Intermittent right flank pain and total gross hematuria | a T-shaped abdominal incision directed towards the right flank, a reducible, slightly tender, solid mass in rt. lumbar area | Negative | laparotomy with partial right colectomy following a sharp injury | Abdominal x-ray, Intravenous urogram (IVU), CT scan | Right side, right kidney | right pyelocaliectasis and ureteropelvic junction obstruction | Hernioplasty |
| Fogarty [19] | 2006 | USA | 76 | Female | nausea, vomiting, right flank pain, and acute renal insufficiency | Not mentioned | abdominal aortic aneurysm | negative | CT scan | Right side, retroperitoneal fat, the right renal pelvis, and ureteropelvic junction | Right hydronephrosis | percutaneous nephrostomy tube, antegrade nephrostography, antegrade internal ureteral stent placement and then hernioplasty after normalization of renal function, and subsequent nephrostomy tube removal |
| Cabello [20] | 2008 | Spain | 79 | Female | painful swelling in the left lumbar region and acute renal colic pain | Not mentioned | hypertension, diabetes, hypercholesterolemia, hypothyroidism, hyperuricemia, hiatus hernia, deep venous thrombosis with pulmonary embolism, chronic bronchitis and morbid obesity | negative | CT scan | bilateral hernia, left side of the renal pelvis and proximal ureter | Left hydronephrosis | Non-surgical |
| Miyazato [21] | 2011 | Japan | 59 | Female | intermittent left back pain for 6-month | left focal back mass and tenderness | right adrenal Cushing's syndrome and left primary aldosteronism | laparoscopic adrenalectomy | Magnetic resonance imaging (MRI) and CT scan | Left side, left kidney and | Not mentioned | Surgery |
| Al Hooti [22] | 2014 | Oman | 60 | Female | right-sided abdominal pain and swelling for 2-month | surgical scar without incisional hernia, non-tender oval palpableswelling, right lumbar area, positive cough sign and reducible | right pelviureteric junction obstruction | (+) open right Anderson Hynes pyeloplasty 10 years before admission | CT sacn, IVU, and Mercaptoacetyltriglycine renal scan | Right side, lower pole of the right kidney | right hydronephrosis | Non-surgical |
| Mehrabi (current report) | 2019 | Iran | 76 | Female | back and right flank pain and a swelling in right flank since 2-month before admission | soft, mildly tender, irreducible and smooth border right lumbar mass | DM, HTN, HLP and overweight | hysterectomy, laparoscopic cholecystectomy and urinary bladder prolapse repair surgery | CT scan | Right sided, retroperitoneal fat, right renal pelvis, ureteropelvic junction and proximal ureter | right hydronephrosis | hernioplasty |

approaches could be done, although open mesh repair is an easier, safer, and more effective method of treating this uncommon surgical illness [23]. In two previous studies, Moreno-Egea et al. evaluated laparoscopic versus open repair in lumbar hernia surgery through some prospective studies [24, 25]. They have found that results did not vary according to morbidity and recurrence rate, although it would reduce postoperative morbidity, pain, and early return to daily routine activities.

In one case, hernioplasty was done following normalization of renal function through percutaneous nephrostomy tube, antegrade nephrostography, antegrade internal ureteral stent placement, and subsequent nephrostomy tube removal.

To our best knowledge, this is one of the first reported cases and also the first literature review on acquired herniation of the renal pelvis and ureteropelvic junction through a Grynfeltt hernia with resultant hydronephrosis.

Kidney herniation through the lumbar triangle is extremely rare, and the diagnosis requires careful clinical evaluation. CT scan is the modality of choice for the assessment. Management through surgery should be done in symptomatic patients. Both laparoscopic and open approach can be done for treating this illness; however, an open approach is an easier and safer method.

#### Abbreviations

CT scan: Computed tomography scan; COPD: Chronic obstructive pulmonary disease; DM: Diabetes mellitus; HTN: Hypertension; HLP: Hyperlipidemia; BMI: Body mass index; IV: Intravenous; IVU: Intravenous urogram; MRI: Magnetic resonance imaging

#### Acknowledgments

We all express our gratitude to the patient who kindly gave consent for this case to be presented in this paper. The authors also wish to thank Dr. Aida Iraji at the Central research laboratory, Shiraz University of Medical Sciences, Shiraz, Iran for her assistance in editing this manuscript.

#### Authors' contributions

Principal author: SM evaluated the patient clinically, operated the patient (main surgeon), read and revised the paper. Co-author: MJYB evaluated the patient clinically, helped to operate the patient (co-surgeon), prepared the first draft and revised the paper. Co-author: MB evaluated the patient clinically, and helped to operate the patient (co-surgeon). All authors read and approved the final manuscript.

#### Competing interests

The authors of this manuscript declare no competing of interests.

#### References

1. van Steensel S, Bloemen A, van den Hil LCL, van den Bos J, Kleinrensink GJ, Bouvy ND. Pitfalls and clinical recommendations for the primary lumbar hernia based on a systematic review of the literature. Hernia. 2019;23(1):107–17. https://doi.org/10.1007/s10029-018-1834-9.
2. Macchi V, Porzionato A, Morra A, Picardi EEE, Stecco C, Loukas M, et al. The triangles of Grynfeltt and petit and the lumbar tunnel: an anatomo-radiologic study. Hernia. 2017;21(3):369–76. https://doi.org/10.1007/s10029-016-1509-3.
3. Suh Y, Gandhi J, Zaidi S, Smith NL, Tan M-Y, Khan SA. Lumbar hernia: A commonly misevaluated condition of the bilateral costoiliac spaces. Transl Res Anat. 2017;8–9:1–5. https://doi.org/10.1016/j.tria.2017.10.002.
4. Zadeh JR, Buicko JL, Patel C, Kozol R, Lopez-Viego MA. Grynfeltt hernia: a deceptive lumbar mass with a Lipoma-like presentation. Case Rep Surg. 2015;2015:954804. https://doi.org/10.1155/2015/954804.
5. Orcutt TW. Ann Surg. 1971;173(2):294–7. https://doi.org/10.1097/00000658-197102000-00018.
6. Scheffler M, Renard J, Bucher P, Botsikas D. Incarcerated Grynfeltt-Lesshaft hernia. J Radiol Case Rep. 2015;9(4):9–13. https://doi.org/10.3941/jrcr.v9i4.2073.
7. Ahmed ST, Ranjan R, Saha SB, Singh B. Lumbar hernia: a diagnostic dilemma. BMJ Case Rep. 2014;2014:bcr2013202085. https://doi.org/10.1136/bcr-2013-202085.
8. Ploneda-Valencia CF, Cordero-Estrada E, Castañeda-González LG, Sainz-Escarrega VH, Varela-Muñoz O, De la Cerda-Trujillo LF, et al. Grynfelt-Lesshaft hernia a case report and review of the literature. Ann Med Surg (Lond). 2016;7:104–6. https://doi.org/10.1016/j.amsu.2016.04.002.
9. Armstrong O, Hamel A, Grignon B, NDoye JM, Hamel O, Robert R, et al. Lumbar hernia: anatomical basis and clinical aspects. Surg Radiol Anat. 2008;30(7):533–7; discussion 609-10. https://doi.org/10.1007/s00276-008-0361-2.
10. Hide IG, Pike EE, Uberoi R. Lumbar hernia: a rare cause of large bowel obstruction. Postgrad Med J. 1999;75(882):231–2. https://doi.org/10.1136/pgmj.75.882.231.
11. Moreno-Egea A, Baena EG, Calle MC, Martínez JA, Albasini JL. Controversies in the current management of lumbar hernias. Arch Surg. 2007;142(1):82–8. https://doi.org/10.1001/archsurg.142.1.82.
12. Mingolla GP, Amelio G. Lumbar hernia misdiagnosed as a subcutaneous lipoma: a case report. J Med Case Rep. 2009;3:9322. https://doi.org/10.1186/1752-1947-3-9322.
13. Kadler B, Shetye A, Patten DK, Al-Nowfal A. A primary inferior lumbar hernia misdiagnosed as a lipoma. Ann R Coll Surg Engl. 2019;101(4):e96–8. https://doi.org/10.1308/rcsann.2019.0009.
14. Stupalkowska W, Powell-Brett SF, Krijgsman B. Grynfeltt-Lesshaft lumbar hernia: a rare cause of bowel obstruction misdiagnosed as a lipoma. J Surg Case Rep. 2017;2017(9):rjx173. https://doi.org/10.1093/jscr/rjx173.
15. Hafner CD, Wylie JH, Brush BE. Petit's lumbar hernia: repair with Marlex mesh. Arch Surg. 1963;86:180–6. https://doi.org/10.1001/archsurg.1963.01310080004002.
16. Mekonnen AG, Gonfa KB. Primary superior lumbar hernia: a rare cause of lumbar swelling. Int Med Case Rep J. 2019;12:67–70. https://doi.org/10.2147/IMCRJ.S178727.
17. Stamatiou D, Skandalakis JE, Skandalakis LJ, Mirilas P. Lumbar hernia: surgical anatomy, embryology, and technique of repair. Am Surg. 2009;75(3):202–7.
18. Presti JC Jr, Narayan P. Lumbar herniation of the kidney. J Urol. 1988;140:586–7. https://doi.org/10.1016/S0022-5347(17)41726-5.
19. Fogarty JD, Hafron JM, Melman A. Renal obstruction caused by herniation of renal pelvis and ureteropelvic junction through superior lumbar triangle hernia (Grynfeltt hernia). Urology. 2006;67(3):620–1. https://doi.org/10.1016/j.urology.2005.09.027.
20. Cabello R, Cancho MJ, Monzó JI, López I, Tabares J, Hernández C. Herniation of renal pelvis and ureteropelvic junction resulting from superior lumbar triangle hernia. Scand J Urol Nephrol. 2008;42(1):81–2. https://doi.org/10.1080/00365590701514589.
21. Miyazato M, Yamada S, Kaiho Y, Ito A, Ishidoya S, Arai Y. Lumbar incisional hernia of the kidney after laparoscopic adrenalectomy in a patient with Cushing's syndrome. Urol Int. 2011;87(3):369–71. https://doi.org/10.1159/000329284.
22. Al Hooti Q, Saleh AA, Mahfooz AB, Aslam M, Moazin M. Kidney herniation through lumbar triangle following open pyeloplasty. J Health Spec. 2014;2:24–5. https://doi.org/10.4103/1658-600X.126061.
23. Vagholkar K, Vagholkar S. Open approach to primary lumbar hernia repair: a lucid option. Case Rep Surg. 2017;2017:5839491. https://doi.org/10.1155/2017/5839491.
24. Moreno-Egea A, Torralba-Martinez JA, Morales G, Fernández T, Girela E, Aguayo-Albasini JL. Open vs laparoscopic repair of secondary lumbar hernias: a prospective nonrandomized study. Surg Endosc. 2005;19(2):184–7. https://doi.org/10.1007/s00464-004-9067-7.
25. Moreno-Egea A, Alcaraz AC, Cuervo MC. Surgical options in lumbar hernia: laparoscopic versus open repair. A long-term prospective study. Surg Innov. 2013;20(4):331–44. https://doi.org/10.1177/1553350612458726.

# 26

# Do partial AZFc deletions affect the sperm retrieval rate in non-mosaic Klinefelter patients undergoing microdissection testicular sperm extraction?

I-Shen Huang[1,2,3,4], Richard J. Fantus[5], Wei-Jen Chen[2,3,4], James Wren[6], Wei-Tang Kao[7,8], Eric Yi-Hsiu Huang[2,3,4], Nelson E. Bennett[6], Robert E. Brannigan[6] and William J. Huang[1,2,3,4*]

**Abstract**

**Background:** The purpose of this study is to evaluate the prognostic factors for sperm retrieval and determine if Y chromosome deletion is associated with deleterious effects on spermatogenesis in non-mosaic Klinefelter patients. Whether Y chromosome deletion determines the sperm retrieval rate in non-mosaic Klinefelter patients has not yet been addressed.

**Methods:** We retrospectively collected medical records of azoospermic patients from Sep 2009 to Dec 2018, and enrolled 66 non-mosaic 47, XXY patients who were receiving mTESE. The predictive values of patients age, serum follicle-stimulating hormone (FSH), luteinizing hormone (LH), testosterone, prolactin, estradiol and Y chromosome deletion were assessed for successful sperm recovery.

**Results:** Testicular sperm recovery was successful in 24 (36.4%) of 66 men. The mean age (36.0 vs. 36.6 years), and levels of FSH (30.0 vs 36.9 IU/L), LH (17.7 vs 21.9 IU/L), testosterone (2.4 vs. 2.1 ng/ml), prolactin (9.1 vs. 8.8 ng/ml), and estradiol (19.4 vs. 22.3 pg/ml) did not show any significant difference when comparing patients with and without successful sperm retrieval. Partial deletion of azoospermic factor c (AZFc) was noted in 5 (20.8%) of 24 patients with successful sperm retrieval, including three *b2/b3* and two *gr/gr* deletion cases, whereas 4 (9.5%) of 42 patients with unsuccessful sperm retrieval were noted to have AZFc partial deletion (one *b2/b3*, one sY1206 and two *gr/gr* deletion), though the difference was not statistically significant ($p = 0.27$).

**Conclusion:** According to present results, age and AZFc partial deletion status should not be a deterrent for azoospermic males with non-mosaic Klinefelter syndrome to undergo mTESE.

**Keywords:** Klinefelter, AZFc deletion, Age, Microdissection testicular sperm extraction

## Background

According to recommendations from the American Society for Reproductive Medicine (ASRM) and European Association of Urology (EAU), cytogenetic analysis is suggested for patients with azoospermia or oligozoospermia. However, the threshold of sperm count recommended for karyotype analysis differs between the two associations: spermatozoa count below 10 million/mL from the EAU and spermatozoa count below 5 million/mL from the ASRM [1, 2]. The main purpose of performing cytogenetic analysis for patients with subfertility or infertility is to provide proper counselling before assisted reproductive technology and inform couples of possible inheritances of paternal genetic disorders in their offspring.

Genetic mutation or chromosome abnormality is more common in infertile males than in the general population, and investigations have shown that the percentage of chromosome abnormalities and Y chromosome

* Correspondence: williamjshuang@gmail.com
[1]Department of Physiology, School of Medicine, National Yang-Ming University, Taipei, Taiwan
[2]Department of Urology, School of Medicine, National Yang-Ming University, Taipei, Taiwan

microdeletions is about 2–6% and 3–5% [3, 4] for oligospermic patients, 13–15% and 6–16% for non-obstructive azoospermia (NOA) patients [5, 6]. Among all chromosome abnormalities, Klinefelter syndrome (KS) is the most common numerical chromosome abnormality found in infertile men with an incidence rate of about 1-in-500 to 1-in-1000 male birth [7]. The majority of cases with 47, XXY non-mosaic Klinefelter karyotype will present as hypergonadotropic hypogonadism and azoospermia, regardless of age, as a sign of primary testicular failure [8]. However, aside from the non-mosaic form, there is a strong probability of finding sperm in semen with mosaic form (46, XY/47, XXY) of KS, depending on the level of XXY cell line mosaicism in the gonads [9]. In general, about 90% of patients have uniform 47, XXY karyotype (pure KS) in which an extra X chromosome is present in somatic and germ cells, while 10% of KS can present with higher-grade of X chromosome aneuploidies (48 or more chromosomes) as well as mosaicism (47, XXY/46, XY) [7]. Mosaic KS men tend to be more androgenized than their non-mosaic KS counterparts in terms of hormone profile and sperm count in ejaculate, representing better fertility potential, especially in low-grade mosaicism form [9].

The azoospermia factor (AZF) region on the Y chromosome long arm is crucial for spermatogenesis and is known for its unique nearly identical direct and indirect repeated palindromic sequences. In addition to KS, the deletion of AZF is another cause for male infertility [10]. Removal of the spermatogenesis candidate gene located in the AZFa or AZFb, which is responsible for production of male gametes, namely the USP9Y, DDX3Y, RBMY and PRY genes, will inevitably lead to spermatogenic failure and therefore is not recommended for microdissection testicular sperm extraction (mTESE) due to the lack of identifiable regions of spermatogenesis in the testes [11]. The result of semen analysis of men with AZFc deletion varies in comparison with azoospermia found in AZFa and AZFb men, ranging from azoospermia to moderate oligozoospermia. Despite causing detrimental effects in sperm production, AZFc deletion is still regarded as a good prognostic factor for azoospermic men; the sperm retrieval rate (SRR) is up to 70% in this population [12].

The incidence of AZFc deletion is higher than incidence of AZFa or AZFb deletion in men, because the Y chromosome AZFc region is predisposed to intrachromosomal non-allelic homologous recombination owing to its composition of large repeat units called "amplicons" [13].

Rearrangement of the AZFc region, including partial deletions, duplications and deletions followed by duplication(s) has been reported [13]. Deletion of the entire AZFc locus on the Y chromosome by means of removing 3.5 Mb segment, including eight multi-copy gene families, is consensually considered a cause for infertility [10, 14]. As for AZFc partial deletion, Gr/gr deletion is the most common type, followed by b2/b3 and b1/b3 deletions. In particular, whether gr/gr deletion causes deleterious effects on spermatogenesis is still an ongoing debate. According to previous literature, the frequency of gr/gr deletion is only higher in certain azoospermia or oligozoospermia populations in Italy and China when compared to the control [15, 16].

Researchers have attempted to find predictors for successful sperm retrieval in KS men; some have demonstrated that testosterone levels after medical treatment, including aromatase inhibitors, clomiphene or human chorionic gonadotropin [17] and age at time of mTESE are reliable prognostic factors [18]. Therefore, they have recommended that patients receive mTESE for sperm retrieval under the age of 35 [18]. To date, due to the limited number of KS men, there are a paucity of articles discussing sperm retrieval rate by mTESE. Moreover, previous study populations did not include Han-Chinese or whether Y chromosome microdeletion may serve as a prognostic factor for possible sperm retrieval. Some clinicians may infer the outcome of sperm retrieval is affected by Y chromosome microdeletion in Klinefelter patients. Our study aimed to analyze predictive factors for sperm retrieval in Han-Chinese KS men and discuss the association for Y chromosome microdeletion with successful sperm retrieval.

## Methods

### Studied populations

We retrospectively reviewed the period between September 2009 to Dec 2018. A total of 66 non-mosaic Klinefelter patients who were receiving microdissection testicular sperm extraction were enrolled in our study. All subjects were genetically ethnic Han-Chinese from Taiwan. Each patient underwent a detailed examination to identify the etiology of azoospermia, including a detailed history, physical examination, two consecutive semen analyses, hormone profile (follicle stimulating hormone (FSH), leutinizing hormone (LH), testosterone and prolactin), chromosome karyotyping, and Y chromosome microdeletion. DNA samples of 107 fertile controls who had fathered at least one child were obtained from 2 medical centers in Taiwan as described by Lin et al. in 2007 [14]. This study was performed according to the Taipei Veterans General Hospital approved Institutional Review Board protocol (IRB number: 2018–03-002CCF).

### DNA extraction

Genomic DNA was extracted from peripheral blood using the QIAamp DNA minikit (Qiagen, Hilden, Germany) according to the manufacturer recommendations. In brief,

20 μl Qiagen protease was pipetted into the bottom of a 1.5 ml microcentrifuge tube, then up to 200 μl whole blood or buffy coat was added to the microcentrifuge tube. After the addition of 200 μl buffer AL to the sample, the sample was thoroughly mixed by vortex mixing and was incubated at 56 °C for 10 min until cell lysis was complete. Two hundred microliters of ethanol (100%) were added to precipitate the DNA. The mixture was carefully applied to the QIAamp spin column, placed inside a 2 ml collection tube, and centrifuged at 8000 rpm, 6000×g for 1 min. The QIAamp Spin column was then placed in a new collection tube, and 500 μl of buffer, AW1 was added and centrifuged. This step was repeated with the buffer AW2 and a high spin was given for 3 min to dry the column membrane. The spin column was subsequently placed in a clean 1.5 ml microcentrifuge tube, and the DNA filtrate was recovered with 200 μl of buffer AE. Following centrifugation, DNA was eluted and stored at – 20 °C until used.

### Cytogenetic analysis

Chromosome analysis was performed using conventional trypsin-Giemsa banding technique. Twenty metaphases were analyzed for each patient, and in cases of suspected mosaicism, the number of metaphases was increased to a total of 50 for analysis. To achieve a more detailed analysis, a 500–550 band level was used for evaluation.

### Yq classical deletions and AZFc subdeletions

Y microdeletion screening in Klinefelter patients was performed by multiplex polymerase chain reaction (PCR) that detects markers in the AZF regions, the sex determining region Y (SRY) gene, and the Y homologous gene pair zinc-finger Y (ZFY) [19]. The sequence-tagged sites (STS) selected are listed in Fig. 1 and Table 1. Six AZFc deletions (sY254, sY1161, sY1191, sY1201, sY1206, and sY1291) were used to identify the type of partial AZFc deletions in all subjects. In addition, DNA from fertile males and female served as positive and negative controls, respectively. Ambiguities in the multiplex PCR assays were resolved by following up with single PCR assays.

### Microdissection testicular sperm extraction

A small incision (3 cm) was made longitudinally on the median raphe, and carried down to the fascia. The testis were mobilized after opening the tunica vaginalis as described in 1999 [20]. We performed a longitudinal incision on the testis instead of open it widely in an equatorial plane along the mid portion of the testis. An operating microscope with 20x~24x magnification allow the surgeon to identify larger and opaquer seminiferous tubules, which are most likely to contain sperm. Tissue with possibility of spermatogenesis was removed and sent for real time analysis by experienced embryologists in our reproductive lab for further intracytoplasmic sperm injection (ICSI).

### Statistical analysis

Outcome variables (age, serum FSH, LH, testosterone, prolactin and estradiol) of azoospermic non-mosaic KS men with successful surgical sperm retrieval were compared to those with unsuccessful sperm retrieval using the Student's t test. The distributions of AZFc partial deletion of Klinefelter patient with or without sperm retrieval and the frequency of AZFc partial deletion comparing azoospermic non-mosaic Klinefelter men with controls were analyzed by the Fisher's exact test. In these tests, values of $p < 0.05$ were regarded as statistically significant.

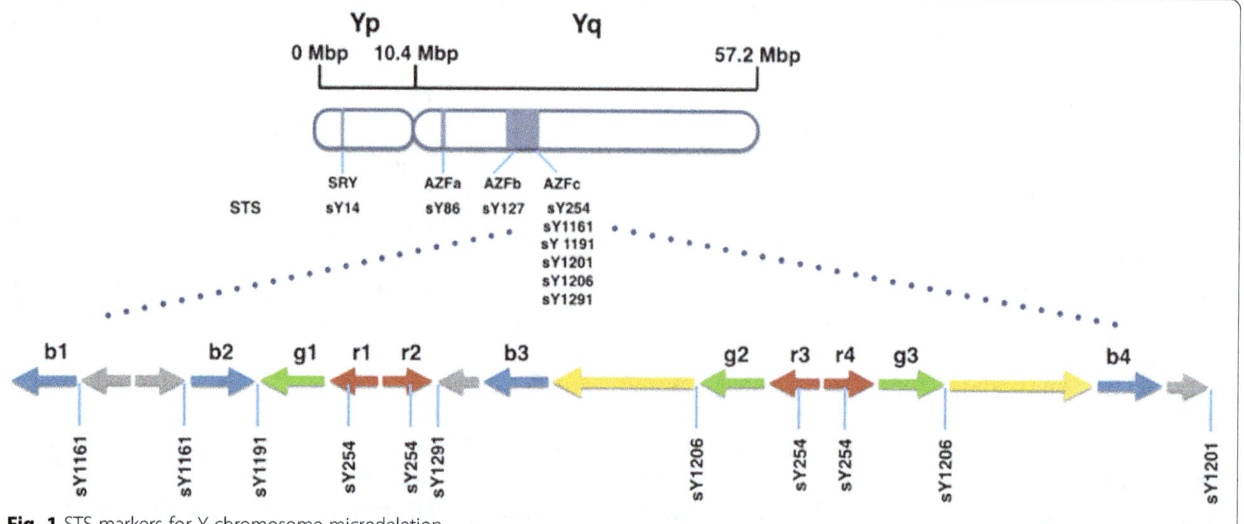


**Fig. 1** STS markers for Y chromosome microdeletion

**Table 1** Sequence of 10 sets of primer employed to identify Y-chromosome microdeletions

| STS/gene | Primer sequence | Product size (bp) | Region |
|---|---|---|---|
| SRY-F | 5' - GAA TAT TCC CGC TCT CCG GA - 3' | 495 | NRY |
| SRY-R | 5' - GCT GGT GCT CCA TTC TTG AG - 3' | | |
| ZFY-F | 5' - ACC RCT GTA CTG ACT GTG ATT ACA C - 3' | 472 | NRY |
| ZFY-R | 5' - GCA CYT CTT TGG TAT CYG AGA AAG T - 3' | | |
| sY86-F | 5' - GTG ACA CAC AGA CTA TGC TTC - 3' | 320 | AZFa |
| sY86-R | 5' - ACA CAC AGA GGG ACA ACC CT - 3' | | |
| sY127-F | 5' - GGC TCA CAA ACG AAA AGA AA - 3' | 274 | AZFb |
| sY127-R | 5' - CTG CAG GCA GTA ATA AGG GA - 3' | | |
| sY254-F | 5' - GGG TGT TAC CAG AAG GCA AA - 3' | 400 | AZFc |
| sY254-R | 5' - GAA CCG TAT CTA CCA AAG CAG C - 3' | | |
| sY1161-F | 5' - CGA CAC TTT TGG GAA GTT TCA - 3' | 377 | AZFc |
| sY1161-R | 5' - TTG TGT CCA GTG GTG GCT TA- 3' | | |
| sY1191-F | 5' – CCA GAC GTT CTA CCC TTT CG - 3' | 385 | AZFc |
| sY1191-R | 5' – GAG CCG AGA TCC AGT TAC CA - 3' | | |
| sY1201-F | 5' – CCG ACT TCC ACA ATG GCT - 3' | 677 | AZFc |
| sY1201-R | 5' – GGG AGA AAA GTT CTG CAA CG - 3' | | |
| sY1206-F | 5' – ATT GAT CTC CTT GGT TCC CC - 3' | 394 | AZFc |
| sY1206-R | 5' – GAC ATG TGT GGC CAA TTT GA - 3 | | |
| sY1291-F | 5' – TAA AAG GCA GAA CTG CCA GG - 3' | 527 | AZFc |
| sY1291-R | 5' – GGG AGA AAA GTT CTG CAA CG - 3' | | |

## Results

### Azoopsermic non-mosaic Klinefelter men and Y chromosome deletion

The cohort of 66 azoospermic non-mosaic Klinefelter men with chromosome 47, XXY had a mean age of 36.4 ± 5.2 years (mean ± SD). Of these 66 men, 9 men (13.6%) had a deletion of one STS marker. More precisely, we identified 5 men with an absence of sY1291 (possible *gr/gr* deletion), 3 men with an absence of sY1191 (possible *b2/b3* deletion) and 1 with an absence of sY1206 only. Of the 24 patients with successful sperm retrieval, 5 (20.8%) had patient AZFc deletion, including 2 possible *gr/gr* deletion and 3 possible *b2/b3* deletion cases (Table 2). Partial AZFc deletion is identified in 4 (9.5%) of 42 patients without sperm retrieval by mTESE, (one possible *b2/b3*, one sY1206, and two possible *gr/gr* deletion), though the difference of Y chromosome deletion was not statistically significant between the successful and non-successful sperm retrieval groups ($p = 0.27$).

### Impact of various parameters on mTESE success

Of the non-mosaic KS patients, mTESE was successful in 24 out of 66 patients, representing 36.4% of cases. Table 2 lists the clinical factors analyzed to predict sperm retrieval, stratified by outcome. Age, partial AZFc deletions, and hormone parameter (LH, FSH, testosterone, prolactin, estradiol) were not predictive factors for successful sperm retrieval.

### Effect of age on sperm retrieval

SRR for mTESE was 34.6% (9/26) at ages below 35 years and 37.5% (15/40) at 35 years and older. Four of 13 KS men older than 40 years of age had successful sperm retrieval; the oldest patient with successful mTESE was 47 years-old (Fig. 2).

**Table 2** Demographic profile of nonmosaic Klinefelter men with positive and negative mTESE outcome

| | Overall Mean ± SD | mTESE (+) Mean ± SD | mTESE (−) Mean ± SD | *p* value |
|---|---|---|---|---|
| Number | *n* = 66 | *n* = 24 | *n* = 42 | |
| Age (yr) | 36.4 ± 5.2 | 36.0 ± 4.9 | 36.6 ± 5.4 | 0.67 |
| FSH (IU/L) | 34.3 ± 17.0 | 30.0 ± 13.1 | 36.9 ± 18.6 | 0.12 |
| LH (IU/L) | 20.4 ± 11.7 | 17.7 ± 9.7 | 21.9 ± 12.6 | 0.16 |
| Testosterone (ng/nl) | 2.2 ± 1.8 | 2.4 ± 2.0 | 2.1 ± 1.6 | 0.47 |
| Prolactin | 9.2 ± 3.7 | 8.7 ± 3.5 | 9.5 ± 3.8 | 0.39 |
| Estradiol (pg/ml) | 21.0 ± 9.9 | 19.5 ± 7.4 | 21.8 ± 11.0 | 0.41 |
| Y partial deletion | 9 (13.6%) | 5 (20.8%) | 4 (9.5%) | 0.27 |
| gr/gr deletion | 4 (6.1%) | 2 (8.3%) | 2 (4.8%) | 0.62 |
| b2/b3 deletion | 4 (6.1%) | 3 (12.5%) | 1 (2.4%) | 0.13 |
| sY1206 deletion | 1 (1.5%) | 0 (0%) | 1 (2.4%) | 1.00 |

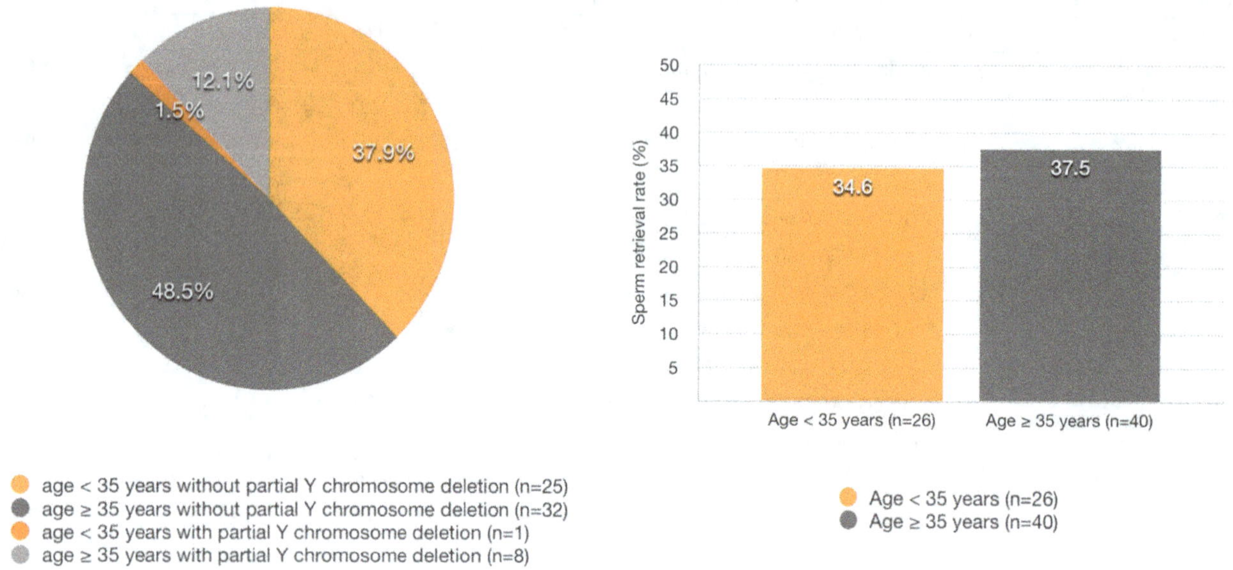


**Fig. 2** Percentage of KS men below and above 35 with Y chromosome deletion and sperm retrieval rate by mTESE

**Partial AZFc deletions distribution between the experimental and control groups**

The frequency of AZFc partial detection was 13.6% (9/66) in KS men and 6.5% (7/107) in the control, although a higher percentage was seen in KS men, however the difference was not statistically significant ($p > 0.05$). The deletion pattern in 9 KS men with AZFc partial deletion included 4 men with possible *gr/gr* deletion, 4 with possible *b2/b3* deletion, and one with sY1206 deletion. Seven men in the control group with AZFc partial deletion included 3 men with possible *gr/gr* deletion and 4 men with possible *b2/b3* deletion. There was no significant difference between the frequencies of specific AZFc partial deletion pattern by means of possible *gr/gr*, possible *b2/b3*, and sY1206 deletion, respectively (Table 3). Y chromosome partial deletion was detected in 5 KS men with successful sperm retrieval.

## Discussion

The extra X chromosome in KS men causes germ cell degeneration and adverse effects to somatic cells, including Leydig and Sertoli cells, resulting in infertility. As a matter of fact, germ cell degeneration take place early in the fetal period, whereas the density and number of seminiferous tubules and mesenchymal tissues remain normal, without obvious pattern change [21]. The hormone levels are unaffected until the onset of puberty, which is when the germ cell depletion, Sertoli cell degeneration, Leydig cell hyperplasia and seminiferous tubule hyalinization initiate and accelerate [22]. Accelerated degeneration of the Sertoli cell is also evidenced by the sign of aberrant nuclear expression of the α-subunit in the Sertoli cells in older teenage KS boys [23]. Based on the concept of early fertility deterioration, sperm banking at a younger age is recommended at puberty, according to their Tanner stage. The results, however, were not promising with regards to KS adolescent semen quality. Sperm in the ejaculate can only be detected in limited cases [8].

If sperm cannot be traced in the semen, using mTESE for testicular sperm retrieval associated with assisted reproductive technology such as ICSI is a recommended option with a satisfactory outcome, and offers these patients the opportunity to father biological children. As shown in several studies, age is a predictive factor for successful sperm retrieval in KS men receiving mTESE; In adult men younger than 35 years old, sperm retrieval rate (SRR) is reported to range from 30 to 77%, with a higher SRR than subjects > 35 years. Consequently, experts recommend performing mTESE under the critical age of 35 or even 30 years to yield a better outcome [18, 24]. However, age as a predictive factor for sperm retrieval was not unanimously proved in other literatures [25, 26]. In our study, age was not a predictive factor for sperm retrieval, and SRR was comparable for KS men under or above the age of 35 (33.3% vs 37.5%, respectively). The mean age of our study population is 36.4

**Table 3** AZFc partial deletion in KS men and controls

| | Fertile control | Klinefelter men | *p* value |
|---|---|---|---|
| Total subjects | 107 | 66 | |
| AZFc partial deletion | 7 | 9 | 0.18 |
| gr/gr deletion | 3 | 4 | 0.43 |
| b2/b3 deletion | 4 | 4 | 0.48 |
| sY1206 deletion | 0 | 1 | 0.38 |

years; only two KS men (age 25 and 27 years) under the age of 30 was evaluated, which will limit the ability to evaluate the influence of age on successful sperm retrieval.

Our Klinefelter cases with older age may be explained by the fact that a majority of cases coming to our center are either referral or consultation for infertility other than delayed puberty, which also implies that most of the Taiwanese KS men remained undiagnosed before marriage. According to Taiwanese government statistics, the average age of marriage for men has increased in the last decade and was 34.2 years in 2015.

*gr/gr* deletion, the most common form of partial AZFc deletion, has been demonstrated a correlation with male infertility in many meta-analysis studies [27, 28]. However, debates rage over whether *gr/gr* deletion and copy number reduction of AZFc genes influence spermatogenesis. The diverse phenotypes in *gr/gr* deletion prevent researchers from drawing definite conclusions on this topic, which is best shown in the Japanese population with 33.9% *gr/gr* deletion men in the control group, and 23.9% in the infertility group, although the controls have unknown fertility status [29]. Based on ethnicity and region, Caucasians (OR = 3.721), people from Europe (OR = 2.465), and people from South Asia (OR = 2.523) with *gr/gr* deletion had a higher risk of male infertility in comparison to those without deletions [28]. But published literatures within the same ethnicity have drawn opposite conclusions. In China, Wu et al. pointed out that *b2/b3* deletion was significantly associated with idiopathic male infertility [30], while in contrast, Yang et al. recorded *gr/gr* deletion, instead of *b2/b3* deletion, serve as a more important anomaly in determining the susceptibility to spermatogenic failure [31].

As a matter of fact, the results may vary without contradiction. Two study populations that were 1500 km apart belonged to different Y chromosome haplogroup, representing distinct paternal lineage. As demonstrated previously, Y lineages as defined by different haplotypes could influence the phenotypical expression of identical *gr/gr* deletion genotype [32]. *Gr/gr* deletions and *b2/b3* have been demonstrated fixed in haplogroup Q1 and haplogroup N; the prevalence of partial deletion will likely mask actual influence from other haplogroups [14, 27, 33, 34]. In the Taiwanese population, Lin et al. found that 14% of men have deletions and duplications of AZFc and that the frequency of deletion vary between different Y haplogroups, ranging from 2.9% in O3e to 100% in N and Q [14]. AZFc partial duplication other than partial deletion increases the risk of spermatogenic failure. Although, in our study, we did not perform quantitative PCR analysis to evaluate DAZ (Deleted in AZoospermia) dosage and duplication in our patients, with regard of the presence of AZFc, partial deletion did not seem to affect SRR.

In Danish and Chinese populations, specific Y haplogroup has been suggested to be an "at risk Y haplogroup" by their over-presentation in the spermatogenic impairment population [31, 35]. Until now, no study has looked into the relationship between different Y haplogroup and SRR in azoospermic cases. Hence, it would be interesting to understand the possible influence of Y haplogroup not only on semen parameters but also on spermatogenesis in the testes.

We examined Y chromosome microdeletions in KS men using 10 sets of primers and detected 9 cases with partial AZFc deletion, including 4 men with possible *gr/gr* deletion, 4 with possible *b2/b3* deletion, and one with sY1206 deletion KS. Our study did not detect complete AZFa, AZFb or AZFc deletion in KS men, which is compatible with the Lin et al. study, suggesting a low percentage of complete deletion pattern in Han Chinese in Taiwan [14]. The incidence of AZFc partial deletion did not differ between the KS men and the fertility control men; the result is consistent with a recent study investigating AZF microdeletion in KS men [36]. However, in a study of Han Chinese KS men in China, the proportion of partial AZFc deletion is higher than our population – 27 (24.3%) of 111 KS men and 11 (11.7%) of the 94 controls compared to our population of 13.6% in KS men and 6.5% in the control [36]. The outcome of our study indicates that the possible *gr/gr* and *b2/b3* deletions are not correlated with KS men in the Taiwan Han-Chinese population, suggesting that although formation of sperm with an extra copy of X chromosome by non-disjunction during meiosis I contributed to paternal error, it did not increase the chance of de novo Y chromosome partial microdeletion.

Previous studies on the preoperative hCG or aromatase inhibitor on KS men have demonstrated varying results, therefore our KS cases were not routinely given hCG or aromatase inhibitors before mTESE [17, 24, 26].. Prior experience with mTESE in KS men with non-obstructive azoospermia reported SRR range from 16 to 70% and cumulative SRR per TESE cycle of 44% [37]. The SRR for KS men above 35 years of age in 3 series were 25, 30 and 50%; it was 37.5% in our study [17, 18, 24].

To our knowledge this is the first article looking into Y chromosome deletion in Klinefelter patients for SRR evaluation. Our results demonstrate that AZFc partial deletion, age, and endocrine variables do not predict sperm retrieval in KS men. Sperm retrieval rate is comparable for men below and above 35 years, and we should not discourage AZFc partial deletion men or men over the age of 35 from accepting mTESE for possible sperm retrieval.

## Conclusion

According to present results, age and AZFc partial deletion status should not be a deterrent for azoospermic males with non-mosaic Klinefelter syndrome to undergo mTESE.

### Abbreviations

ASRM: American Society for Reproductive Medicine; AZF: Azoospermia factor; DAZ: Deleted in AZoospermia; EAU: European Association of Urology; FSH: Follicle stimulating hormone; ICSI: Intracytoplasmic sperm injection; KS: Klinefelter syndrome; LH: Leutinizing hormone; mTESE: Microsurgical testicular sperm extraction; NAHR: Non-allelic homologous recombination; NOA: Non-obstructive azoospermia; PCR: Polymerase chain reaction; SRR: Sperm retrieval rate; SRY: Sex determining region Y; STS: Sequence-tagged sites; ZFY: Zinc-finger Y

### Acknowledgements

Not applicable.

### Authors' contributions

IH contributed to study conception and design. WC, JW, WK, EH contributed to data acquisition. IH contributed to analysis and interpretation of data. IH, RF contributed to drafting the manuscript. NB, RB, WH were involved in revising the manuscript. All authors have read and approved the manuscript.

### Competing interests

The authors declare that they have no competing interests.

### Author details

[1]Department of Physiology, School of Medicine, National Yang-Ming University, Taipei, Taiwan. [2]Department of Urology, School of Medicine, National Yang-Ming University, Taipei, Taiwan. [3]Department of Urology, Taipei Veterans General Hospital, No 201, Section 2, Shipai Rd, Taipei 112, Taiwan, Republic of China. [4]Department of Urology, School of Medicine, Shu-Tien Urological Research Center, National Yang-Ming University, Taipei, Taiwan. [5]Section of Urology, Department of Surgery, University of Chicago Medicine, 5841 S. Maryland Avenue, Chicago, IL 60637, USA. [6]Division of Male Reproductive Surgery and Men's Health, Department of Urology, Northwestern University Feinberg School of Medicine, NMH/Arkes Family Pavilion Suite 2300, 676 N Saint Clair, Chicago, IL 60611, USA. [7]Department of Urology, Shuang Ho Hospital, Taipei Medical University, No.291, Zhongzheng Rd., Zhonghe District, New Taipei City 23561, Taiwan. [8]Graduate Institute of Clinical Medicine, Taipei Medical University, New Taipei City, Taiwan.

### References

1. Medicine PCoASfR. Diagnostic evaluation of the infertile male: a committee opinion. Fertil Steril. 2012;98(2):294–301.
2. Jungwirth A, Giwercman A, Tournaye H, Diemer T, Kopa Z, Dohle G, et al. European Association of Urology guidelines on male infertility: the 2012 update. Eur Urol. 2012;62(2):324–32.
3. Van Assche E, Bonduelle M, Tournaye H, Joris H, Verheyen G, Devroey P, et al. Cytogenetics of infertile men. Hum Reprod. 1996;11(Suppl 4):1–24 discussion 5-6.
4. Fu L, Xiong DK, Ding XP, Li C, Zhang LY, Ding M, et al. Genetic screening for chromosomal abnormalities and Y chromosome microdeletions in Chinese infertile men. J Assist Reprod Genet. 2012;29(6):521–7.
5. Oliva R, Margarit E, Ballescá JL, Carrió A, Sánchez A, Milà M, et al. Prevalence of Y chromosome microdeletions in oligospermic and azoospermic candidates for intracytoplasmic sperm injection. Fertil Steril. 1998;70(3):506–10.
6. Oates RD, Silber S, Brown LG, Page DC. Clinical characterization of 42 oligospermic or azoospermic men with microdeletion of the AZFc region of the Y chromosome, and of 18 children conceived via ICSI. Hum Reprod. 2002;17(11):2813–24.
7. Bojesen A, Juul S, Gravholt CH. Prenatal and postnatal prevalence of Klinefelter syndrome: a national registry study. J Clin Endocrinol Metab. 2003;88(2):622–6.
8. Rives N, Milazzo JP, Perdrix A, Castanet M, Joly-Hélas G, Sibert L, et al. The feasibility of fertility preservation in adolescents with Klinefelter syndrome. Hum Reprod. 2013;28(6):1468 79.
9. Samplaski MK, Lo KC, Grober ED, Millar A, Dimitromanolakis A, Jarvi KA. Phenotypic differences in mosaic Klinefelter patients as compared with non-mosaic Klinefelter patients. Fertil Steril. 2014;101(4):950–5.
10. Kuroda-Kawaguchi T, Skaletsky H, Brown LG, Minx PJ, Cordum HS, Waterston RH, et al. The AZFc region of the Y chromosome features massive palindromes and uniform recurrent deletions in infertile men. Nat Genet. 2001;29(3):279–86.
11. Kleiman SE, Almog R, Yogev L, Hauser R, Lehavi O, Paz G, et al. Screening for partial AZFa microdeletions in the Y chromosome of infertile men: is it of clinical relevance? Fertil Steril. 2012;98(1):43–7.
12. Stahl PJ, Masson P, Mielnik A, Marean MB, Schlegel PN, Paduch DA. A decade of experience emphasizes that testing for Y microdeletions is essential in American men with azoospermia and severe oligozoospermia. Fertil Steril. 2010;94(5):1753–6.
13. Repping S, Skaletsky H, Lange J, Silber S, Van Der Veen F, Oates RD, et al. Recombination between palindromes P5 and P1 on the human Y chromosome causes massive deletions and spermatogenic failure. Am J Hum Genet. 2002;71(4):906–22.
14. Lin YW, Hsu LC, Kuo PL, Huang WJ, Chiang HS, Yeh SD, et al. Partial duplication at AZFc on the Y chromosome is a risk factor for impaired spermatogenesis in Han Chinese in Taiwan. Hum Mutat. 2007;28(5):486–94.
15. Giachini C, Laface I, Guarducci E, Balercia G, Forti G, Krausz C. Partial AZFc deletions and duplications: clinical correlates in the Italian population. Hum Genet. 2008;124(4):399–410.
16. Yang Y, Ma M, Li L, Su D, Chen P, Ma Y, et al. Differential effect of specific gr/gr deletion subtypes on spermatogenesis in the Chinese Han population. Int J Androl. 2010;33(5):745–54.
17. Ramasamy R, Ricci JA, Palermo GD, Gosden LV, Rosenwaks Z, Schlegel PN. Successful fertility treatment for Klinefelter's syndrome. J Urol. 2009;182(3): 1108–13.
18. Okada H, Goda K, Yamamoto Y, Sofikitis N, Miyagawa I, Mio Y, et al. Age as a limiting factor for successful sperm retrieval in patients with nonmosaic Klinefelter's syndrome. Fertil Steril. 2005;84(6):1662–4.
19. Krausz C, Hoefsloot L, Simoni M, Tüttelmann F, Andrology EAo, network EMGQ. EAA/EMQN best practice guidelines for molecular diagnosis of Y-chromosomal microdeletions: state-of-the-art 2013. Andrology. 2014;2(1):5–19.
20. Schlegel PN. Testicular sperm extraction: microdissection improves sperm yield with minimal tissue excision. Hum Reprod. 1999;14(1):131–5.
21. Coerdt W, Rehder H, Gausmann I, Johannisson R, Gropp A. Quantitative histology of human fetal testes in chromosomal disease. Pediatr Pathol. 1985;3(2–4):245–59.
22. Aksglaede L, Wikström AM, Rajpert-De Meyts E, Dunkel L, Skakkebaek NE, Juul A. Natural history of seminiferous tubule degeneration in Klinefelter syndrome. Hum Reprod Update. 2006;12(1):39–48.
23. Wikström AM, Hoei-Hansen CE, Dunkel L, Rajpert-De ME. Immunoexpression of androgen receptor and nine markers of maturation in the testes of adolescent boys with Klinefelter syndrome: evidence for degeneration of germ cells at the onset of meiosis. J Clin Endocrinol Metab. 2007;92(2):714–9.
24. Rohayem J, Fricke R, Czeloth K, Mallidis C, Wistuba J, Krallmann C, et al. Age and markers of Leydig cell function, but not of Sertoli cell function predict the success of sperm retrieval in adolescents and adults with Klinefelter's syndrome. Andrology. 2015;3(5):868–75.
25. Koga M, Tsujimura A, Takeyama M, Kiuchi H, Takao T, Miyagawa Y, et al. Clinical comparison of successful and failed microdissection testicular sperm extraction in patients with nonmosaic Klinefelter syndrome. Urology. 2007; 70(2):341–5.
26. Schiff JD, Palermo GD, Veeck LL, Goldstein M, Rosenwaks Z, Schlegel PN. Success of testicular sperm extraction [corrected] and intracytoplasmic sperm injection in men with Klinefelter syndrome. J Clin Endocrinol Metab. 2005;90(11):6263–7.
27. Navarro-Costa P, Gonçalves J, Plancha CE. The AZFc region of the Y chromosome: at the crossroads between genetic diversity and male infertility. Hum Reprod Update. 2010;16(5):525–42.
28. Bansal SK, Jaiswal D, Gupta N, Singh K, Dada R, Sankhwar SN, et al. Gr/gr deletions on Y-chromosome correlate with male infertility: an original study, meta-analyses, and trial sequential analyses. Sci Rep. 2016;6:19798.

29. de Carvalho CM, Zuccherato LW, Fujisawa M, Shirakawa T, Ribeiro-dos-Santos AK, Santos SE, et al. Study of AZFc partial deletion gr/gr in fertile and infertile Japanese males. J Hum Genet. 2006;51(9):794–9.
30. Wu B, Lu NX, Xia YK, Gu AH, Lu CC, Wang W, et al. A frequent Y chromosome b2/b3 subdeletion shows strong association with male infertility in Han-Chinese population. Hum Reprod. 2007;22(4):1107–13.
31. Yang Y, Ma M, Li L, Zhang W, Xiao C, Li S, et al. Evidence for the association of Y-chromosome haplogroups with susceptibility to spermatogenic failure in a Chinese Han population. J Med Genet. 2008;45(4):210–5.
32. Navarro-Costa P, Pereira L, Alves C, Gusmão L, Proença C, Marques-Vidal P, et al. Characterizing partial AZFc deletions of the Y chromosome with amplicon-specific sequence markers. BMC Genomics. 2007;8:342.
33. Zhang F, Lu C, Li Z, Xie P, Xia Y, Zhu X, et al. Partial deletions are associated with an increased risk of complete deletion in AZFc: a new insight into the role of partial AZFc deletions in male infertility. J Med Genet. 2007;44(7):437–44.
34. Repping S, van Daalen SK, Korver CM, Brown LG, Marszalek JD, Gianotten J, et al. A family of human Y chromosomes has dispersed throughout northern Eurasia despite a 1.8-Mb deletion in the azoospermia factor c region. Genomics. 2004;83(6):1046–52.
35. Krausz C, Quintana-Murci L, Forti G. Y chromosome polymorphisms in medicine. Ann Med. 2004;36(8):573–83.
36. Li LX, Dai HY, Ding XP, Zhang YP, Zhang XH, Ren HY, et al. Investigation of AZF microdeletions in patients with Klinefelter syndrome. Genet Mol Res. 2015;14(4):15140–7.
37. Corona G, Pizzocaro A, Lanfranco F, Garolla A, Pelliccione F, Vignozzi L, et al. Sperm recovery and ICSI outcomes in Klinefelter syndrome: a systematic review and meta-analysis. Hum Reprod Update. 2017;23(3):265–75.

27

# Can clinical and urodynamic parameters predict the occurrence of neutralizing antibodies in therapy failure of intradetrusor onabotulinumtoxin A injections in patients with spinal cord injury?

Christian Tiburtius[1*†], Ralf Böthig[1†], Birgitt Kowald[2], Sven Hirschfeld[3] and Roland Thietje[3]

**Abstract**

**Background:** The aim of the study was to clarify whether clinical and/or urodynamic parameters could be used to infer the probability of neutralizing antibody (NAb) formation as a possible cause of therapy failure (non-response, NR) in patients with neurogenic detrusor overactivity (NDO) due to acquired spinal cord injury/disease (SCI/D) treated with intradetrusor botulinum neurotoxin A (BoNT-A) injections.

**Methods:** A retrospective chart review was performed of all patients with SCI/D who underwent both intradetrusor onabotulinumtoxin A injections and the determination of neutralizing antibodies against BoNT-A between January 1, 2002, and December 31, 2018. NR was defined as urodynamically confirmed persistent or reappearing NDO.

**Results:** A total of 2700 BoNT-A injections in 414 patients were ascertained. In 69 patients with primary NR after the first BoNT-A injection ($n = 6$) or with secondary NR after more than one BoNT-A injection ($n = 63$), an antibody analysis was performed. Antibody examination showed 36 (52.2%) negative, 5 (7.2%) borderline and 14 (each 20.3%) each of positive and highly positive values. Subgroup analysis indicated a correlation between NAb formation and the duration of BoNT-A therapy ($p = 0.015$), the mean number of BoNT-A injections ($p = 0.011$) and the time interval between BoNT-A applications (< 7 months, $p = 0.022$). Urodynamic data analysis indicate significant differences with cut-off values of MCC (< 225 ml, $p = 0.038$) and MDP (> 45 cm$H_2O$, $p = 0.040$). However, in the regression analysis models, the predictive value for the occurrence of NAb was too low (MCC: ROC AUC 0.62, MDP: ROC AUC 0.52) to distinguish with sufficient certainty between NAb-positive and NAb-negative NR patients.

(Continued on next page)

* Correspondence: c.tiburtius@bgk-hamburg.de
†Christian Tiburtius and Ralf Böthig contributed equally to this work.
[1]Centre for Spinal Injuries, Department Neuro-Urology, BG Trauma Hospital Hamburg, Bergedorfer Str. 10 Germany, 21033 Hamburg, Germany

(Continued from previous page)

**Conclusions:** Despite significant correlations, clinical and urodynamic parameters are only partially suitable for predicting antibody formation against BoNT-A.

**Keywords:** Neurogenic bladder, Spinal cord injury, Botulinum neurotoxin a, Therapy failure, Overactive detrusor function

## Background

Patients with spinal cord injury/disease (SCI/D) frequently develop neurogenic lower urinary tract dysfunction (NLUTD). Depending on the level of the lesion, up to 95% of patients suffer from neurogenic detrusor overactivity (NDO) [1]. NDO can cause neurogenic urinary incontinence and other adverse events, such as recurrent urinary tract infection, bladder stones, hydronephrosis and vesicoureteral reflux, contributing to a risk of deteriorated renal function and impaired quality of life [2, 3]. Oral antimuscarinics are effective and commonly used as first-line mono- or combination therapy for NDO [4, 5]. Nevertheless, numerous patients discontinue antimuscarinic treatment due to insufficient responses with the consecutive need for higher drug doses or because patients suffer from intolerable side effects such as dry mouth, constipation or sight disorder [6, 7]. Intradetrusor botulinum neurotoxin A (BoNT-A) injections have basically changed the treatment options in patients with refractory NDO and have become a well-established and widely accepted second-line treatment for these patients [8–10]. The European Association of Urology (EAU) Guidelines strongly recommend the use of BoNT-A injection in the detrusor to reduce NDO in SCI/D patients if antimuscarinic therapy is ineffective [3].

Although BoNT-A has been very successfully used for the treatment of refractory NDO for approximately two decades, there is a considerable number of cases of treatment discontinuation and non-response (NR). Recent studies have investigated the long-term outcomes and reasons for the discontinuation of BoNT-A injections [11, 12]. However, the detailed mechanisms of therapy failure are unclear; biochemical processes such as antibody formation and structural changes in the detrusor muscle have been discussed [13], as well as technical issues and catheterization-related difficulties [14]. If neutralizing antibodies (NAbs) against BoNT-A can be detected, they are considered the cause of treatment failure. Nevertheless, only a few studies have investigated the role of NAbs in patients with therapy failure [15, 16], especially in SCI/D patients with NDO.

Recently, various possibilities have been discussed to improve the long-term success rate of BoNT-A therapy. Among others, a change from onabotulinumtoxin A to abobotulinumtoxin A or vice versa has shown certain chances of success [17]. Otherwise, only considerably more invasive surgical treatment options are often considered. In these cases, for individual therapy recommendations, it would be important to know which patients are better suited for each therapy option.

Currently, the question of whether antibody formation is a possible cause of non-response has become particularly important. However, antibody determination is expensive and complex.

It therefore seems important to investigate whether clinical or urodynamic data can predict antibody formation as a possible cause of therapy failure in the case of BoNT-A injection for NDO due to SCI/D.

## Methods

At the Spinal Cord Injury Centre, BG Klinikum Hamburg, Germany, we processed a monocentric retrospective chart review of SCI/D patients treated with BoNT-A injections and searched for patients who underwent single or repeated antibody examinations due to primary (PNR) or secondary (SNR) NR. NR was defined as persistent or reappearing NDO.

Prior to each BoNT-A injection, the preoperative assessment included urinalysis and culture. In the case of positive urine culture, patients received antibiotic treatment according to an antibiogram. Patients with negative urine culture received a single shot of antibiotic prophylaxis with a second-generation cephalosporin. All BoNT-A injections were performed under cystoscopic control by consultants under local or general anaesthesia according to current recommendations [18, 19]. All patients received 200 U or 300 U onabotulinumtoxin A. We only used the newer formulation of the Botox® preparation (Allergan, Inc., Irvine, California) with increased specific activity (i.e., less BoNT protein per unit of activity of 5 ng/100 U). After approval of 200 U Botox® in 2011 for the diagnosis "urinary incontinence in adults with neurogenic detrusor hyperactivity in the neurogenic bladder due to stable subcervical spinal cord injury or multiple sclerosis", a dose of 200 U was initially started if patients fitted into the approval. Patients mostly received low-dose antimuscarinic therapy accompanied by BoNT-A injections to extend the injection intervals, except when there were intolerable side effects due to antimuscarinic therapy.

For the clinical signs of persistent or reappearing NDO after BoNT-A injection therapy, we evaluated the occurrence of self-reported incontinence episodes between aseptic intermittent catheterization or, with preserved sensitivity, a remarkable increase in catheterization frequency in combination with a decrease in catheterization volume within the first 3 months after BoNT-A injection. All patients with these clinical signs of therapy failure within 3 months after BoNT-A injection (after exclusion or treatment for a causative urinary tract infection (UTI)) were screened for the presence of neutralizing antibodies and received a urodynamic examination for the confirmation of NDO [20] within this period. Antibody tests were performed with a commercially available Mouse Phrenic Nerve Hemidiaphragm Assay for measuring neutralizing antibodies (Toxogen®, Toxogen GmbH, Hannover, Germany). The results of this test were grouped as "negative", "borderline", "positive" or "highly positive". For theoretical and clinical reasons, the analyses of the negative tests were compared with the other groups.

Urodynamic studies were performed according to International Continence Society standards [21, 22] after the exclusion of UTI by urinalysis and culture. We evaluated the following two urodynamic parameters as essential criteria for a lack of effectiveness: maximum cystometric capacity (MCC, in the absence of sensation, the clinician decided to terminate filling in accordance with high detrusor filling pressure due to involuntary detrusor contraction/NDO) and maximum detrusor pressure (MDP) during filling cystometry [23].

The inclusion criteria of the study were as follows: SCI/D, age ≥ 14 years, no previous reconstructive surgery, clinical or "self-reported" signs of PNR or SNR with subsequent urodynamic evaluation and antibody testing after at least one BoNT-A injection due to NDO, independent of any possible antimuscarinic concomitant medication. Further botulinum toxin therapy as a result of non-urological indications, e.g., spasticity, was considered an exclusion criterion.

The data were entered into a database and anonymized during entry. The data are presented as the mean and standard deviation (SD) or as the median with 25 and 75% interquartile ranges (IQRs), depending on the presence of a normal distribution. The statistical significance level was set to $p < 0.05$ for all tests. By means of the Shapiro-Wilk test, the existence of a normal distribution of the data was tested. In the case of two groups with normally distributed data, Student's t-test was used. For non-normalized data, the Wilcoxon rank sum test was used. Logistic regression analysis was used to investigate which features influenced the likelihood of antibody formation. Fisher's Chi-square test or Fisher's exact test was used to show a relationship between qualitative characteristics. Statistical analyses were conducted using SAS 9.2 software (SAS Institute Inc., Cary, NC, USA).

The neurological level of SCI/D was classified according to the ISNCSCI and the severity (degree of impairment) in accordance with the American Spinal Injury Association (ASIA) Impairment Scale (AIS) [24].

The Institutional Review Board (IRB, Hauptgeschäftsführer der Berufsgenossenschaft für Gesundheitsdienst und Wohlfahrtspflege, Pappelallee 33, 22,089 Hamburg) approved the present study, and all applicable institutional and governmental regulations concerning the ethical use of the data were followed.

We certify that all applicable institutional and governmental regulations concerning the ethical use of human volunteers were followed during the course of this research.

## Results

Between January 1, 2002, and December 31, 2018, a total of 2700 BoNT-A injections were performed in 414 SCI/D patients at the Spinal Cord Injury Centre, BG Klinikum Hamburg, Germany. All patients suffered from intolerable side effects or were clinically and urodynamically refractory to primary oral or intravesical antimuscarinic treatment prior to BoNT-A therapy. All patients underwent aseptic intermittent catheterization. Overall, 69 patients (16.7%) met the study inclusion criteria. Table 1 shows the demographic and SCI/D-related characteristics of all 69 NR patients.

Among all 69 NR patients, 6 had PNR (8.7%) after the first BoNT-A injection, and 63 had SNR (91.3%). Thus, 91.3% of all 69 NR patients had received more than one onabotulinumtoxin A injection (SNR).

Antibody examination showed the following results: 36/69 (52.2%) patients with clinically and urodynamically confirmed NR had no antibodies, and 14/69 (20.3%) had highly positive and 14/69 (20.3%) had positive antibody levels. A total of 5/69 (7.2%) patients were grouped as borderline (Table 2). A total of 5/6 patients with PNR had no antibody detection, and one patient was classified as borderline. The mean age at non-response was 44.91 years. The median period of time between the date of SCI/D and the first BoNT-A injection was 6.56 years. The median duration between the first BoNT-A injection and NR was 4.91 years. The median interval between BoNT-A injections was 7.85 months. The median number of intradetrusor BoNT-A injections until NR added up to 8.

Of all 414 BoNT-A patients, 28 (6.7%) developed antibodies, 14 (3.4%) with highly positive and 14 (3.4%) with positive levels against onabotulinumtoxin A, including the borderline group ($n = 5$), 7.9% did.

### A – results of demographic and clinical data comparison

To clarify whether it is possible to find correlations between the formation of antibodies against BoNT-A and

**Table 1** patient's characteristics

| Patient's characteristics | |
|---|---|
| No. pts. | 414 |
| No. pts. with Non-Response | 69 |
| male (%) | 53 (77) |
| female (%) | 16 (23) |
| Tetraplegic n (%) | 24 (35) |
| Paraplegic n (%) | 45 (65) |
| AIS A *n* (%) | 49 (71) |
| AIS B *n* (%) | 9 (13) |
| AIS C *n* (%) | 7 (10) |
| AIS D *n* (%) | 4 (6) |
| C1 – C4, AIS A, B, C *n* (%) | 8 (12) |
| C5– C8, AIS A, B, C *n* (%) | 13 (19) |
| T1 – S5, AIS A, B, C *n* (%) | 44 (64) |
| any level, AIS D *n* (%) | 4 (5) |
| Age at SCI/D (mean; SD; range), years | 31.76; 13.99; 4–73 |
| Age at first BoNT-A injection (mean; SD; range), years | 39.56; 14.33; 14–85 |

(*NR* Non response, *AIS* American Spinal Injury Association Impairment Scale, *SCI/D* Spinal cord injury/disease, *BoNT-A* botulinum neurotoxin A)

demographic and clinical data, we statistically examined the following groups of NR patients: patients with highly positive, positive and borderline antibody titres ($n = 33$) versus patients with negative ($n = 36$) antibody titres (Table 3).

We found no significant differences between the sexes or between patients with primary or secondary therapy failure. The extent of neurological deficits (senso-motoric complete or incomplete paralysis) and the severity of SCI/D had no significant influence on the probability of antibody formation. Tetraplegics with NR did not produce antibodies more frequently than paraplegics or vice versa. The probability of antibody formation did not differ with respect to the age of the patients at the time of paralysis onset, the first BoNT-A injection or therapy failure. Additionally, the time interval between the onset of paralysis and the first injection of BoNT-A did not influence the probability of antibody formation as the cause of therapy failure.

On the other hand, with increasing duration of BoNT-A therapy until the occurrence of NR, the probability of NAb formation seemed to increase significantly (NAb neg. vs. pos.: 4.34 years. ± 3.14 vs. 6.37 yrs. ± 3.71; $p = 0.015$, Fig. 1). The median value of the number of

**Table 2** Patients with non-response

| Patients with Non-Response | ***n*** = 69 |
|---|---|
| Primary Non-Response (%) | 6 (9) |
| Secondary Non-Response n (%) | 63 (91) |
| Antibody high positive n (%) | 14 (20) |
| Antibody positive *n* (%) | 14 (20) |
| Antibody borderline *n* (%) | 5 (8) |
| Antibody negative *n* (%) | 36 (52) |
| Age at Non-Response (mean ± SD; range), years | 44.91 ± 14.75; 15–86 |
| Time from SCI/D onset to first BoNT-A (median; 25%/75%; range), years | 6.57; 2.66/10.84; 0–34 |
| Time from first BoNT-A injection to Non-Response (median; 25%/75%; range), years | 4.91; 2.94/7.26; 0–14 |
| Number of BoNT-A injections (median; 25%/75%; range) | 8; 4/11; 1–24 |
| Time interval between BoNT-A injections (median; 25%/75%; range), month | 7.85; 6.4/8.97; 1–18 |

(*SCI/D* Spinal cord injury/disease, *BoNT-A* botulinum neurotoxin A)

**Table 3** demographic and clinical correlations for antibody formation

| | Evaluation | Statistical Test, ***P***-value | Significance |
|---|---|---|---|
| 1 | Male vs. female | $Chi^2 = 0.710$ | non-significant |
| 2 | PNR vs. SNR | exact Fisher = 0.108 | non-significant |
| 3 | Motor. + sensor. Complete vs. incomplete lesion (AIS A vs. AIS B, C, D) | $Chi^2 = 0.764$ | non-significant |
| 4 | Motor. complete vs. motor. Incomplete lesion (AIS A, B vs. AIS C, D) | $Chi^2 = 0.406$ | non-significant |
| 5 | Severity of SCI/D | exact Fisher = 0.190 | non-significant |
| 6 | Age at SCI/D | exact Fisher = 0.257 | non-significant |
| 7 | Age at first BoNT-A injection | exact Fisher = 0.212 | non-significant |
| 8 | Age at Non-Response | exact Fisher = 0.529 | non-significant |
| 9 | Time interval onset SCI/D to first BoNT-A injection | Mann-Whitney-U = 0.788 | non-significant |
| 10 | Mean time interval first BoNT-A injection to Non-Response | T-Test = 0.015 | significant |
| 11 | Number of BoNT-A injections<br>Number of BoNT-A injections, Cut off > 5 | Mann-Whitney-U = 0.011<br>$Chi^2 = 0.024$ | significant<br>significant |
| 12 | Median time interval between BoNT-A injections<br>Median time interval between BoNT-A injections, Cut off < 7 month | Mann-Whitney-U = 0.320<br>$Chi^2 = 0.022$ | non-significant<br>significant |

(*PNR* Primary non response, *SNR* Secondary non response, *AIS* American Spinal Injury Association Impairment Scale, *SCI/D* Spinal cord injury/disease, *BoNT-A* botulinum neurotoxin A)

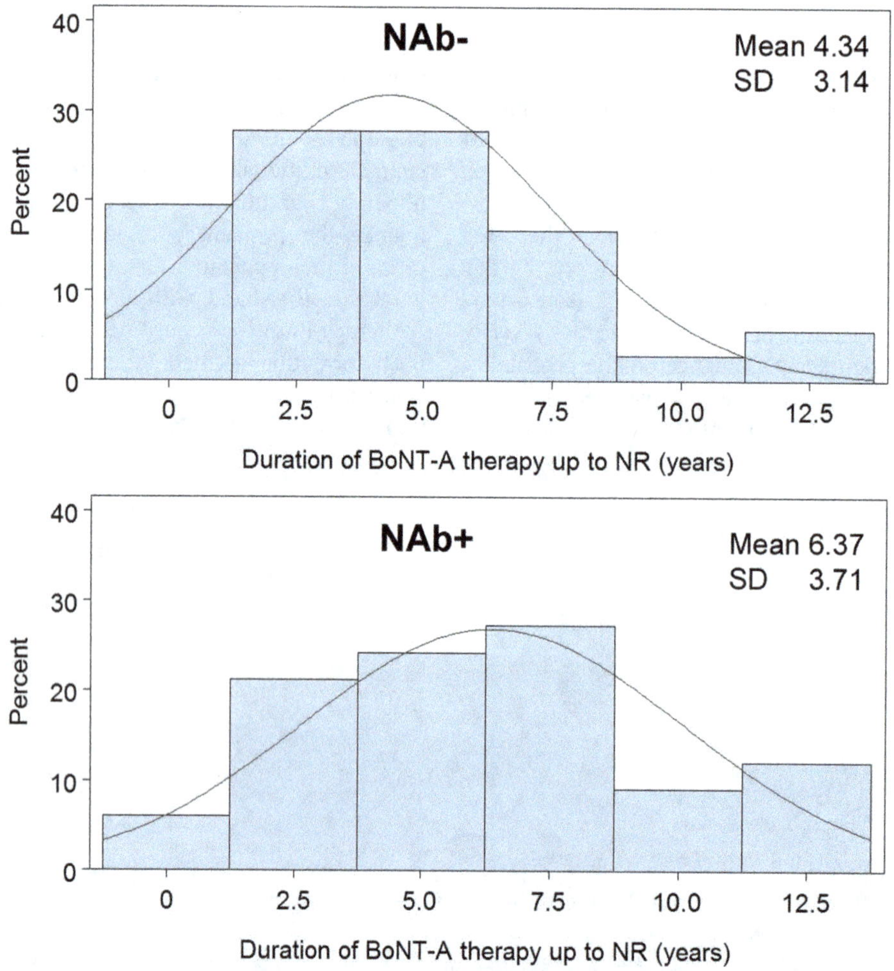


**Fig. 1** Mean duration of BoNT-A therapy up to the time of NR in NAb+ and Nab patients, $p = 0.0153$

BoNT-A injections also differed significantly between NR patients with and without NAb formation (NAB neg. vs. pos.: 6, 3–9 vs. 9 7–12; $p = 0.011$). The probability of antibody formation increased significantly after the 5th BoNT-A injection (Chi$^2$, $p = 0.024$, Fig. 2a). The time interval between BoNT-A injections also showed an influence on the probability of NAb formation. Although there was no significant difference between the mean values of the intervals of BoNT-A injections in patients with and without NAb formation (NAB neg. vs. pos.: 7.84 months, 7.03–8.64 vs. 7.91 months, 6.18–9.99; $p = 0.320$), a mean interval between BoNT-A injections of less than 7 months significantly increased the risk of positive antibody detection (Chi$^2$, $p = 0.022$, Fig. 2b).

In summary, the data show that the mean number of BoNT-A injections, a cut-off value of more than 5 injections, a longer mean duration of BoNT-A therapy up to non-response and intervals between BoNT-A injections less than 7 months are significantly correlated with a higher probability of antibody formation. This leads to a time shift of therapy failure to the right of the curve in NR patients who produce antibodies (Fig. 3).

However, the cut-off value of the "number of BoNT-A injections" determined by means of an adapted logistic function could only distinguish very poorly between patients with and without antibody formation (ROC AUC 0.66, Fig. 4a).

### B – results of urodynamic data comparison

To confirm the presence of NR, a urodynamic study was performed in each patient with clinical signs of non-response.

For the two urodynamic parameters MCC and MDP, there were no significant differences in the probability of antibody formation in the statistical comparison of the medians (MCC: NAb neg. vs. pos.: 293.5 ml, ± 111.5 vs. 256.6 ml, ±105.8; $p = 0.164$ and MDP: NAb neg. vs. pos.: 31.56 cm $H_2O$, ± 9.23 vs. 32.42 cm $H_2O$, ± 15.81; $p = 0.784$). However, in subgroup analysis, significantly more frequent antibody formation could be detected with a cut-off value for MCC < = 225 ml (Chi$^2$, $p = 0.038$) and for MDP > 45 cm$H_2O$ (Fisher's exact test, $p = 0.040$) (Table 4). However, both cut-off values determined by an adapted logistic function could not discriminate with sufficient accuracy between patients with and without antibodies: the ROC AUC for MCC was 0.62 (Fig. 4b), and the ROC AUC for MDP was 0.52 (Fig. 4c).

### Discussion

To the best of our knowledge, the present study represents the largest population of SCI patients with therapy failure after BoNT-A injections into the detrusor in which the determination of neutralizing antibodies against onabotulinumtoxin A was performed. Using clinical, demographic and urodynamic data, correlations with the probability of antibody formation were analysed. Although significant correlations were found among the duration of BoNT-A therapy, the number of injections, the mean therapy interval and urodynamic parameters (MCC and MDP), the "adapted logistic function" did not allow the definition of cut-off points that could distinguish with sufficient certainty between NAb-positive and NAb-negative NR patients.

Although BoNT-A injections have been used very successfully and safely for many years for the treatment of refractory NDO in patients with SCI/D [25], there are a significant number of treatment failures and a relatively large number of treatment discontinuations during long-term follow-up. In 2009, Pannek et al. reported an approximate long-term success rate of 74% [26]. In a recent review [27], summarizing 18 studies with a total of 1533 patients, discontinuation rates between 12.1 and 45.2% were described. A 10-year observation period in

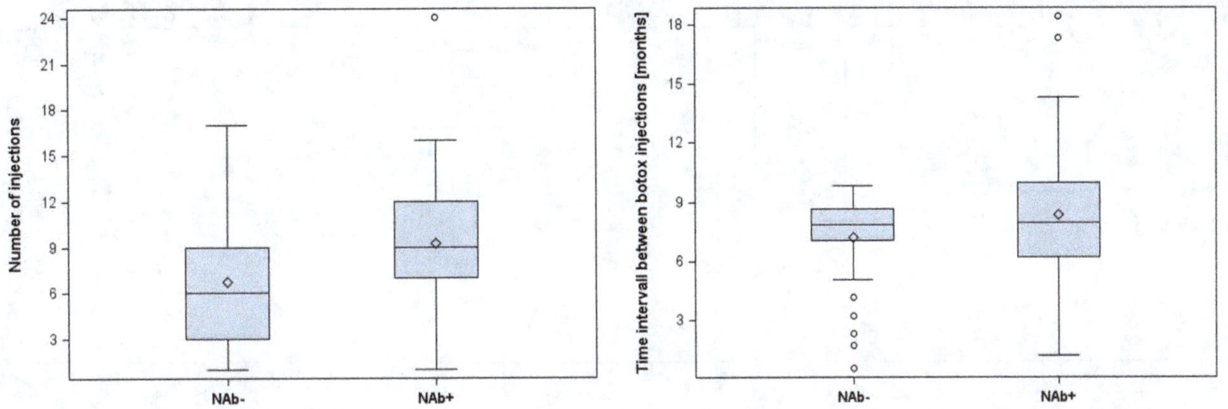


**Fig. 2** **a** Median number of BoNT-A injections; $p = 0.0108$; **b** Median interval between BoNT-A injections; $p = 0.3201$

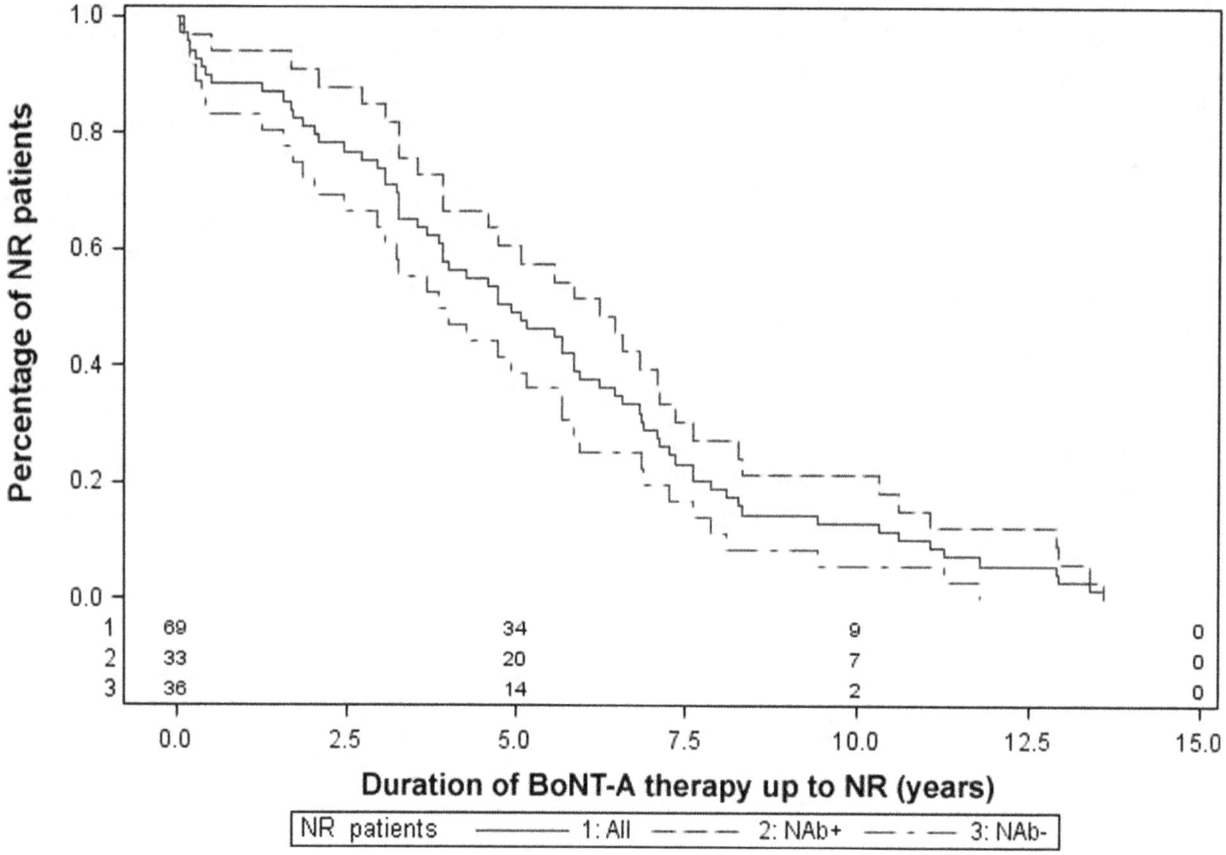


**Fig. 3** Time course of non-response in NAb+ and NAb- patients

140 patients showed an estimated 10-year discontinuation-free survival rate of 49.1% [13] and a discontinuation rate of 40% [12]. In addition to personal decisions and technical problems, antibody formation or structural changes in the detrusor are considered the main cause of treatment discontinuation. Nevertheless, the role of NAbs in therapy failure of refractory NDO has not been ultimately clarified. Until now, only a few studies and limited data have existed regarding the risk of NAb formation in patients with NDO. In previous studies in urological patients, in contrast to striated muscular injection treatments due to spasticity, no antibodies were detected [9, 28]. In contrast, a recent meta-analysis of NAbs in BoNT-A treatment showed the following results [16]: in five studies with data from 294 patients with urological indications, the frequency of

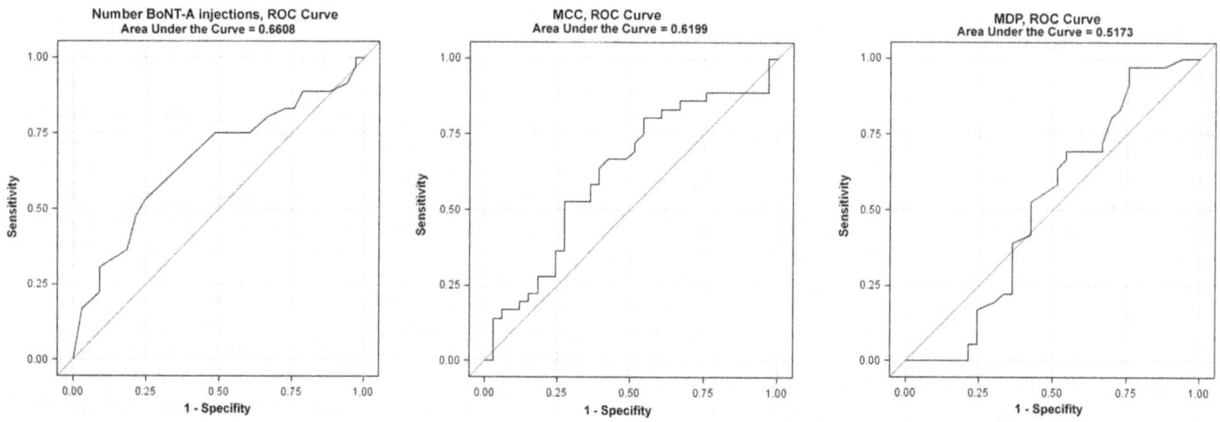


**Fig. 4** **a** Number of BoNT-A injections, ROC curve, AUC = 0.661; **b** MCC, ROC curve, AUC = 0.612; **c** MDP, ROC curve, AUC = 0.520

**Table 4** urodynamic correlations for antibody formation

| Evaluation | mean; SD; range | Statistical Test, ***P***-value | Significance |
|---|---|---|---|
| MCC (ml) | NAb - 293.5; 111.5; 64–468<br>NAB + 256.6; 105.8; 58–482 | t-Test = 0.164 | non-significant |
| MCC cut off <= 225 ml | | $Chi^2$ = 0.038 | significant |
| MDP ($cmH_2O$) | NAB - 31.5556; 9.2256; 15–55<br>NAb + 32.4242; 15.8055; 7–61 | t-Test = 0.784 | non-significant |
| MDP cut off > 45 $cmH_2O$ | | exact Fisher = 0.040 | significant |

(*MCC* maximum cystometric capacity, *MDP* maximum detrusor pressure)sss

NAbs was reported to be 2.7% (95% confidence interval (95% CI) 0.009–0.064); in clinically responding urological patients, the NAb frequency was 3.8% (95% CI 0.011–0.123); and no studies that examined NAbs in SNR patients for urologic indications were identified. In 2008, Schulte-Baukloh et al. [29] reported on NAbs in 8 of 25 patients (4 positives, 4 borderline) after intradetrusor BoNT-A injection, with complete therapy failure in 3 of 4 patients with positive titres. However, the authors found no correlation among the number of BoNT-A injections ($p = 0.124$), the injection interval ($p = 0.815$), or the total amount of BoNT-A applied ($p = 0.090$). Hegele et al. [15] showed NAb formation in 5 patients (16.1%) out of 31 patients treated with intradetrusor BoNT-A injections due to an overactive bladder. In a 3-year, open-label extension study of two 52-week, phase III studies (DIGNITY) in 117 centres in North America, Europe, Latin America, South Africa, and the Asia-Pacific region [30, 31], 8 of 381 patients (all SCI, 2.1%) seroconverted to positive NAbs. Four of these 8 patients continued to experience clinical benefits even after seroconversion. It was striking that the patients with seroconversion had shorter intervals (4.9 months) between BoNT-A injections than the total population (9.1 months).

It should be noted that in all the studies mentioned and in our own patients, only the newer formulation of Botox® with lower antigenicity was used. Allergan changed the composition of Botox® in 1997: the protein content decreased from 25 ng/100 U to 5 ng/100 U. Afterwards, the risk of antibody formation in patients with cervical dystonia decreased by a factor of 6 [32].

In our own 17-year study, we found a total failure rate of 16.7% (69/414), 1.4% with PNR (6/414) and 15.2% with SNR (63/414). Slightly more than half of NR patients did not show NAbs against BoNT-A (52.2%, 36/69), each 20.3% (14/69) showed positive or highly positive antibody levels, and 7.2% (5/69) were grouped as borderline. An analysis of the risk factors for NAb formation in NR showed a significant increase in the probability of positive NAb detection with both an increasing duration of therapy and an increasing number of BoNT-A injections of more than 5 repeated BoNT-A injections. In accordance with this finding, a gradually decreased therapeutic effect after the 4th BoNT-A injection in SCI/D patients with NDO was reported [33]. Furthermore, a significant decrease in quality of life in patients who received five or more injections was described [27].

Perhaps the two risk factors for antibody formation mentioned above describe the same phenomenon: antigenicity that leads to a higher probability of antibody formation as a cause of NR due to the duration of therapy and the number of injections. Our data showed that treatment failure occurred significantly later in patients with Nab formation than in NR patients without NAb formation.

We identified a second risk factor for the formation of NAb in NR with a mean interval between BoNT-A injections < 7 months. This was also shown in a large extension study [31], in which all 8 NAb-positive SCI/D patients had significantly shorter therapy intervals.

Recent studies from France reported a benefit of approximately 50% in patients with intradetrusor injection failure in NDO with botulinum toxin switching from onabotulinumtoxin A to abobotulinumtoxin A or the reverse order [34]. The clinical and urodynamic success rates were 51.7, 57.7 and 56.14% [17, 35, 36]. This corresponds to the proportion of NAb-"non-negative" patients with therapy failure in our study. Unfortunately, no antibody determinations were made in the studies mentioned above. Here, it would be of great interest to look for a correlation between antibody formation and a successful toxin switch.

From a theoretical point of view, it could be assumed that NAb-positive NR patients are more likely to benefit from a toxin change than patients without antibody formation who do not (or no longer) respond to BoNT-A injections because in NAb-positive NR patients, the cause of therapy failure is probably due to the immunogenicity of the BoNT-A preparation. The cause of therapy failure in NAb-negative NR patients is currently not well understood. Histological examinations of the detrusor [37] or the urothelium and suburothelium [38] cannot detect the suspected ultra-structural changes in the bladder wall after (repeated) BoNT-A injections. In contrast, after BoNT-A injections, there was significantly less fibrosis of the bladder wall than in untreated patients. Furthermore, a comparison of samples from patients who responded to BoNT-A therapy and from patients who did not respond showed no difference in inflammation. Responders to BoNT-A therapy tend to show less fibrosis and oedema of the bladder wall than non-responders [39].

For patients who do not benefit from a toxin switch, surgical therapy alternatives must often be considered. It would therefore be valuable if, even without antibody testing, clinical and urodynamic evidence could be used to distinguish between NR patients with and without NAb formation. The identification of NR patients without antibody formation (corresponding to a "negative" result on the NAb test) could be helpful for the clinical decision-making process.

In this context, the present study also examined whether urodynamic parameters are suitable to predict the formation of NAb as a cause of NR. The statistical evaluations show that the probability of positive antibody detection increases significantly in NR patients with low MCC (< 225 ml) and high MDP (> 45 $cmH_2O$). Therefore, it seems plausible that patients with smaller MCC and higher MDP values might have early recurrence of NDO and would benefit from an earlier BoNT-A injection than those who without these values. This would be a possible explanation for why these patients produce antibodies more frequently. However, neither these urodynamic nor the clinical criteria presented above are sufficiently successful in our analysis to identify or exclude with sufficient certainty NR patients with antibody formation or to identify NAb-negative NR patients. In this regard, further studies are needed to better understand this potential context.

It is important to recognize that the present study has some limitations. First, this is due to the retrospective nature of data collection with a limited number of participants, but to our knowledge, there is no larger long-term study with NAb determination in the literature. Second, no additional data on concomitant medication, e.g., oral or intravesical antimuscarinics, are available. Finally, no difference was made between injections of 200 or 300 MU onabotulinumtoxin A. These limitations may cause some biases that must be considered in the interpretation of our results. These problems can only be solved by future prospective studies with a strict study protocol and larger study groups. Nevertheless, the authors believe that the presented results may provide some important basic information about possible associations between clinical and urodynamic data and the probability of NAb formation in NLUTD patients with therapy failure after intradetrusor BoNT-A injections.

## Conclusions

The present study shows that despite some significant correlations (duration of BoNT-A therapy, number of BoNT-A injections, interval between injections, and urodynamic parameters such as MCC and MDP), the probability of the occurrence of antibodies against BoNT-A in the case of therapy failure cannot be determined with sufficient certainty using clinical and urodynamic data alone. The predictive value of these parameters is too low to indicate antibody formation as the cause of NR. A recommendation for the subsequent therapy of non-responders to BoNT-A can therefore not be derived from these investigations.

Further studies are necessary to improve the evidence of follow-up therapy in the case of therapy failure against BoNT-A.

### Abbreviations

AIS: American Spinal Injury Association impairment scale;; ASIA: American Spinal Injury Association; AUC: Area under curve; BoNT-A: Botulinum neurotoxin A; CI: Confidence interval; IQR: Interquartile range; MCC: Maximum cystometric capacity; MDP: Maximum detrusor pressure; NAb: Neutralizing antibodies;; NDO: Neurogenic detrusor overactivity; NLUTD: Neurogenic lower urinary tract dysfunction; NR: Non response; PNR: Primary non response; ROC Curve: Receiver operating characteristic curve; SCI/D: Spinal cord injury/disease; SNR: Secondary non response

### Acknowledgments

Not applicable.

### Authors´ contributions

CT and RB have full access to all the data in the study and take responsibility for the integrity of the data and the accuracy of the data analysis. The study concept and study design was created by CT and RB. Acquisition of data was performed by CT and RB. Analysis and interpretation of data was performed by BK, CT and RB. Drafting of the manuscript was done by RB and CT. RT and SH are responsible for the critical revision of the manuscript and for important intellectual content. Statistical analysis was performed by BK, RB and CT. Administrative, technical, or material support and supervision was done by RT and SH. All authors have read and approved the final manuscript.

### Competing interests

The authors declare that they have no competing interests.

### Author details

[1]Centre for Spinal Injuries, Department Neuro-Urology, BG Trauma Hospital Hamburg, Bergedorfer Str. 10 Germany, 21033 Hamburg, Germany. [2]Biomechanical Laboratory, BG Trauma Hospital Hamburg, Hamburg, Germany. [3]Centre for Spinal Injuries, BG Trauma Hospital Hamburg, Hamburg, Germany.

### References

1. Weld KJ. Dmochowski. Association of level of injury and bladder behavior in patients with post-traumatic spinal cord injury. Urology. 2000;55:490–4.
2. Gao Y, Danforth T, Ginsberg DA. Urologic management and complications in spinal cord injury patients: a 40- to 50-year follow-up study. Urology. 2017;104:52–8.
3. Groen J, Pannek J, Castro Diaz D, Del Popolo G, Gross T, Hamid R, et al. Summary of European Association of Urology (EAU) guidelines on Neuro-urology. Eur Urol. 2016;69:324–33.
4. Madersbacher H, Mürtz G, Stöhrer M. Neurogenic detrusor overactivity in adults: a review on efficacy, tolerability and safety of oral antimuscarinics. Spinal Cord. 2013;51(6):432–41.

5. Kessler TM, Bachmann LM, Minder C, Löhrer D, Umbehr M, Schünemann HJ, et al. Adverse event assessment of antimuscarinics for treating overactive bladder: a network meta-analytic approach. PLoS One. 2011;6:e16718.
6. Buser N, Ivic S, Kessler TM, Kessels AG, Bachmann LM. Efficacy and adverse events of antimuscarinics for treating overactive bladder: network meta-analyses. Eur Urol. 2012;62(6):1040–60.
7. Madhuvrata P, Singh M, Hasafa Z, Abdel-Fattah M. Anticholinergic drugs for adult neurogenic detrusor overactivity: a systematic review and meta-analyses. Eur Urol. 2012;62(5):816–30.
8. Mangera A, Andersson KE, Apostolidis A, Chapple C, Dasgupta P, Giannantoni A, et al. Contemporary management of lower urinary tract disease with botulinum toxin a: a systematic review of botox (onabotulinumtoxinA) and dysport (abobotulinumtoxinA). Eur Urol. 2011; 60(4):784–95.
9. Cruz F, Herschorn S, Aliotta P, Brin M, Thompson C, Lam W, et al. Efficacy and safety of onabotulinumtoxin in patients with urinary incontinence due to neurogenic detrusor overactivity: a randomised, double-blind, placebo-controlled trial. Eur Urol. 2011;60:742–50.
10. Ginsberg D, Gousse A, Keppenne V, Sievert KD, Thompson C, Lam W, et al. Phase 3 efficacy and tolerability study of onabotulinumtoxinA for urinary incontinence from neurogenic detrusor overactivity. J Urol. 2012;187:2131–9.
11. Rovner E, Kohan A, Chartier-Kastler E, Jünemann KP, Del Popolo G, Herschorn S, et al. Long-term efficacy and safety of OnabotulinumtoxinA in patients with neurogenic detrusor Overactivity who completed 4 years of treatment. J Urol. 2016;196(3):801–8.
12. Leitner L, Guggenbühl-Roy S, Knüpfer SC, Walter M, Schneider MP, Tornic J, et al. More than 15 years of experience with Intradetrusor OnabotulinumtoxinA injections for treating refractory neurogenic detrusor Overactivity: lessons to be learned. Eur Urol. 2016;70(3):522–8.
13. Baron M, Peyronnet B, Auble A, Hascoet J, Castel-Lacanal E, Miget G, et al. Long-term discontinuation of Botulinum toxin a Intradetrusor injections for neurogenic detrusor Overactivity: a multicenter study. J Urol. 2019;201(4): 769–76.
14. Joussain C, Popoff M, Phe V, Even A, Bosset PO, Pottier S, et al. Long-term outcomes and risks factors for failure of intradetrusor onabotulinumtoxin a injections for the treatment of refractory neurogenic detrusor overactivity. Neurourol Urodyn. 2018;37:799–806.
15. Hegele A, Frohme C, Varga Z, Olbert P, Kranz J, Hofmann R. Antibodies after Botulinum toxin a injection into Musculus detrusor Vesicae: incidence and clinical relevance. Urol Int. 2011;87:439–44.
16. Fabbri M, Leodori G, Fernandes RM, Bhidayasiri R, Marti MJ, Colosimo C, et al. Neutralizing antibody and Botulinum toxin therapy: a systematic review and meta-analysis. Neurotox Res. 2016;29(1):105–17.
17. Peyronnet B, Castel-Lacanal E, Manunta A, Roumiguié M, Marque P, Rischmann P, et al. Failure of botulinum toxin injection for neurogenic detrusor overactivity: switch of toxin versus second injection of the same toxin. Int J Urol. 2015;22(12):1160–5.
18. Peyronnet B, Gamé X, Vurture G, Nitti VW, Brucker BM. Botulinum toxin use in Neurourology. Rev Urol. 2018;20(2):84–93.
19. Karsenty G, Baverstock R, Carlson K, Diaz DC, Cruz F, Dmochowski R, et al. Technical aspects of botulinum toxin type a injection in the bladder to treat urinary incontinence: reviewing the procedure. Int J Clin Pract. 2014;68(6): 731–42.
20. Koschorke M, Leitner L, Sadri H, Knüpfer SC, Mehnert U, Kessler TM. Intradetrusor onabotulinumtoxinA injections for refractory neurogenic detrusor overactivity incontinence: do we need urodynamic investigation for outcome assessment? BJU Int. 2017;120(6):848–54.
21. Rosier PFWM, Kuo HC, De Gennaro M, Gammie A, Finazzi Agro E, Kakizaki H, et al. International consultation on in-continence 2016; executive summary: urodynamic testing. Neurourol Urodyn. 2019;38(2):545–52.
22. D'Ancona C, Haylen B, Oelke M, Abranches-Monteiro L, Arnold E, Goldman H, et al. Standardisation steering committee ICS and the ICS working group on terminology for male lower Urinary Tract & Pelvic Floor Symptoms and dysfunction the international continence society (ICS) re-port on the terminology for adult male lower urinary tract and pelvic floor symptoms and dysfunction. Neurourol Urodyn. 2019;38(2):433–77.
23. Pannek J, Kennelly M, Kessler TM, Linsenmeyer T, Wyndaele JJ, Biering-Sørensen F. International spinal cord injury urodynamic basic data set (version 2.0). Spinal Cord Ser Cases. 2018; doi: https://doi.org/10.1038/s41394-018-0133-0. eCollection.
24. Kirshblum SC, Burns SP, Biering-Sorensen F, Donovan W, Graves DE, Jha A, et al. International standards for neurological classification of spinal cord injury (revised 2011). J Spinal Cord Med. 2011;34(6):535–46.
25. Li GP, Wang XY, Zhang Y. Efficacy and safety of OnabotulinumtoxinA in patients with neurogenic detrusor Overactivity caused by spinal cord injury: a systematic review and meta-analysis. Int Neurourol J. 2018;22(4):275–86.
26. Pannek J, Göcking K, Bersch U. Long-term effects of repeated intradetrusor botulinum neurotoxin a injections on detrusor function in patients with neurogenic bladder dysfunction. BJU Int. 2009;104(9):1246–50.
27. Ni J, Wang X, Cao N, Si J, Gu B. Is repeat Botulinum toxin a injection valuable for neurogenic detrusor overactivity-a systematic review and meta-analysis. Neurourol Urodyn. 2018;37(2):542–53.
28. Schurch B, de Sèze M, Denys P, Chartier-Kastler E, Haab F, Everaert K, et al. Botox detrusor Hyperreflexia study team. Botulinum toxin type a is a safe and effective treatment for neurogenic urinary incontinence: results of a single treatment, randomized, placebo controlled 6-month study. J Urol. 2005;174(1):196–200.
29. Schulte-Baukloh H, Bigalke H, Miller K, Heine G, Pape D, Lehmann J, et al. Botulinum neurotoxin type a in urology: antibodies as a cause of therapy failure. Int J Urol. 2008;15(5):407–15.
30. Kennelly M, Dmochowski R, Ethans K, Karsenty G, Schulte-Baukloh H, Jenkins B, et al. Long-term efficacy and safety of onabotulinumtoxinA in patients with urinary incontinence due to neurogenic detrusor overactivity: an interim analysis. Urology. 2013;81(3):491–7.
31. Kennelly M, Dmochowski R, Schulte-Baukloh H, Ethans K, Del Popolo G, Moore C, et al. On behalf of 191622-094 investigators. Efficacy and safety of onabotulinumtoxinA therapy are sustained over 4 years of treatment in patients with neurogenic detrusor overactivity: final results of a long-term extension study. Neurourol Urodyn. 2017;36(2):368–75.
32. Jankovic J, Vuong KD, Ahsan J. Comparison of efficacy and immunogenicity of original versus current botulinum toxin in cervical dystonia. Neurology. 2003;60(7):1186–8.
33. Chen SF, Kuo HC. Therapeutic outcome and patient adherence to repeated onabotulinumtoxinA detrusor injections in chronic spinal cord-injured patients and neurogenic detrusor overactivity. J Formos Med Assoc. 2015; 114(7):583–9.
34. Peyronnet B, Gamé X. Failures and long-term discontinuations of intradetrusor botulinum toxin injections for neurogenic detrusor overactivity: a new challenge in neurourology. Neurourol Urodyn. 2018; 37(3):1182–3.
35. Peyronnet B, Roumiguié M, Castel-Lacanal E, Guillotreau J, Malavaud B, Marque P, et al. Preliminary results of botulinum toxin a switch after first detrusor injection failure as a treatment of neurogenic detrusor overactivity. Neurourol Urodyn. 2016;35(2):267–70.
36. Bottet F, Peyronnet B, Boissier R, Reiss B, Previnaire JG, Manunta A, et al. Groupe d'Etude de Neuro-Urologie de langue Française (GENULF) and the committee of NeuroUrology of the French Association of Urology (AFU). Switch to Abobotulinum toxin a may be useful in the treatment of neurogenic detrusor overactivity when intradetrusor injections of Onabotulinum toxin a failed. Neurourol Urodyn. 2018;37(1):291–7.
37. Haferkamp A, Schurch B, Reitz A, Krengel U, Grosse J, Kramer G, et al. Lack of ultrastructural detrusor changes following endoscopic injection of botulinum toxin type a in overactive neurogenic bladder. Eur Urol. 2004; 46(6):784–91.
38. Apostolidis A, Jacques TS, Freeman A, Kalsi V, Popat R, Gonzales G, et al. Histological changes in the urothelium and suburothelium of human overactive bladder following intradetrusor injections of botulinum neurotoxin type a for the treatment of neurogenic or idiopathic detrusor overactivity. Eur Urol. 2008;53(6):1245–53.
39. Compérat E, Reitz A, Delcourt A, Capron F, Denys P, Chartier-Kastler E. Histologic features in the urinary bladder wall affected from neurogenic overactivity—a comparison of inflammation, oedema and fibrosis with and without injection of botulinum toxin type a. Eur Urol. 2006;50(5):1058–64.

# 28

# Observation of intracellular bacterial communities in urinary sediment using brightfield microscopy

Carlos Martínez-Figueroa[1], Karen Cortés-Sarabia[1], Luz del Carmen Alarcón-Romero[1], Hilda Guadalupe Catalán-Nájera[2], Micaela Martínez-Alarcón[2] and Amalia Vences-Velázquez[1*]

**Abstract**

**Background:** Urinary tract infections (UTIs) are usually related to the presence of *Escherichia coli*, a microorganism that adopts an intracellular life-style during the pathogenesis of cystitis. Evidence of the underlying mechanism in urothelial cells from urine samples has been reported. However, intracellular communities have not yet been described in squamous cells in fresh samples stained with Sternheimer-Malbin method, thus, we have provided these descriptions in this case report.

**Case presentation:** Number 1 was a male patient with symptoms of UTI, his urinalysis revealed hematuria and nitrites. In the urine sediment, we found urothelial cells with internal endosomes filled with short rods. Case number 2, female patient with recurrent UTI by *E. coli*, her urinalysis showed positive nitrites, glycosuria, bacteriuria and squamous cells with endosomes filled with short rods. Both patients were positive for *E. coli* isolation.

**Conclusions:** These case reports provide evidence of the presence of intracellular bacterial communities in urothelial and squamous cells (not previously reported) in fresh urine samples stained with Sternheimer-Malbin using brightfield microscopy. The clinical impact and pathogenic mechanisms involved in the invasion of the squamous epithelium need further investigation.

**Keywords:** Urinary tract infections, *Escherichia coli*, Intracellular bacterial communities, Urinary sediment, Case report

## Background

*Escherichia coli* is the main etiological agent associated with urinary tract infections (UTIs). This microorganism is perfectly adapted to the environment of the urinary system. During the pathogenesis of cystitis, this bacteria use the intracellular route to form an intracellular biofilm, named as intracellular bacterial community (IBC), that has been studied in both in vivo and in vitro models [1, 2]. IBCs are formed in superficial urothelial cells, they go through several maturation stages leading to biofilm reorganization before differentiating into the filamentous and coccoid morphotypes commonly found in the late intracellular community [2, 3]. Only a few cases on the presence of IBCs in urothelial cells of patients with UTI have been reported. Here, we report two new cases involving not only urothelial cells but also squamous cells.

* Correspondence: ameliavences.v@uagro.mx
[1]Laboratorio de Inmunobiología y Diagnóstico Molecular, Facultad de Ciencias Químico Biológicas, Universidad Autónoma de Guerrero, Av. Lázaro Cárdenas s/n, University City, C.P.39090 Chilpancingo, Guerrero, Mexico

## Case presentation

### Patients information

#### *Case number 1*

A 50-year-old male patient, without any background of chronic or infectious diseases, urinary stones, or anatomical abnormalities, came to the hospital's emergency room with pelvic pain but no fever, vomiting or chills.

Reported symptoms included dysuria, polaquiuria, hematuria and foul smelling urine.

### *Case number 2*

A 64-year-old patient, with a background of diabetes mellitus, hypertension and hyperthyroidism, came to the bacteriological service area of the hospital's emergency room for controlling a recurrent UTI. No additional symptoms were reported. During the follow up, the patient showed a few episodes of healing and relapse.

### Diagnostic assessment

For urinalysis, 10 mL of urine were aliquoted in a 16 × 150 mm tube. Chemical tests were performed using test strips (SPINREACT URIN-10). After chemical testing, urine was centrifuged for 5 min at 450 g, supernatant was aspirated using a pipette until 0.5 mL was left and 50 μL of Sternheimer-Malbin dye was added. The Sternheimer-Malbin stain is a supravital dye composed by safranin O and cristal violet, is used to contrast the formed elements and to stain structures that have lost their vitality. Finally, sediments were examined under a brightfield microscope at 40× magnification.

### *Case number 1*

Nitrites and hematuria (> 100 erythrocytes/field) were confirmed by chemical and microscopic analyses of the patient's urine sample. In the sediments, superficial urothelial cells, along with scarce squamous cells, monohydrate calcium oxalate, and moderate bacteriuria including two bacterial morphotypes (short rods and filamentous forms) were observed, whereas no-leukocytes were found. In the interior of an endosome from a superficial urothelial cell, we observed the presence of moving short rod bacteria (Fig. 1) (supplementary material 1).

### *Case number 2*

Nitrites and glycosuria were confirmed by chemical analysis of the patient's urine sample. In the sediment test, we observed bacteriuria, leukocyturia (5–10/field), and squamous cells with endosome-containing bacteria. Moving along different focus planes in the microscope, we were able to determine that short rods were in the interior of the cells and not in their surface. This location was confirmed in at least ten squamous cells along the sediment preparation (Fig. 2).

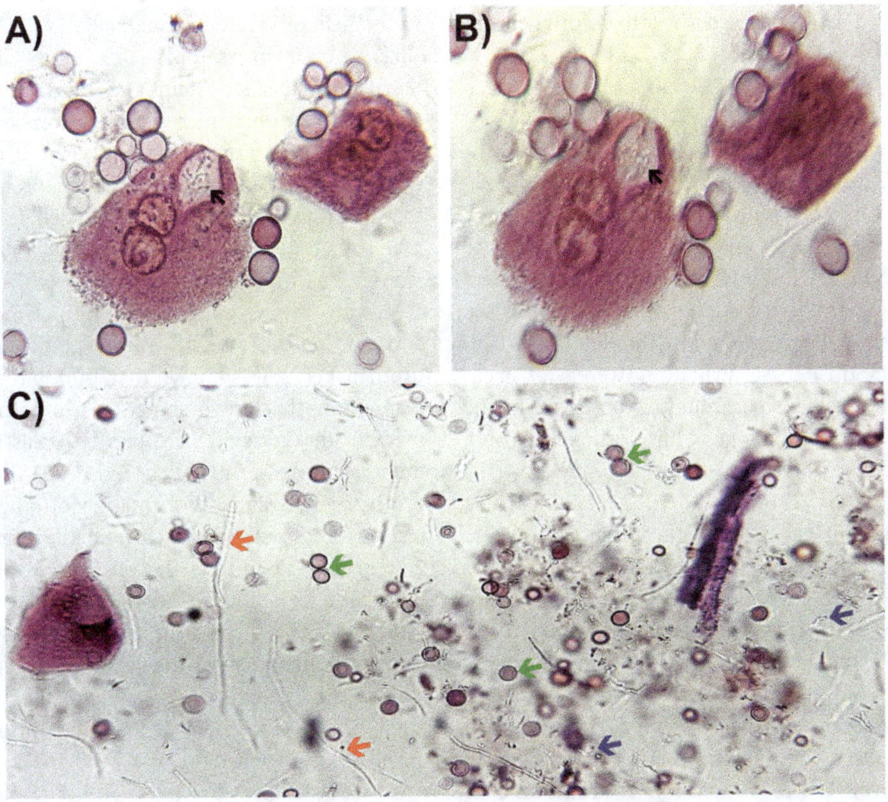


**Fig. 1** Representative image of the urinary sediment of a patient with *E. coli* infection. **a** Clear field microscopy and **b** clear field microscopy with cylinder-type illumination images. Note the presence of urothelial cells with bacteria inside an endosome (black arrows). **c** Bright field microscope image showing different bacterial morphotypes, short (blue arrows) and long (red arrows) rods, and hematuria (green arrows). Images are at a 40× magnification

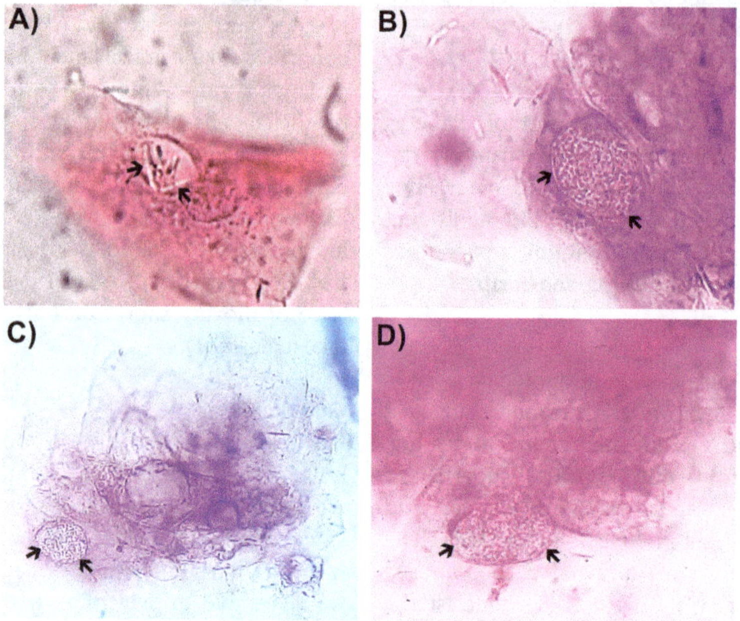


**Fig. 2** Intracellular bacteria in the urinary sediment. **a-d** Bright field microscope image showing squamous cells with bacteria inside an endosome (black arrows). The sample was stained using the Sternheimer-Malbin method. The image is at 40× magnification

### Diagnostic

For both cases, we isolated *E. coli* with colony counts greater that > 100,000 UFC/mL.

## Discussion and conclusions

IBC formation is a protective mechanism of invasion of the bladder by *E. coli*. It has been reported that biofilm formation is related with the evasion of the host innate immune response, antibiotic resistance, and urinary tract persistence [3, 4]. However, there are just a few reports about the presence of IBCs in the urine of patients with cystitis. Rosen et al. (2007), reported the existence of IBC-like structures in women with cystitis, these structures were similar to those exfoliated intracellular communities observed in the urine of mice with cystitis, and that this pathogenic route could be implicated in the recurrence of the infection [5]. Whereas, Robino et al. (2014) found IBCs in 36.8% of a population of children with urinary tract infections by *E. coli*. The presence of these IBCs was associated with recurrent infections in patients without morphological or structural abnormalities in their urinary tracts [6].

The squamous epithelium is found in the bladder trigone and the urethra in both sexes. The presence of IBCs in squamous cells could indicate that there is an infection in any of these sites, an infection that may have not been previously described. In the contrary, IBC formation in urothelial cells is generally related to know infections. Consequently, further investigation to establish pathogenic mechanism mediating IBC formation in squamous cells and its contribution to the development of cystitis is needed [2, 7].

According to our findings, the contributions of this study to the field of UTIs are listed as follows: A) The presence of IBCs in fresh samples can be determined using Sternheimer-Malbin stain and brightfield microscopy, instead of electronic microscopy of confocal microscopy and Giemsa stain, as reported previously; B) IBC may form in squamous cells (case 2), a bacterial protection mechanism that had only been found in urothelial cells [1, 2], indicating that squamous epithelium could be infected; and C) The filamentous morphotype of *E. coli*, which has been associated with phagocytosis evasion by polymorphonuclear cells and an increase in adherence points, can be found in urothelial cells. It is known that, during the pathogenic cycle, filamentous bacteria fragmentate to form short rods that mediate the invasion of superficial cells and contribute to the recurrence of the infection through the invasion of basal urothelial cells and the formation of quiescent intracellular reservoirs associated with chronic infections [2, 8, 9].

A urinary sediment analysis is conventionally used to search for crystals, cylinders, and cells in urine samples. However, it may also be a useful tool in the search of the mechanism of pathogenesis of different microorganism because results, such as intracellular invasion could explain the recurrence of an infection and the failure of an antibiotic treatment. It would be important to determine the prognostic value of IBCs and bacterial morphotypes in urinary tract infections and their clinical significance as well as to explore those intracellular pathways that allow the adaptation of IBCs to squamous cells.

**Abbreviations**

*E. coli*: *Escherichia coli*; IBC: intracellular bacterial communities; UTI: Urinary tract infections

**Acknowledgements**

We are very grateful to María Ruiz Rosas for all the contributions and technical support.

**Authors' contributions**

CMF and LDCAR evaluated urine sediments, made contributions to data collection, literature search and they wrote the report. KCS and AW reviewed and edited the manuscript, also participated in study design. HGCN and MMA literature research, and performed microbiological diagnosis. We state that all authors have read and approved the manuscript.

**Competing interests**

The authors declare that they have no competing interests.

**Author details**

[1]Laboratorio de Inmunobiología y Diagnóstico Molecular, Facultad de Ciencias Químico Biológicas, Universidad Autónoma de Guerrero, Av. Lázaro Cárdenas s/n, University City, C.P.39090 Chilpancingo, Guerrero, Mexico. [2]Servicio de urgencias, Laboratorio clínico, Clínica Hospital ISSSTE, Iguala, Guerrero, Mexico.

**References**

1. Justice SS, Hung C, Theriot JA, Fletcher DA, Anderson GG, Footer MJ, et al. Differentiation and developmental pathways of uropathogenic *Escherichia coli* in urinary tract pathogenesis. Proc Natl Acad Sci. 2004;101(5):1333–8.
2. Andersen TE, Khandige S, Madelung M, Brewer J, Kolmos HJ, Møller-Jensen J. *Escherichia coli* Uropathogenesis in vitro: invasion, cellular escape, and secondary infection analyzed in a human bladder cell infection model. Infect Immun. 2012;80(5):1858–67.
3. Anderson GG, Palermo JJ, Schilling JD, Roth R, Heuser J, Hultgren SJ. Intracellular Bacterial Biofilm-Like Pods in Urinary Tract Infections. Science. 2003;301(5629):105–7.
4. Mulvey MA, Schilling JD, Hultgren SJ. Establishment of a persistent *Escherichia coli* reservoir during the acute phase of a bladder infection. Infect Immun. 2001;69(7):4572–9.
5. Rosen DA, Hooton TM, Stamm WE, Humphrey PA, Hultgren SJ. Detection of intracellular bacterial communities in human urinary tract infection. PLoS Med. 2007;4(12):e329.
6. Robino L, Scavone P, Araujo L, Algorta G, Zunino P, Pírez MC, et al. Intracellular bacteria in the pathogenesis of *Escherichia coli* urinary tract infection in children. Clin Infect Dis. 2014;59(11):e158–64.
7. Pawnila W. Ross Histología Texto y Atlas: correlación con biología molecular y celular. 7th ed. China: Wolters Kluwer; 2015.
8. Justice SS, Hunstad DA, Seed PC, Hultgren SJ. Filamentation by *Escherichia coli* subverts innate defenses during urinary tract infection. Proc Natl Acad Sci. 2006;103(52):19884–9.
9. Schwartz DJ, Chen SL, Hultgren SJ, Seed PC. Population dynamics and niche distribution of uropathogenic *Escherichia coli* during acute and chronic urinary tract infection. Infect Immun. 2011;79(10):4250–9.

29

# Risk assessment of neuromuscular stimulation by energy-based transurethral resection devices: An ex vivo test standard

Ulrich Biber[1*], Ovidiu Jurjut[1], Markus D. Enderle[1] and Wilhelm K. Aicher[2]

**Abstract**

**Background:** During transurethral resection of bladder tumours (TURB), radio-frequency (RF) currents can lead to adverse neuromuscular stimulation (NMS). Here we present a novel ex vivo method to determine the risk of RF generators and their bipolar TURB modes to cause NMS. We aimed to develop an experimental platform for safety evaluation of new RF generators and their modes with a newly established test standard, suitable for replacement or reduction of animal testing.

**Methods:** We tested four contemporary RF generators with their bipolar modes for TURB in saline. A two-stage ex vivo approach was pursued: First, we recorded voltages at possible positions of the obturator nerve behind a porcine bladder wall in a TURB model using 18 RF applications per generator. Second, these voltage records were used as stimuli to evoke nerve compound action potentials (CAPs) in isolated porcine axillary nerves. The NMS potential was defined as the ratio between the observed area under the CAPs and the theoretical CAP area at maximum response and a firing rate of 250 Hz, which would reliably induce tetanic muscle responses in most human subjects. The measurement protocol was tailored to optimise reproducibility of the obtained NMS potentials and longevity of the nerve specimens.

**Results:** As prerequisite for the clinical translation of our results, the robustness of our test method and reproducibility of the NMS potential are demonstrated with an excellent correlation ($r = 0.93$) between two sets of identical stimuli ($n = 72$ each) obtained from 16 nerve segments with similar diameters ($4.2 \pm 0.37$ mm) in the nerve model. The RF generators differed significantly ($p < 0.0001$) regarding NMS potential (medians: 0–3%).

**Conclusions:** Our test method is suitable for quantifying the NMS potential of different electrosurgical systems ex vivo with high selectivity at a reasonable degree of standardization and with justifiable effort. Our results suggest that the clinical incidence of NMS is considerably influenced by the type of RF generator. Future generations of RF generators take advantage from the proposed test standard through higher safety and less animal testing. Health professionals and treated patients will benefit most from improved RF surgery using generators with a low NMS risk.

**Keywords:** Electrical stimulation, Electrosurgical unit, Radio-frequency current, Compound action potential, Bipolar loop electrode, Bladder, Prostate, Obturator nerve, TURB, TURP

* Correspondence: ulrich.biber@erbe-med.com
[1]Erbe Elektromedizin GmbH, Waldhoernlestrasse 17, 72072 Tuebingen, Germany

## Background

The surgical application of RF current can lead to adverse NMS. This is commonly attributed to the so called faradic effect created by unwanted frequencies below 20 kHz (pp. 518–519 in [1]). In urology, adverse NMS events have been reported during transurethral resection of bladder (TURB) [2–5] and prostatic tumours (TURP) [4, 6]. Moreover, in gynaecology, the hysteroscopic transcervical resection should be mentioned. TURB is the most common surgical technique (gold standard) for the definitive diagnosis and initial treatment of bladder cancer [5], which is one of the most common urinary tract malignancies [7]. Potential intraoperative complications of TURB include bleeding and bladder perforation, typically as a consequence of stimulation of the obturator nerve, which may be associated with sudden, strong contractions of leg adductors. These contractions can lead to uncontrolled movements of the instruments introduced into the bladder, possibly leading to a bladder perforation, which requires conversion to open surgery. Current in vivo or clinical techniques for evaluating NMS typically include documenting the incidence of adverse NMS events such as obturator nerve reflex/adductor muscle contraction or bladder injury/perforation rate [2, 3, 5, 8, 9]. In some studies, the severity of intraoperative NMS events is evaluated on a rating scale, such as "no", "weak/moderate" and "strong/severe" [10, 11]. Moreover, compound muscle action potentials from adductor muscles were examined in patients undergoing TUR surgery [12, 13]. To reduce the risk of NMS, several measures were described: First, a pharmacological block of the obturator nerve [8, 11–14]. Second, intubation anaesthesia and relaxation of skeletal muscles of the patient (chpts. 11.3 & 11.3.4 in [15]). Third, a low-power setting, e.g. 50 W for cutting and 40 W for coagulation instead of a typically higher setting [2]. Fourth, the use of bipolar instead of monopolar RF current: Some studies reported advantages of bipolar over monopolar TURB, including a lower recurrence rate, better quality of biopsy specimens for the pathologist, less haemorrhage, lower incidence of the TUR syndrome and also reduced risk of NMS [2, 10]. A recent meta-analysis including seven clinical trials suggests that the incidence of obturator reflex and bladder wall perforation for monopolar vs. bipolar TURB is 14.8% vs. 3.7% ($p <$ 0.0001) and 4.3% vs. 0.3% ($p = 0.003$) [3]. However, there are also studies showing that bipolar is not superior to monopolar TURB with respect to these complications [5, 9, 16, 17]. Consequently, the EAU guideline (Update 2016) to "Non-muscle-invasive Bladder Cancer" states that the results concerning resection techniques for TURB remain controversial (chpt. 5.11.3 in [18]). Overall, the measures described to reduce the incidence of NMS do not really solve the problem, as they either pose a different risk to the patient or impair performance of the RF application. A satisfactory solution would be RF generators which, due to technical advances, trigger less NMS. Therefore, we developed an ex vivo test system to assess the unfavourable NMS risk of different RF generators. This was previously only possible with in vivo animal testing or clinical trials.

## Methods

A two-stage ex vivo approach was pursued: First, during the application of RF energy in an ex vivo TURB model, we recorded voltage curves at possible positions of the obturator nerve behind a porcine bladder wall (Fig. 1a). Second, these voltage records were used as stimuli in another ex vivo model with peripheral porcine nerves (Fig. 1b). The influence of these stimuli on nerve activity, i. e. the generation of evoked nerve compound action potentials (CAP) was recorded. A CAP is the spatial sum of action potentials generated by all stimulated axons of a whole nerve or a large population of axons recorded extracellularly. Thus, in this study, the firing rate and strength of CAPs represent a surrogate measure for the risk of NMS. We refer to this measure as "NMS potential", which is defined mathematically in subsection "Data analysis". The tested RF generators (250–450 kHz base frequency) were used with the control algorithm/mode for cutting with bipolar instruments in saline solution. Activation is divided into an ignition phase, in which spark formation is triggered at relatively high current flow (e.g. 8 A), and a cut phase, in which sparking is maintained at relatively low currents (e.g. 4 A). The ignition phase is fixed, whereas during the cut phase the intensity can be adjusted via the generator setting. Since the hardware components and modes differ, the exact electric parameters and instrument-specific adaptations are quite different between manufacturers. Thus, the recorded voltage curves represented a spectrum of different manufacturers and generator settings.

### Experimental design

We tested four different contemporary RF generators (Erbe Elektromedizin GmbH, Bowa-electronic GmbH, Olympus Corporation) combined with a resection electrode loop (24 Fr, WA22507D, Olympus), hereafter called instrument, at their minimum, default and maximum effect settings. Each combination of RF generator and effect setting was applied six times in the ex vivo TURB model. The resultant 72 stimuli were applied twice in the ex vivo nerve model, i. e. 144 values representing an NMS potential were obtained.

### Experimental setup – ex vivo TURB model

This first stage of the ex vivo model was designed to mimic the essential components of TURB surgery (Fig.

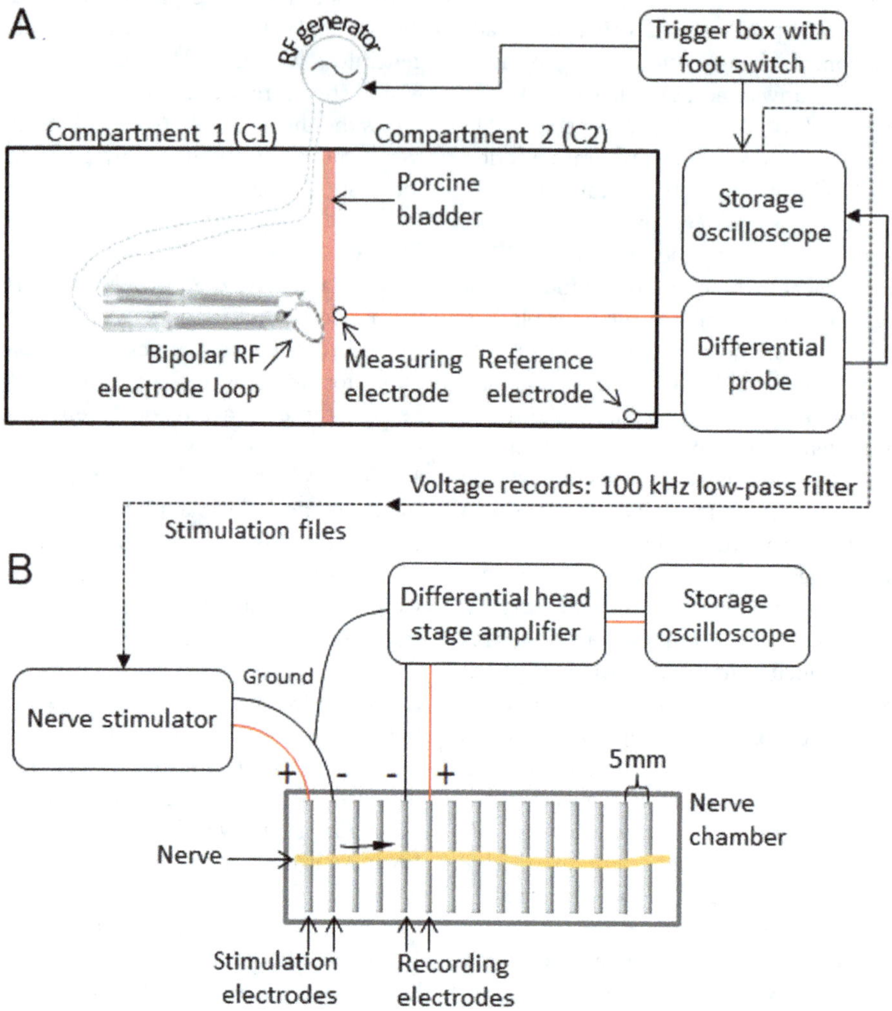


**Fig. 1** Experimental setup. **a** Ex vivo TURB model – C1 represents the inside and C2 the exterior of the bladder. The tank for the two compartments was made of transparent material and included an exchangeable two-piece tissue holder frame (aperture: 13.5 cm) creating a waterproof seal between C1 and C2 using sealing hoses. Voltage recording was performed at 5 MS/s with a storage oscilloscope. Activation of the instrument and data logging were synchronised with a trigger box which in turn was activated by a foot switch. **b** Ex vivo nerve model – CAP recording at a distance of 1.5 cm from the stimulation site using a differential head stage amplifier and a storage oscilloscope. The nerve chamber's electrodes were installed at a fixed distance of 5 mm

1a). We recorded voltage curves at possible positions of the obturator nerve. Porcine bladder tissue separated two relevant functional compartments: One compartment for the instrument (C1), representing the inside of the bladder (mucous layer), which was filled with normal saline solution as during bipolar TURB. The other compartment (C2), representing the exterior of the bladder (adventitia/serous layer), was filled with normal saline as well. In C1 the bladder tissue was cut vertically. The measuring electrode was positioned in C2 contacting the exterior bladder tissue. The distance between instrument and measuring electrode was set to ~ 3 mm in the same horizontal plane given a typical mean bladder tissue thickness of 2.5 mm. However, this distance varied due to the cutting movements (~ 1 cm) of the instrument (in theory ~ 3–6 mm). The distance of ~ 3 mm (or more) was chosen for two reasons: First, it represents a relative safety distance regarding the risk to cause thermal damage to nervous structures [19]. Second, this distance represents a reasonable compromise between sufficient and too much voltage amplitude measured with our equipment. The instrument was fixed to a height gauge for positioning and for cutting the bladder tissue by manual traction. For more accurate positioning of the instrument in C1 a LED light source with an optical fibre was fixed below the measuring electrode in C2, pointing towards the bladder tissue. The spot light shined through the bladder wall allowing for accurate initial instrument positioning in C1. The differential probe for voltage recording (TA058, Pico Technology) was connected to the measuring electrode (point electrode, diameter: 1 mm, surface material: gold) and to a reference electrode, which was fixed at the edge of C2 (Fig. 1a).

**Conduction of test – ex vivo TURB model**

Fresh abattoir porcine bladder was stretched evenly in a tissue holder frame. The thickness of the stretched bladder in the retractor frame was measured with a calliper. If necessary, this procedure was repeated to achieve a final thickness of 2–3 mm across the entire aperture. For each RF application, instrument and measuring electrode were repositioned to start over with unused tissue. The instrument was placed in an upright position (electrode tip facing downwards) tilted by 20 ± 5° with respect to the plane of the bladder and was activated with contact to the bladder. The activation time was 900 ± 20 ms with a vertical cut length of ~ 1 cm resulting in an average cut speed of 1.1 cm/s. The cut depth was adjusted to avoid perforation of the bladder while at the same time ensuring a not too superficial cut with a clearly visible trace. In case of perforation the bladder tissue was replaced and the respective measurement was excluded. In case of poor cut quality (no or too superficial cut) the respective measurement was also excluded. RF generator type and effect setting were documented and the voltage record was saved. A "stimulus ID" was assigned to measurements selected for nerve stimulation.

**Pre-processing of voltage records for ex vivo nerve model**

Voltage records obtained in the ex vivo TURB model were processed with Scilab software v.6.0.1 (94,528 Rungis, France) for nerve stimulation. Frequencies above 100 kHz that cannot evoke CAPs [20, 21] were removed with a second order low-pass Butterworth filter (Scilab functions: 'analpf', 'dscr', 'flts'). This includes the RF generator's base frequency components, which would have introduced a detrimental noise source and also could have caused thermal damage to the nerves. The processed voltage records, hereafter called stimuli, were sorted in ascending order with respect to peak to peak voltage and divided into groups of six. Additionally, a snippet of a specific stimulus was chosen as reference stimulus, which clearly evoked a CAP and marked the 80% quantile of peak to peak voltages of all stimuli.

**Experimental setup – ex vivo nerve model**

The second stage of the ex vivo model used standard electrophysiological methods (Fig. 1b). Isolated peripheral porcine axillary nerve trunks were harvested immediately post mortem and stored in Ringer's solution (Fresenius Kabi). They were used for CAP recording after an initial storage period of at least two hours but no longer than 32 h. The isolated nerve specimens were placed on electrodes in a nerve chamber that could be closed with a lid to preserve humidity inside. The electrodes in the nerve chamber were used either as stimulation or recording locations. The stimulation electrodes were connected to an arbitrary waveform generator (Keysight 33512B), serving as nerve stimulator. The recording electrodes were connected to a differential head stage amplifier (npi electronic EXT-02F/2). In turn, this amplifier was connected to a storage oscilloscope for CAP recording.

**Conduction of test – ex vivo nerve model**

The measurements were performed at ambient temperature. Fixed settings for the differential head stage amplifier were used: 100 Hz high-pass, 20 kHz low-pass and 500× gain. The storage oscilloscope was also used with fixed settings: 1 s sampling duration, 1 MS/s sampling rate. The measurement protocol for the CAP recording consisted of the following steps:

1. Determination of maximal CAP amplitude:
   a. Stimulation using a conventional rectangular pulse with a duration of 100 µs at a stimulus amplitude of 7 V (about 2× higher than the typical stimulus intensity required to evoke the maximal CAP amplitude)
   b. If the maximal CAP amplitude was < 4 mV, the recording location was changed
2. Determination of stimulus amplitude (threshold) to evoke a just measurable CAP (~ 40 µV)
   a. Stimulation by conventional rectangular pulse with a duration of 100 µs
   b. Adjustment of stimulus amplitude starting with 100 mV
   c. If the threshold was > 200 mV, the recording location was changed
3. Calculation of 80% of the maximal CAP amplitude $CAP_{80}$
4. Adjustment of reference stimulus to evoke $CAP_{80}$ to obtain a scaling factor (SF):
   a. For example: $SF = \frac{\text{Reference stimulus amplitude to evoke } CAP_{80}\text{:7.1 V}}{\text{Original reference stimulus amplitude:5.7 V}} \approx 1.25$
5. Stimulation with one set of six stimuli scaled by the SF calculated in Step 4
6. Stimulation with reference stimulus scaled by the SF of Step 4 to check if
   a. CAP amplitude > 80% × $CAP_{80}$ continuation with Step 5
   b. CAP amplitude < 80% × $CAP_{80}$ continuation with Step 7
7. Placement of nerve specimen in Ringer's solution for at least 1 min
8. Placement of nerve specimen in nerve chamber at former position as exactly as possible

9. Continuation with Step 1 until all stimuli were recorded

The measurement protocol was conducted twice with all 72 stimuli. Additionally, for control and background measurements, the same stimuli were applied on non-functional nerve specimens with the respective scaling factors calculated in Step 4 of the measurement protocol. To render a nerve specimen non-functional it was squeezed with tweezers between stimulation and recording locations. After each measurement "stimulus ID" and amplitude were documented and the CAP recording was saved.

### Data analysis

Data was analysed with Scilab. The NMS potential was calculated for each stimulation in the nerve model: First, DC offset was removed and the records were high-pass filtered at 100 Hz (linear phase FIR-filter, Scilab functions 'wfir', 'syslin' and 'flts') and low-pass filtered at 3 kHz (Second order Butterworth, Scilab functions 'analpf', 'dscr' and 'flts'). Second, background measurements were subtracted from the respective test measurements to eliminate signal distortions due to stimulus artefacts. Third, these optimized CAP records were used for the automated CAP detection (Figure S1). The areas under the CAPs were used to calculate the NMS potential of each individual stimulation:

$$NMS\ potential = \sum_{n=1}^{No.\ of\ CAPs} \frac{1}{N\_MAX_{CAPs}} \times \frac{Area\ of\ CAP(n)}{Area\ of\ max.\ amplitude\ CAP}$$

The NMS potential was defined relative to the CAP, which is a well-established measure for nerve activity [22–25]. An NMS potential of 100% corresponds to the maximum CAP area at a firing rate of 250 Hz, which would reliably induce tetanic muscle responses in most human subjects ([26], see their Fig. 5), although 50 Hz are typically sufficient for a single muscle fibre [27]. We have therefore assumed 250 Hz as worst-case firing rate of the CAPs, i. e. the worst-case number of CAPs during the analysed time window of 850 ms ($N\_Max_{CAPs}$) was set to 213. The actual number of evoked CAPs for a stimulus (*No. of CAPs*) and their areas were set in relation to $N\_MAX_{CAPs}$. This was achieved by adding up the areas of the evoked CAPs (*Area of CAP(n)*) and dividing it by the area that corresponds to 213 ($N\_MAX_{CAPs}$) CAPs with maximal amplitude. Finally, the NMS potential was expressed as percentage to emphasize the relation to the worst-case stimulation. Thus, the NMS potential ranged from 0 to 100% and has no unit. In theory, NMS potentials higher than 100% could occur but it surely includes the worst-case stimulation for the stimuli applied. The highest NMS potential actually obtained was 17%.

Statistical calculations were performed with GraphPad Prism software v.7.01 (GraphPad Software, California, U.S.A.). Median, range and confidence limits were calculated for descriptive purposes. Differences between continuous data of more than two samples were detected using one factor analysis of variance with post hoc multiple comparisons. The normal distribution was confirmed or disconfirmed with the Kolmogorov-Smirnov-Test for small sample size. Differences between NMS potentials were detected using the Kruskal-Wallis test since it was not normally distributed. For analysing differences between specific groups corrected Dunn's test was used. Linear regression analysis was used to describe correlations (NMS potentials from identical stimuli).

## Results

### CAPs in different phases of RF activation

In a simplified view the activation of bipolar RF instruments in saline is characterised by two distinct phases: In the first phase the ignition of a spark is triggered by relatively high current flow and during the second phase, where cutting takes place, the spark is sustained at a relatively lower current flow. The ignition and cut phases can be distinguished in the stimulus traces corresponding to the RF activations, e.g. in Fig. 2. Both during the ignition and the cut phase CAPs were detected. For this, the stimulus shown in Fig. 2 represents a typical example where one or a few relatively strong CAPs occur when the spark is ignited and several, usually weaker CAPs occur when the electrode loop is brought closer to the possible nerve position. In the definition of the NMS potential, this distinction is not made but it is important to take into consideration that these two contributions are included.

### Inter data-set reliability

An important feature of our two-stage approach is that stimuli obtained from the first stage might be applied multiple times in the second stage. Applying exactly the same stimuli multiple times allows demonstrating reproducibility of the NMS potential. Furthermore, with respect to standardisation and reproducibility two variables that define the physiological status of the nerve specimens are most important: First, the number of undamaged fibres and, second, the responsiveness of these fibres. Therefore, it was important to harvest the nerve specimens carefully without imposing mechanical loads and to use similar nerve diameters (target diameter: 4 mm). The 16 nerve segments used actually had an average diameter of 4.2 ± 0.37 mm. Consequently, a similar amount of undamaged nerve fibres per specimen can be

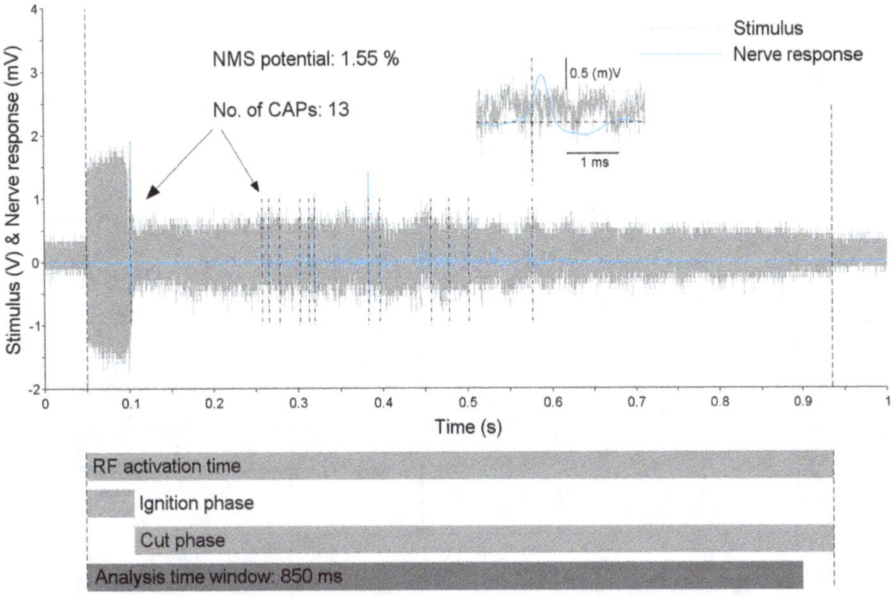


**Fig. 2** Typical example of nerve response (blue) to a single stimulus (grey) that was applied to an isolated porcine axillary nerve and originates from an RF activation with a bipolar resection electrode loop. Amount and strength of detected CAPs within the analysed time window defined the NMS potential. See Figure S1 for details on the CAP detection algorithm. CAPs were detected both during the ignition and the cut phase of the RF activation corresponding to the stimulus. The zoom view shows the last CAP detected in this stimulation

assumed. Moreover, the responsiveness of the specimens was monitored according to Step 1 and Step 2 of the measurement protocol. A correlation plot of the two data sets (Fig. 3), in which exactly the same stimuli ($n$ = 72) were applied twice, shows a high degree of correlation (Spearman $r = 0.93$) and a very robust goodness of fit to a linear regression ($r^2 = 0.87$). The slope of the regression line (1.03) was not significantly different from one ($p = 0.60$) and the y-intercept was close to zero (0.64%).

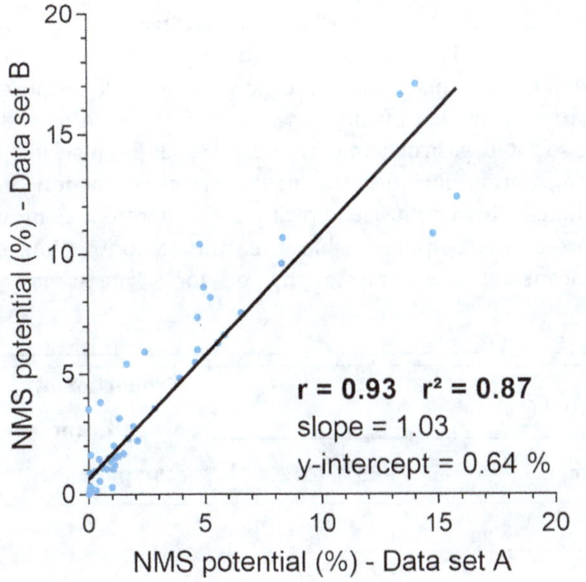


**Fig. 3** Correlation of NMS potentials obtained from 16 porcine axillary nerve segments in response to two identical sets of stimuli ($n = 72$ per data set) originating from RF activations with a bipolar resection electrode loop. ~ 76% (55/72) of the stimuli resulted in a NMS potential larger than 0%

### NMS potential of different RF generators

In the ex vivo nerve model we tested 72 stimuli from four contemporary RF generators, i. e. 18 stimuli from each generator. Each stimulus was tested twice on separate nerves. Therefore, 144 NMS potential readings were obtained. We found significant differences in NMS potentials (Fig. 4) between the four commercial RF generators (Kruskal-Wallis test $p < 0.0001$) with medians between 0% (RF generator A) and ~ 3% (RF generator D) (Table 1).

## Discussion

The basis for the validity of the ex vivo TURB model was to mimic the essential components of this clinical application. The usage of normal saline in compartment C1 is equivalent to the clinical setting of TURB. The usage of normal saline in compartment C2 is a simplification based on multiple considerations: First, the electrical conductivity of normal saline solution is quite similar to that of extracellular human blood plasma or interstitial fluid outside the bladder wall (~ 1.9 S/m and 1.7 S/m at 25 °C). Second, exactly matching the conductivities is not mandatory because the extracellular fluid conductivity may vary, e. g. as a consequence of various

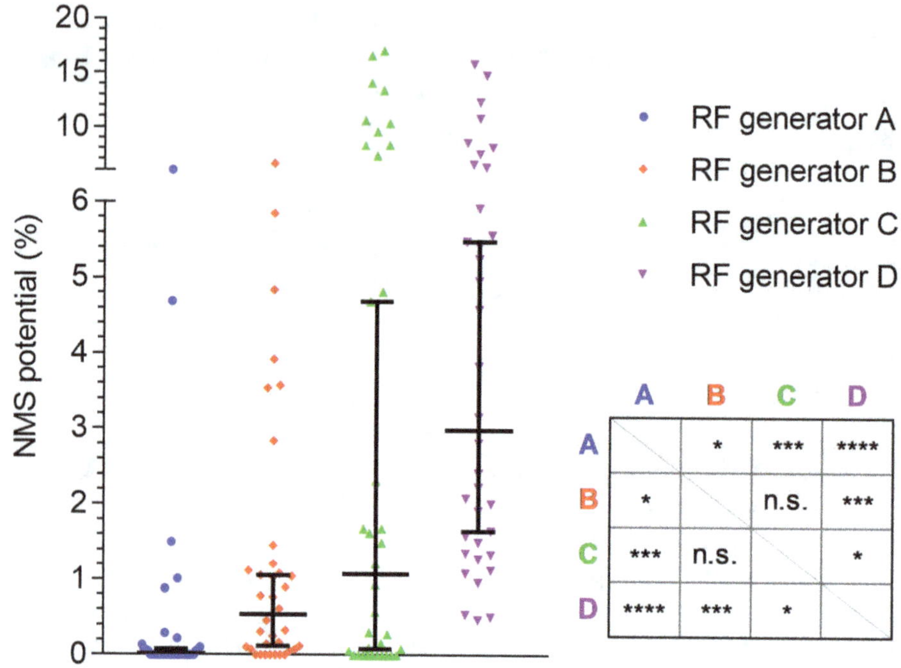


**Fig. 4** NMS potentials of four contemporary RF generators ($n = 36$ per generator) with medians and 95% CI (error bars) and post-hoc table (Dunn's test). The NMS potentials of each generator originate from RF activations with a bipolar resection electrode loop used in saline with minimum, default and maximum effect settings in equal shares ($n = 12$ per effect setting)

pathological states [28]. Third, assuming the relatively high conductivity of normal saline solution within C2 is an appropriate worst-case estimate, in which a fluid behind the bladder wall makes direct contact to the obturator nerve without further tissue in between. In comparison, muscle or connective tissue is approximately five times less conductive (0.3–0.4 S/m). The usage of porcine bladder is the most appropriate substitute for human bladder since pigs have been established as a model for research of human diseases due to similarities, which includes size, organ structure and function, physiology and organ development [29, 30]. A high sampling rate (5 MS/s) for the differential probe was chosen to assure faithful reproduction of the signal in the nerve model. Extracellular recording of CAPs from peripheral nerve trunks is a well-established method to study nerve activity that is utilised both in teaching at universities and in preclinical studies [22–25]. A similar test method is used clinically e. g. by recording CAPs of the auditory nerve in cochlear implant patients (for a review see [31]). Another potential ex vivo test method suitable for this study could be a nerve-skeletal muscle preparation that encompasses the sciatic nerve and the associated gastrocnemius muscle [32–34]. This kind of preparation includes the neuromuscular junction and the effector or muscle allowing for a more direct measure of the output variable, i. e. muscle contraction, by means of electromyography or force measurement.

**Table 1** NMS potential of four contemporary RF generators

| RF generator[a] | NMS potential (%) | | | Proportion of significant comparisons |
|---|---|---|---|---|
| | Median | Range | 95% C.I. | |
| A | 0 | 0 – 6 | 0 – 0.06 | 5/6 (83%) |
| B | 0.53 | 0 – 6.6 | 0.12 – 1.1 | |
| C | 1.08 | 0 – 17 | 0.08 – 4.7 | |
| D | 2.98 | 0 – 16 | 1.6 – 5.5 | |

[a]with bipolar resection electrode loop in saline solution with minimum, default and maximum effect settings

However, this increases the overall complexity of the test method and the effort of dissection compared to the usage of an isolated peripheral nerve trunk. It would be much more challenging to standardise measurements at this level of complexity and there is no well-established ex vivo methodology incorporating a mammalian nerve-skeletal muscle preparation. Moreover, porcine nerves are very similar to human nerves regarding anatomy and physiology [29, 30]. Employing fresh tissue samples spares use of live animals, does not require animal testing application for the study, nor ethical animal husbandry or other additional efforts. Taken together, the porcine nerve trunk model seems to be the most parsimonious yet reliable ex vivo test method to address the aims of this study. A high inter-data set correlation (Fig. 3) demonstrates reproducibility of the outcome measure, which is due to the standardisation of the test method.

The justification for the two-stage setup is as follows: First, CAP recording during RF activation is not possible due to RF interference. Second, voltage recording enables multiple tests with the same stimulus in the nerve model, thereby demonstrating reproducibility. Regarding the position of the voltage measurement in the TURB model, we have pre-tested several positions. Only at a distance of ~ 3 mm from the RF application was the signal strength sufficient, and it was also far enough away not to damage the measuring electrode and theoretically a nerve [19]. The choice of position thus represents a clinical worst-case for nerve stimulation without nerve damage. In addition, the voltage recordings were processed (100 kHz low pass & scaling) to serve as input for the nerve model while minimising damage to the nerve samples and maximising nerve response. Therefore, the original strength of the voltage recordings was not the decisive parameter for the obtained NMS potentials. Instead, the scaling of the stimulation signals to adapt to the individual responsiveness and impedance of each nerve sample was crucial to obtain comparable NMS potentials across the entire measurement series. In parallel, scaling compensated for the reduced nerve excitability that occurs ex vivo during prolonged and repeated stimulations.

Another point of discussion is why generator voltage should not be used as input for a nerve model or for the immediate evaluation of NMS. At first glance, the voltage recordings of the TURB model look like an attenuated version of the generator voltage (data not shown). However, there are important differences: First, different tissue layers of the bladder attenuate the signal depending on frequency and thus act as a complex filter. Second, NMS may be caused by DC loops around the high-density or "active" electrode, which are caused by sparks and cannot be detected in the outer chain of generator, electrodes and connecting wires [35]. Thus, an application model with the relevant tissue components is necessary for the evaluation of NMS.

Regarding the outcome measure, we observed obvious differences between the RF generators in terms of their NMS potential (Fig. 4). Thus, the percentage of significant comparisons between the generators (~ 87%, Table 1) is an indicator for the selectivity of our test method. The differences in NMS potential have at least two reasons: First, differences of the effect settings, i. e. the minimum, default and maximum effect settings of each vendor are not in complete correspondence with respect to basic electrical parameters such as applied voltage and maximum power output. Second, differences in the programming of the RF generators and the components used in these generators could be the cause. Our test method is suitable for quantifying the NMS potential of different electrosurgical systems ex vivo but it does not reveal causes behind the differences observed. An additional study limitation is that the NMS potential does not translate into a relevant clinical parameter such as the incidence of obturator reflex or bladder perforation. However, the observed differences in NMS potential should clinically lead to more or less adverse NMS events. Of course, other influencing factors that are not represented by our model, such as the experience of the surgeon, patient-specific differences such as weight, pathological changes, etc. must also be taken into account. Furthermore, clinically investigated influencing factors, such as the monopolar versus bipolar technique or the use of a pharmacological block, were not addressed in our ex vivo model. These system-level questions are likely to remain a task of in vivo testing. Nonetheless, the comparison of new electrosurgical systems with well-established and safe equipment allows for a meaningful safety evaluation. To our knowledge, the test method described here is the first to address the ex vivo risk assessment of NMS for transurethral resection devices. In the future, this test method can easily be adapted to test bipolar TURP as well as monopolar TURB and TURP, e.g. the TURB model can be adapted to emulate TURP using prostatic instead of bladder tissue.

## Conclusions

Our test method is suitable for quantifying the NMS potential of different electrosurgical systems ex vivo with high selectivity at a reasonable degree of standardisation and with justifiable effort. Our results suggest that the clinical incidence of NMS is considerably influenced by the type of RF generator. The development of future generations of RF generators takes advantage from the proposed test standard through higher safety and by replacement or reduction of the extent of animal testing. Most important, health professionals and treated patients will benefit from improved RF surgery using generators with a low risk of NMS.

## Abbreviations

CAP: (Evoked nerve) Compound action potential; NMS: Neuromuscular stimulation; RF: Radio-frequency; TURB: Transurethral resection of bladder (tumour); TURP: Transurethral resection of the prostate


## Acknowledgements

We thank I. Sigle, L. Blobel, P. Selig and M. Zenker for their excellent technical assistance.


## Authors' contributions

UB, OJ and MDE conceived and designed the study. UB was responsible for the data acquisition. OJ checked and verified data input by UB. UB and OJ performed statistical analyses. The data was interpreted by all authors. UB drafted and WKA critically reviewed the manuscript. OJ and MDE revised the manuscript. All authors read and approved the final manuscript.

## Competing interests

UB, OJ and MDE are employees of Erbe Elektromedizin GmbH (Sponsor). Otherwise, the authors declare that they have no competing interests.


## Author details

[1]Erbe Elektromedizin GmbH, Waldhoernlestrasse 17, 72072 Tuebingen, Germany. [2]Department of Urology, University Hospital Tuebingen, Tuebingen, Germany.


## References


1. Hug B, Haag R. Hochfrequenzchirurgie. In: Kramme R, editor. Medizintechnik: Verfahren, Systeme, Informationsverarbeitung; mit 170 Tabellen. 3rd ed. Heidelberg: Springer; 2007. p. 515–38.
2. Gupta NP, Saini AK, Dogra PN, Seth A, Kumar R. Bipolar energy for transurethral resection of bladder tumours at low-power settings: initial experience. BJU Int. 2011;108:553–6. https://doi.org/10.1111/j.1464-410X.2010.09903.x.
3. Zhao C, Tang K, Yang H, Xia D, Chen Z. Bipolar versus Monopolar transurethral resection of nonmuscle-invasive bladder Cancer: a meta-analysis. J Endourol. 2016;30:5–12. https://doi.org/10.1089/end.2015.0410.
4. Prentiss RJ, Harvey GW, Bethard WF, Boatwright DE, Pennington RD. Massive adductor muscle contraction in transurethral surgery: cause and prevention; development of new electrical circuitry. Trans Am Assoc Genitourin Surg. 1964;56:64–72.
5. Ozer K, Horsanali MO, Gorgel SN, Ozbek E. Bladder injury secondary to obturator reflex is more common with plasmakinetic transurethral resection than monopolar transurethral resection of bladder cancer. Cent European J Urol. 2015;68:284–8. https://doi.org/10.5173/ceju.2015.565.
6. Shulman MS, Vellayappan U, Monaghan TG, Coukos WJ, Krenis LJ. Simultaneous bilateral obturator nerve stimulation during transurethral electrovaporization of the prostate. J Clin Anesth. 1998;10:518–21.
7. Ferlay J, Autier P, Boniol M, Heanue M, Colombet M, Boyle P. Estimates of the cancer incidence and mortality in Europe in 2006. Ann Oncol. 2007;18:581–92. https://doi.org/10.1093/annonc/mdl498.
8. Khorrami M, Hadi M, Javid A, Izadpahani M-H, Mohammadi Sichani M, Zargham M, Alizadeh F. A comparison between blind and nerve stimulation guided obturator nerve block in transurethral resection of bladder tumor. J Endourol. 2012;26:1319–22. https://doi.org/10.1089/end.2012.0037.
9. Sugihara T, Yasunaga H, Horiguchi H, Matsui H, Nishimatsu H, Nakagawa T, et al. Comparison of perioperative outcomes including severe bladder injury between monopolar and bipolar transurethral resection of bladder tumors: a population based comparison. J Urol. 2014;192:1355–9. https://doi.org/10.1016/j.juro.2014.05.100.
10. Shiozawa H, Aizawa T, Ito T, Miki M. A new transurethral resection system: operating in saline environment precludes obturator nerve reflexes. J Urol. 2002;168:2665–7. https://doi.org/10.1097/01.ju.0000031402.89232.e1.
11. Bolat D, Aydogdu O, Tekgul ZT, Polat S, Yonguc T, Bozkurt IH, et al. Impact of nerve stimulator-guided obturator nerve block on the short-term outcomes and complications of transurethral resection of bladder tumour: a prospective randomized controlled study. Can Urol Assoc J. 2015;9:E780–4. https://doi.org/10.5489/cuaj.3149.
12. Atanassoff PG, Weiss BM, Brull SJ, Horst A, Külling D, Stein R, Theiler I. Electromyographic comparison of obturator nerve block to three-in-one block. Anesth Analg. 1995;81:529–33.
13. Atanassoff PG, Weiss BM, Brull SJ, Horst A, Külling D, Stein R, Theiler I. Compound motor action potential recording distinguishes differential onset of motor block of the obturator nerve in response to etidocaine or bupivacaine. Anesth Analg. 1996;82:317–20.
14. Magora F, Rozin R, Ben-Menachem Y, Magora A. Obturator nerve block: an evaluation of technique. Br J Anaesth. 1969;41:695–8. https://doi.org/10.1093/bja/41.8.695.
15. Burger M, Wieland W-F. Transurethrale Resektion der Blase. In: Hofmann R, editor. Endoskopische Urologie. Berlin: Springer Berlin Heidelberg; 2009. p. 151–63. https://doi.org/10.1007/978-3-642-01167-2_12.
16. Venkatramani V, Panda A, Manojkumar R, Kekre NS. Monopolar versus bipolar transurethral resection of bladder tumors: a single center, parallel arm, randomized, controlled trial. J Urol. 2014;191:1703–7. https://doi.org/10.1016/j.juro.2013.12.004.
17. Mashni J, Godoy G, Haarer C, Dalbagni G, Reuter VE, Al-Ahmadie H, Bochner BH. Prospective evaluation of plasma kinetic bipolar resection of bladder cancer: comparison to monopolar resection and pathologic findings. Int Urol Nephrol. 2014;46:1699–705. https://doi.org/10.1007/s11255-014-0719-9.
18. Babjuk M, Bohle A, Burger M, Capoun O, Cohen D, Comperat EM, et al. EAU guidelines on non-muscle-invasive Urothelial carcinoma of the bladder: update 2016. Eur Urol. 2017;71:447–61. https://doi.org/10.1016/j.eururo.2016.05.041.
19. Tirelli G, Camilot D, Bonini P, Del Piero GC, Biasotto M, Quatela E. Harmonic scalpel and Electrothermal bipolar vessel sealing system in head and neck surgery: a prospective study on tissue heating and histological damage on nerves. Ann Otol Rhinol Laryngol. 2015;124:852–8. https://doi.org/10.1177/0003489415588556.
20. Lacourse JR, Miller WT, Vogt M, Selikowitz SM. Effect of high-frequency current on nerve and muscle tissue. IEEE Trans Biomed Eng. 1985;32:82–6. https://doi.org/10.1109/TBME.1985.325636.
21. Lapicque L. Recherches quantitatives sur l'excitation électrique des nerfs traitée comme une polarization. J Physiol Pathol Gen. 1907;9:620–35.
22. Zafeiridou G, Spilioti M, Kagiava A, Krikonis K, Kosmidis EK, Karlovasitou A, Kimiskidis VK. Differential effects of lacosamide, phenytoin and topiramate on peripheral nerve excitability: an ex vivo electrophysiological study. Neurotoxicology. 2016;52:57–63. https://doi.org/10.1016/j.neuro.2015.10.016.
23. Kagiava A, Theophilidis G. Assessing the permeability of the rat sciatic nerve epineural sheath against compounds with local anesthetic activity: an ex vivo electrophysiological study. Toxicol Mech Methods. 2013;23:634–40. https://doi.org/10.3109/15376516.2013.825826.
24. Li J, Shi R. A device for the electrophysiological recording of peripheral nerves in response to stretch. J Neurosci Methods. 2006;154:102–8. https://doi.org/10.1016/j.jneumeth.2005.12.007.
25. Kagiava A, Aligizaki K, Katikou P, Nikolaidis G, Theophilidis G. Assessing the neurotoxic effects of palytoxin and ouabain, both $Na^+/K^+$-ATPase inhibitors, on the myelinated sciatic nerve fibres of the mouse: an ex vivo electrophysiological study. Toxicon. 2012;59:416–26. https://doi.org/10.1016/j.toxicon.2011.12.007.
26. Dideriksen JL, Leerskov K, Czyzewska M, Rasmussen R. The relation between the frequency of short-pulse electrical stimulation of afferent nerve fibers and evoked muscle force. IEEE Trans Biomed Eng. 2017. https://doi.org/10.1109/TBME.2017.2671853.
27. Blinks JR, Rudel R, Taylor SR. Calcium transients in isolated amphibian skeletal muscle fibres: detection with aequorin. J Physiol. 1978;277:291–323.
28. Dobiszewski KF, Deek MP, Ghaly A, Prodan C, Hill AA. Extracellular fluid conductivity analysis by dielectric spectroscopy for in vitro determination of cortical tissue vitality. Physiol Meas. 2012;33:1249–60. https://doi.org/10.1088/0967-3334/33/7/1249
29. Schook LB, Tumbleson ME. Advances in swine in biomedical research. New York: Plenum Press; 1996.
30. Lunney JK. Advances in swine biomedical model genomics. Int J Biol Sci. 2007;3:179–84. https://doi.org/10.7150/ijbs.3.179.
31. He S, Teagle HFB, Buchman CA. The electrically evoked compound action potential: from laboratory to clinic. Front Neurosci. 2017;11:339. https://doi.org/10.3389/fnins.2017.00339.

32. Sáez JC, Norris B, Concha J. Effect of colchicine on the electrophysiological properties of the toad sciatic-gastrocnemius preparations in vivo. Pharmacology. 1982;25:278–85. https://doi.org/10.1159/000137752.
33. Biró G. Excitatory effects of the electrical activity of muscle on the contiguous nerve. Acta Biochim Biophys Acad Sci Hung. 1977;12:403–10.
34. Maleque MA, Adhikary PK, Pavuluri S, Kopsombut P, Rucker HK. Potentiation of cholinergic activity with pyridino1,2-aimidazo5,4-bindole: in vitro studies. Gen Pharmacol. 1990;21:199–203.
35. Slager CJ, Schuurbiers JC, Oomen JA, Bom N. Electrical nerve and muscle stimulation by radio frequency surgery: role of direct current loops around the active electrode. IEEE Trans Biomed Eng. 1993;40:182–7. https://doi.org/10.1109/10.212058.

# A prospective observational cohort study of posterior tibial nerve stimulation in patients with multiple sclerosis: Design and methods

Giulia I. Lane[1*], Yang Mao-Draayer[2], Paholo Barboglio-Romo[1], J. Quentin Clemens[1], Priyanka Gupta[1], Rod Dunn[1], Yongmei Qin[1], Anne P. Cameron[1] and John T. Stoffel[1]

**Abstract**

**Background:** Posterior tibial nerve stimulation (PTNS) is a promising treatment for lower urinary tract symptoms (LUTS) in patients with MS. However, long term data focusing on PTNS impact on health-related quality of life (HRQOL), bowel and bladder symptoms are lacking. This paper describes a study protocol that examines the extended efficacy of PTNS on MS related bladder and bowel symptoms and resulting HRQOL.

**Methods/Design:** This is a single-centered, prospective, longitudinal, observational cohort study of patients with MS who suffer from LUTS and are refractory to two prior treatment modalities. Participants who have elected to pursue PTNS therapy for LUTS will be eligible. The primary outcome is the median number of urinary frequency and incontinence episodes on a 3-day voiding diary at 3, 12 and 24 months compared to baseline. Secondary outcome measures will include change in total AUA-SS, M-ISI, NBSS, SF-12, SSS and BCS scores from baseline The Expanded Disability Status Scale and magnetic resonance imaging will be evaluated at baseline and annually throughout the study.

**Discussion:** This research protocol aims to expand on the existing literature regarding outcomes of PTNS in MS. Specifically, it will provide long term follow-up data on bladder, bowel, sexual and HRQOL outcomes. The completion of this study will provide longitudinal efficacy data of the impact of PTNS in MS patients.

**Keywords:** Quality of life, Urinary incontinence, Neuromodulation, Multiple sclerosis, Prospective studies, Tibial nerve, Urinary bladder, Neurogenic

## Background

Multiple Sclerosis (MS) is the most common autoimmune neuro-inflammatory disease of the central nervous system and affects approximately 31 per 100,000 Americans annually, with 700,000 Americans living with MS in 2010 [1].

MS is characterized by four primary disease courses: clinically isolated syndrome (CIS), relapsing remitting (RRMS), secondary progressive (SPMS) and primary progressive (PPMS) [2, 3]. Clinically isolated syndrome is a pre-MS syndrome and is described as the initial episode of neurologic deficit which may progress to MS. [2] In some patients, CIS precedes the diagnosis of relapsing-remitting

* Correspondence: giuliala@med.umich.edu
[1]Department of Urology, University of Michigan, 1500 East Medical Drive, Taubman Center 3875, Ann Arbor, MI 48109, USA

MS (RR-MS). Relapsing-remitting MS (RRMS) is characterized by discrete episodes of neurological dysfunction or relapses, with no interim disease progression. Patients may fully recover from a relapse or may experience residual deficits. Secondary progressive MS patients have gradual neurological deterioration (progression) with increasing physical debilitation following a period of relapsing remitting disease [4]. Finally, primary-progressive MS (PPMS) is defined as steady disease progression from its onset and may include periods of stable disease or temporary symptomatic improvement [5].

Lower urinary symptoms (LUTS) including overactive bladder (OAB) are reported in 75–90% of all MS patients, and can be very bothersome to patients [6]. However, stage and type of disease may impact perception and severity of urinary symptoms in MS patients. Utilizing urodynamic data, others showed that there is high prevalence of urinary symptoms even in clinically isolated syndrome (CIS), before greater neurologic impact from the disease is found [7]. Once patients have established disease, urinary symptoms may be perceived differently based on rapidity of disease progress.

Current management of MS related LUTS follows the overactive bladder pathway: first line lifestyle modifications, second line adjunctive pharmacotherapy, third line neuromodulation (sacral or posterior tibial) or chemodenervation of the bladder (onabotulinum toxin) and fourth line invasive surgical reconstruction [8–10]. The implementation of intermittent or indwelling catheter can be an adjunct to these therapies (Fig. 1).

Each intervention can have significant quality of life implications. For example, second line pharmacotherapy with anticholinergic is often poorly tolerated because it can exacerbate symptoms of dry mouth, constipation and central nervous system side effects like confusion [8]. Likewise, the addition of intermittent catheterization can add complexity to the patient's lifestyle with unclear impact on decreasing LUTS [11]. In regards to third line therapy, intradetrusor onabotulinumtoxin (Botox) can be effective at controlling symptoms, but it requires cystoscopy to administer, the treatment needs to be repeated every 6–12 months, and each administration carries a risk of urinary tract infection and urinary retention [12].

Neuromodulation, another third line therapy, includes both sacral neuromodulation and posterior tibial nerve stimulation. Sacral neuromodulation involves 1 or 2 surgeries for placement of a neuromodulation lead and an implantable pulse generator to stimulate the S3 nerve root. Limited data suggest sacral neuromodulation may be effective for MS related LUTS, however the sacral neuromodulation leads are not MRI compatible [8, 13, 14]. Since many patients with MS require frequent MRI for surveillance, this poses a barrier for use of current implantable sacral neuromodulation technology. In these patients, percutaneous posterior tibial nerve stimulation (PTNS) offers a minimally invasive alternative to relieve bladder symptoms via similar pathways as sacral neuromodulation.

Posterior tibial nerve stimulation, involves placement of a solid stainless-steel needle into the posterior tibial

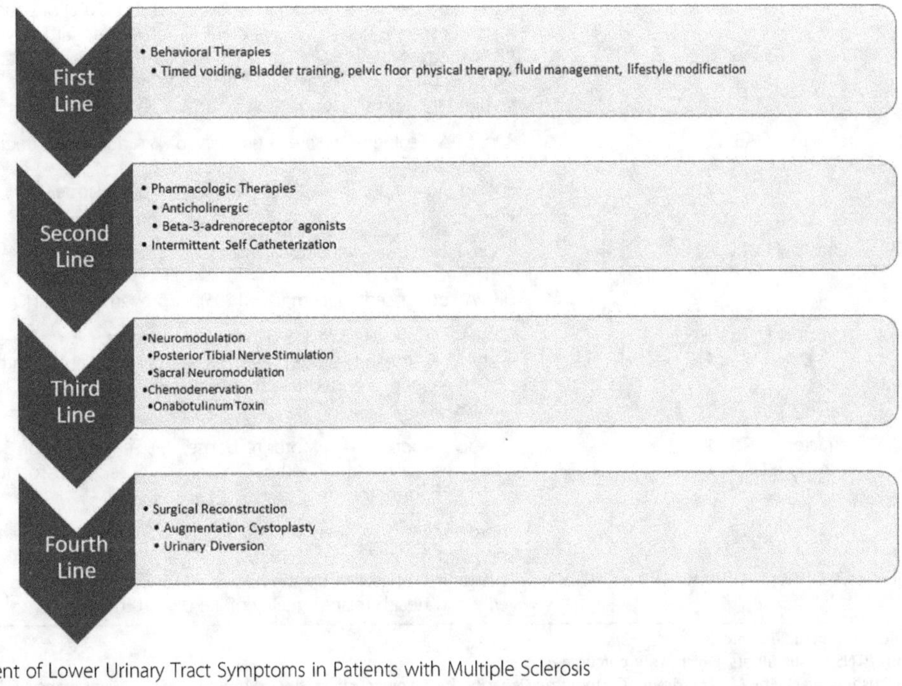


**Fig. 1** Management of Lower Urinary Tract Symptoms in Patients with Multiple Sclerosis

nerve and uses this to conduct a fixed electrical pulse through the nerve. The posterior tibial nerve derives from the L4-S3 nerve roots, neuromodulation of this nerve has been shown to improve overactive bladder symptoms [15]. The office-based therapy is performed weekly for 12 weeks during 30-min sessions; patients who have improvement in symptoms can proceed to maintenance treatments at regularly scheduled intervals.

Only seven clinical studies have been published regarding the use of PTNS in patients with MS and refractory LUTS [16–22]. (Table 1) Of these studies, four represent prospective case series evaluating the efficacy of PTNS for LUTS in MS, with a total of 131 patients [18–20, 22]. These studies reported significant improvement in LUTS with overall the rate of improvement (defined as greater than 50% improvement in symptoms) between 33 and 89% (Table 1).

Despite these findings, the studies were limited by their short term follow up (range 3–12 months), strict inclusion criteria, and lack of important quality of life outcomes. Outcomes beyond 12 months and the impact of standard maintenance therapy have only been studied in one prior study [20]. Moreover, there is limited research on the effects of PTNS on related pelvic organ dysfunction such as bowel and sexual function among patients with MS. [23, 24] As PTNS requires significant investment on the part of patients and clinicians, further studies generating more robust evidence regarding the long term impact of this therapy are warranted. Furthermore, we believe it is important to follow PTNS treatment outcomes longitudinally to determine if it is effective in a progressive disease such as MS. Previous published PTNS studies did not address how efficacy could be affected by the type of MS, disability status or whether the efficacy could be maintained long term in the setting of a progressive disease.

Therefore, the aim of this study is to describe short- and long-term clinical outcomes, including quality of life, bladder, bowel and sexual function, in MS patients who undergo PTNS treatment for refractory LUTS.

**Table 1** Literature review of Posterior Tibial Nerve Stimulation in Multiple Sclerosis

| Author | Year | N | Inclusion Criteria* | Follow-up (months) | Primary Outcome Results |
|---|---|---|---|---|---|
| Fjorback [1] | '07 | 8 | UDS: DO and MCC < 300 mL | n/a | • PTNS unable to suppress detrusor contraction.<br>• No reduction of urgency<br>• No difference in peak detrusor pressure<br>• Median volume at first contraction was 36% higher with stimulation. ($p = 0.0078$) |
| Kabay [2] | '08 | 29 | storage symptoms | n/a | • Mean volume first involuntary contraction increased from 183 to 230 mL. ($p < 0.001$)<br>• Mean maximum cystometric capacity increased from 193 to 286 mL. ($p < 0.001$) |
| Kabay [3] | '09 | 19 | LUTS | 3 | • Complete Response rates > 50% improvement: urgency (33%), incontinence (40%), frequency (58%), nocturia (75%), pad test (90%) of patients<br>• Partial Response between 25 and 50% improvement:urgency (53%), incontinence (50%), frequency (26%), nocturia (25%), pad test (10%) of patients<br>• UDS response: DSD resolved in 3/5, significant improvement after PTNS in first involuntary detrusor contraction volume, MCC, Qmax, PVR ($p < 0.05$) |
| de Seze [4]** | '11 | 70 | refractory OAB symptoms | 3 | • 30d: 51% resolution of severe urgency, 67% reduction in frequency by 3 episodes/day<br>• 90d: improvement in 83.3% of patients in 3 day bladder diary, MHU or warning time |
| Gobbi [5] | '11 | 18 | refractory LUTS | 3 | • Improved frequency, nocturia, Increased voided volume,<br>• PPBC decreased by 3 points ($p = 0.003$), PPIUS decreased by 2 points ($p = 0.005$), UB-VAS decreased by 4 cm ($p = 0.005$), improvement in KHQ ($p < 0.05$) |
| Zecca [6] | '14 | initial: 83 Maint: 74 | refractory LUTS, UDS with DO, UAB or DSD | 24 | • 60% (44/74) required maintenance every 2 weeks, 4% required maintenance every week, mean treatment was: 1.79 sessions/patient/month<br>• 82% of patients reported treatment satisfaction on TS-VAS, GRA, and PPBC at 24 months |
| Zecca [7] | '14 | 83 | refractory LUTS, UDS with Dom UAB or DSD | 3 | • Sensory response: 64%, Motor response: 6%, Sensory-Motor: 30%; Sensory response with or without motor response was associated with better outcome than motor alone ($p < 0.001$) |
| Canbaz-Kabay [23] | '17 | initial: 29 Maint: 21 | refractory OAB | 12 | • Improvement in frequency, nocturia, urgency (all $p < 0.001$) and voided volume improved mean 72 cc ($p < 0.05$).<br>• Change from baseline on the ICIQ-SF, OABv8 and OAB-q: decreased symptom severity and health related quality of life ($P < 0.001$) |

*all studies included adults with multiple sclerosis

**Study of Transcutaneous PTNS versus others, which were percutaneous

*UDS* urodynamics, *DO* detrusor overactivity, *MCC* Maximum Cystometric Capacity, *LUTS* Lower urinary tract symptoms, *Maint* Maintenance, *NR* Not reported

## Methods/Design

### Study design and population

The study is registered with clinicaltrials.gov, NCT04063852. This study is designed as a single-centered, prospective, longitudinal cohort study with plans to follow participants for up to 24 months. Adult patients at the University of Michigan outpatient urology clinic presenting with multiple sclerosis and lower urinary tract symptoms (LUTS) including urinary frequency, urgency, incontinence refractory to two prior treatments who have elected to pursue percutaneous PTNS will be invited to participate (Table 2). Refractory symptoms are defined as bothersome LUTS that have not responded to at least two prior therapies including behavior modification, pharmacotherapy, pelvic floor physical therapy or bladder onabotulinum toxin. Full inclusion and exclusion criteria are listed in Table 2.

The PTNS procedure will be performed per the manufacturer's specifications using a Neuromodulation System (Urgent® PC, Minnetonka, MN), as previously described [15]. Participants will undergo treatment for 30 min, once per week for 12 weeks. After 12 weeks, those with more than 50% improvement in symptoms based on a visual analog scale, will be offered maintenance PTNS sessions for 30 min every 28 days for a total of 24 months.

**Table 2** Inclusion and Exclusion criteria

| **Inclusion Criteria** |
|---|
| Adults (age greater than or equal to 18 years old) |
| Diagnosis of Multiple Sclerosis |
| Lower urinary tract symptoms (urinary frequency, urgency and/or incontinence) |
| Failed prior first and second line therapy (behavioral and pharmacotherapy) |
| Electing for Posterior Tibial Nerve Stimulation therapy for urinary symptoms.<br>Patients performing Intermittent Catheterization are Eligible |
| **Exclusion Criteria** |
| Age less than 18 years |
| Indwelling catheters (urethral or suprapubic) |
| currently pregnant or planning pregnancy |
| Unable to attend weekly office visits for PTNS |
| urodynamic findings of bladder outlet obstruction |
| History of: |
| bladder reconstruction (augmentation cystoplasty, catheterizable channel) |
| cystectomy |
| bladder stones |
| pacemaker or defibrillator |
| malignancy of bladder |
| sacral neuromodulation |
| intravesical injection of onabotulinum toxin within 9 months |

### Recruitment

Participants will be recruited via a three-pronged approach. First, neurourology clinics at a tertiary care referral center will be screened for eligible patients. Eligible patients will be mailed letters regarding the study. Second, neurology and physical medicine and rehabilitation physicians at the same institution will be notified of the study. Finally, advertisements for the study will be posted on social media networks.

### Screening and enrollment

Patients who meet inclusion criteria will be evaluated at baseline. Demographic and social information, and complete history and physical and neurologic evaluation with the Expanded Disability Status Scale (EDSS) will be evaluated at this time. Information from prior brain and spine MRI studies will be collected, if available. Participants will complete baseline questionnaires outlined below and summarized in Table 3.

### Follow-up and retention

Efforts will be made to follow-up all patients through 24 months after time 0 (initiation of PTNS). This is inclusive of patients who do not have an improvement of symptoms with initial 12 weeks of PTNS and do not pursue maintenance PTNS. In order to promote follow-up and retention, participants will be offered the opportunity to complete questionnaires in person or electronically, via a Research Electronic Data Capture (REDCap) [25]. Furthermore, participants will be compensated at the time of return of a 3-day voiding diary at times 0, 12, and 24 months.

**Table 3** Outcome measurements and time points

| | Time Points (month) | | | |
|---|---|---|---|---|
| | 0* | 3** | 12 | 24 |
| **Demographic Intake Form** | x | | | |
| **LUTS Measurements:** | | | | |
| **3 Day Voiding Diary** | x | x | x | x |
| **AUA-SS** | x | x | x | x |
| **M-ISI** | x | x | x | x |
| **NBSS** | x | x | x | x |
| **Visual Analog Scale** | | x | | |
| **Sexual Satisfaction Scale** | x | x | x | x |
| **Bowel Control Scale** | x | x | x | x |
| **SF-12** | x | x | x | x |
| **Expanded Disability Scale** | x | | x | x |

*Time 0: start of PTNS therapy; **Time 3 months: end of weekly PTNS therapy; *AUA-SS* American Urological Association Symptom Score, *M-ISI* Michigan Incontinence Symptom Index, *NBSS* Neurogenic Bladder Symptom Score

**Collection of study data**
Study data will be collected and managed using REDCap hosted at the University of Michigan [25]. REDCap is a secure, web-based application designed to support data capture for research studies [25].

**Study measurements**
Eligible persons will be evaluated at baseline (time of first PTNS treatment) and then at months 3, 12 and 24 from baseline (Table 3). Patients will be administered instruments assessing LUTS, HRQOL, Bowel and Sexual symptoms. Data collection instruments are summarized in Table 4.

**Description of urinary symptom assessment tools** For evaluation of LUTS the following instruments will be utilized: 1) 3-day voiding diary, 2) American Urological Association Symptom Score (AUA-SS), 3) Michigan Incontinence Symptom Index (M-ISI), and 4) Neurogenic Bladder Symptom Score. Voiding diaries are recommended in the routine evaluation of patients with neurogenic overactive bladder and the 3 day diary has been shown to be reliable in the evaluation of urge urinary incontinence [26, 27]. The AUA-SS was validated in 1992 and has been widely used in urologic literature including in the assessment of patients with MS. [11, 28, 29] Scores range from 0 to 35 with greater scores indicating more severe symptoms. The M-ISI is a 10 item questionnaire was developed and validated to discern between type of incontinence and the severity and bother caused by incontinence [30]. Greater scores indicate increased symptoms and the minimally important difference for urge urinary incontinence subdomain is 2 points [30]. The M-ISI has been utilized in prior literature in the context of MS. [11] The Neurogenic Bladder Symptom Score is a 22 item survey developed and validated for use in patients with spinal cord injury, MS and spina bifida [31]. The NBSS is a symptom scale which captures data regarding urinary incontinence, storage and voiding symptoms and complications of neurogenic bladder [31]. (Table 4).

**Description of adjunct assessment tools** Additional information regarding sexual activity and bowel symptoms will be assessed via selected tools which are part of the Multiple Sclerosis Quality of Life Index (MSQLI) [32, 33]. The MSQLI serves as a comprehensive assessment of HRQOL in patients with MS and consists of a Health Status Questionnaire (SF-36) and 9 subscales including bowel and sexual domains [32, 33]. For the purposes of this study the SF-12, Bowel Control Scale and Sexual Satisfaction Scale from the MSQLI are selectively utilized. The SF-12 is a 12-item version of the SF-36, the SF-12, was chosen to assess health status in order to decrease survey fatigue [34]. Literature has shown comparable results between SF-36 and SF-12 in the MS population [34, 35]. The Bowel Control Scale is a 5 item scale evaluating constipation, bowel accidents, bowel urgency and the impact of bowel symptoms of lifestyle on a 25 point scale with higher scores indicating greater bowel problems [33]. The Sexual Satisfaction Scale is a 5-item index addressing overall sexual adjustment in patients with MS and was adapted by the MSQLI from the Sexual History Form, scores range from 4 to 24 with higher scores indicating greater problems with sexual satisfaction [32, 33]. Both the Sexual Satisfaction Scale and the Bowel Control Scale have been widely used and

**Table 4** Description of data collection instruments

| | Name | Description |
|---|---|---|
| **Urinary Measures** | 3-day Voiding Diary | Patient completed 3 day assessment of fluid intake, output, incontinence episodes and pad changes. |
| | American Urological Association Symptom Score (AUA-SS) | Validated symptom score for the evaluation of Lower Urinary Tract Symptoms in Benign Prostatic Hyperplasia. Has been used in MS related research in the past. |
| | Michigan Incontinence Symptom Score (M-ISI) | Validated score developed to discern between type of incontinence and the severity and bother caused by urinary incontinence |
| | Neurogenic Bladder Symptom Score (NBSS) | Objective and validated assessment of bladder symptoms specifically created for use in patients with neurogenic bladder |
| **Bowel and Sexual Measures** | Sexual Satisfaction Scale | Validated, 5 item index addressing overall sexual adjustment in patients with MS and was adapted by the MSQLI from the Sexual History Form, scores range from 4 to 24 with higher scores indicating greater problems with sexual satisfaction. |
| | Bowel Control Scale | validated, 5 item scale evaluating constipation, bowel accidents, bowel urgency and the impact of bowel symptoms of lifestyle on a 25 point scale with higher scores indicating greater bowel problems |
| **General HRQOL** | SF-12 | Validated 12 item quality of life survey for use in patients with chronic conditions. |
| **MS Impact** | Expanded Disability Scale | Physician Completed assessment of impact of MS |

*HRQOL* Health Related Quality of Life. *MS* Multiple Sclerosis

validated as part of the MSQLI in the MS literature [32, 33]. (Table 4).

**Description of neurologic disability assessment tools**
Neurologic impact of multiple sclerosis in participants will be evaluated using the Expanded Disability Status Scale (EDSS) at baseline and annually by a neurologist, resulting in 3 measurements over the 24-month study time frame [36]. Additionally, we will evaluate participants for change in Magnetic Resonance Imaging (MRI) over the 24-month period, including T2 lesion number and location. The EDSS was developed in the 1950s and has long been the standard for assessing MS progression in phase III clinical trials [36]. The EDSS assesses eight neurological exam functional systems; EDSS 0 means normal and 10, death. Aside from EDSS, MRI will provide objective measures of MS disease burden as reflected on T2 lesion load (Table 4).

### Study outcomes

The primary outcome will be change in the median number of urinary frequency and urinary incontinence episodes on a 3-day voiding diary [37]. Secondary outcomes will be change in AUA symptom score (AUA-SS) and bothersome score, Michigan Incontinence Symptom Index (M-ISI), Neurogenic Bladder Symptom Score (NBSS), and from the Multiple Sclerosis Quality of Life Index (MSQLI) the Health Status Questionnaire (SF-12), Sexual Satisfaction Scale (SSS), and Bowel Control Scale (BCS) [28, 30–33].

### Sample size

In this descriptive study, we aim to enroll at least 50 participants. While it is likely that the count of episodes in each of the time frames follows a Poisson distribution, the difference statistic could very well be expected to follow a normal distribution. If not, appropriate transformations would be applied to create an approximately normal distribution. Allowing for up to a 10% dropout rate, this sample size will provide a 95% chance to have a 95% confidence interval for our change statistic that is within +/− 1/3 of a standard deviation. In other words, if we have an underlying standard deviation of 3 for the difference in counts, simulation results indicate that over 95% of the time, the 95% confidence interval for the change statistic would fall within the mean +/− 1. This will provide sufficient precision for our outcomes of interest.

## Statistical analysis

Baseline descriptive demographic data will be presented for the entire cohort. The primary outcome of median number of urinary frequency and incontinence episodes on a 3-day voiding diary at 3, 12 and 24 months will be compared to baseline for each patient using paired analysis. Secondary outcome measures including total AUA-SS, M-ISI, NBSS, SF-12, SSS and BCS scores at 3, 12 and 24 months will be compared to baseline for each patient using paired analysis. Continuous variables will be evaluated using paired t-test and categorical data will be analyzed using McNemar's test. Paired data will be evaluated using a 2-sided paired t-test. Median values will be analyzed using a Wilcoxon signed rank test. Statistical significance will be considered with $p < 0.05$.

In order to assess for predictors of improvement of symptoms response to PTNS, planned subgroup analysis will be performed stratifying patients based on gender, EDSS score, and burden of disease on MRI. Furthermore, an interim analysis at evaluating outcomes at 3 and 12 months after PTNS is planned.

## Discussion

The current literature regarding outcomes of PTNS in patients with MS who suffer from refractory lower urinary tract symptoms is favorable and is summarized in Table 1 [16–22, 38]. In 2009 Kabay published 3-month clinical outcomes in 19 patients showing significant decrease in mean overactive bladder questionnaire (OAB-V8) scores (15.7 vs 7.6, $p < 0.05$) [18]. Additionally they found a 40% complete response for urinary incontinence, and 58% complete response for urinary frequency on bladder diaries [18]. In 2011, Gobbi reported 3 month results in 18 patients from a multicenter, open label trial which found that there was statistically significant improvement in frequency (9 vs 6 voids, $p = 0.04$) and nocturia (3 vs 1 episodes, $p = 0.002$), additionally there was a 70% treatment satisfaction and significant improvement in the patient perception of bladder condition (PPBC) and patient perception of intensity of urgency scales (PPIUS) as well as the King's Health Questionnaire (KHQ) [19]. The same group published long term outcomes (mean 24 months, range 15–41) which included variable maintenance PTNS every 2–4 weeks, in 83 patients [20]. They reported 89% had greater than 50% improvement on the PPBC at 12 months and 82% had treatment satisfaction and improvement in PPBC at 24 months [20]. Of the 74 patients undergoing maintenance, the mean monthly treatment frequency was 1.8 sessions [20]. Most recently, Canbaz Kabay published 12-month outcomes in 29 patients, with 21 patients undergoing maintenance PTNS at variable intervals between 2 and 4 weeks [22]. Similar to prior studies, they found significant improvements in frequency, nocturia, urgency, and incontinence at 3, 6, 9 and 12 months of follow-up [22]. Furthermore, they found that there was significant improvement on International Consultation on Incontinence Questionnaire-Short Form (ICIQ-SF), OAB-V8 and OAB-q at 12 months [22].

Prior literature suggests that PTNS will improve LUTS in patients with MS, and that results may be sustained up to 24 months with maintenance therapy. However, the literature is limited in several ways. First, only two prior studies report outcomes beyond 3 months, in a total of 95 patients [20, 22]. Next, the published maintenance schedules for PTNS in MS have varied between every 2–4 weeks, which makes it difficult to assess whether monthly maintenance PTNS is adequate for sustained efficacy [20, 22]. Furthermore, all prior studies have excluded patients with EDSS greater than 7 [16–22, 38]. Since patients with greater EDSS scores have increased disability, the impact of progressive MS patients who require assistive devices or wheelchairs for mobility is unknown. Finally, prior studies did not assess how early MS would respond to treatment. In light of ours and others' studies showing RRMS are associated with more bothersome urinary symptoms, it will interesting to see how the treatment will affect early MS with EDSS less than 2 and if disease progression impacts PTNS efficacy [7, 23].

Another significant knowledge gap is that health related quality of life (HRQOL) has been reported in only one study and no prior studies have reported on potential improvements in bowel and sexual function with PTNS [19]. Evaluating the impact on HRQOL provides data to guide clinicians and patients on whether the investment in PTNS is worthwhile for overall health. Assessment of bowel and sexual function outcomes may expand the applications for PTNS in this population. Finally, none of the previous PTNS studies have incorporated MRI measures. As another novel exploratory measure, our protocol will also incorporate retrospective MRI data of the participants, obtained for routine neurologic surveillance, before and after PTNS in order to evaluate whether brain and spinal cord lesion location, T2 lesion number and volume changes, and disease burden impact track with PTNS treatments.

## Conclusion

This research protocol aims to expand on the existing literature regarding outcomes of PTNS in MS. Specifically, it will provide 24-month follow-up data on bladder, bowel, sexual and HRQOL outcomes. Further, it will be investigational data correlating EDSS and MRI results to PTNS, to evaluate whether lesion location or burden of disease is predictive of response to PTNS.

### Abbreviations

AUA-SS: American Urological Association Symptom Score; BCS: Bowel Control Scale; CIS: Clinically isolated syndrome; EDSS: Expanded Disability Status Scale; HRQOL: Health related quality of life; KHQ: King's Health Questionnaire; LUTS: Lower urinary tract symptoms; M-ISI: Michigan Incontinence Symptom Index; MRI: Magnetic resonance imaging; MS: Multiple Sclerosis; MSQLI: Multiple Sclerosis Quality of Life Index; NBSS: Neurogenic Bladder Symptom Score; OAB: Overactive bladder; PPBC: Patient perception of bladder condition; PPIUS: Patient perception of intensity of urgency scales; PPMS: Primary progressive multiple sclerosis; PTNS: Posterior tibial nerve stimulation; RRMS: Relapsing remitting multiple sclerosis; SF-12: Health Status Questionnaire; SPMS: Secondary progressive multiple sclerosis; SSS: Sexual Satisfaction Scale

### Acknowledgements

Not applicable.

### Authors' contributions

GL: developing research plan, writing manuscript, read and approved final manuscript. YMD: developing research plan, writing manuscript, read and approved final manuscript. PBR: developing research plan, read and approved final manuscript. QC: developing research plan, read and approved final manuscript. PG: developing research plan, read and approved final manuscript. RD: developing statistical analytic plan, read and approved final manuscript. YQ: developing statistical analytic plan, read and approved final manuscript. AC: developing research plan, read and approved final manuscript. JS: developing research plan, writing manuscript, read and approved final manuscript.

### Competing interests

GL: no competing interests. YMD has served as a consultant and/or received grant support from: Acorda, Bayer Pharmaceutical, Biogen Idec, EMD Serono, Genzyme, Novartis, Questor, Chugai Pharmaceuticals, and Teva Neuroscience. Dr. Mao-Draayer is currently supported by grants from the NIH NIAID Autoimmune Center of Excellence: UM1-AI110557; NIH NINDS R01-NS080821, PCORI, Chugai, Novartis and Genzyme. PBR: no competing interests. QC: no competing interests. PG: no competing interests. RD: no competing interests. YQ: no competing interests. AC: reports personal fees from Wellspect, grants from Medtronic, outside of the submitted work. JS is supported by grants from the Department of Defense; received grant support from Ipsen, Uroplasty.

### Author details

[1]Department of Urology, University of Michigan, 1500 East Medical Drive, Taubman Center 3875, Ann Arbor, MI 48109, USA. [2]Department of Neurology, University of Michigan, Ann Arbor, MI, USA.

### References

1. Wallin MT, Culpepper WJ, Campbell JD, Nelson LM, Langer-Gould A, Marrie RA, et al. The prevalence of MS in the United States: a population-based estimate using health claims data. Neurology. 2019;92(10):e1029–40.
2. Types of MS. National Multiple Sclerosis Society. Available from: https://www.nationalmssociety.org/What-is-MS/Types-of-MS. Cited 2019 May 20.
3. Compston A, Coles A. Multiple sclerosis. Lancet. 2002;359(9313):1221–31.
4. Koch M, Kingwell E, Rieckmann P, Tremlett H, UBC MS. Clinic neurologists. The natural history of secondary progressive multiple sclerosis. J Neurol Neurosurg Psychiatry. 2010;81(9):1039–43.
5. Lublin FD, Reingold SC, Cohen JA, Cutter GR, Sørensen PS, Thompson AJ, et al. Defining the clinical course of multiple sclerosis: the 2013 revisions. Neurology. 2014;83(3):278–86.
6. Khalaf KM, Coyne KS, Globe DR, Armstrong EP, Malone DC, Burks J. Lower urinary tract symptom prevalence and management among patients with multiple sclerosis. Int J MS Care. 2015;17(1):14–25.
7. Di Filippo M, Proietti S, Gaetani L, Gubbiotti M, Di Gregorio M, Eusebi P, et al. Lower urinary tract symptoms and urodynamic dysfunction in clinically isolated syndromes suggestive of multiple sclerosis. Eur J Neurol. 2014;21(4):648–53.
8. Stoffel JT. Contemporary management of the neurogenic bladder for multiple sclerosis patients. Urol Clin North Am. 2010;37(4):547–57.
9. Overactive Bladder (OAB) Guideline - American Urological Association. Available from: https://www.auanet.org/guidelines/overactive-bladder-(oab)-guideline. Cited 2019 May 15.
10. Gormley EA, Lightner DJ, Burgio KL, Chai TC, Clemens JQ, Culkin DJ, et al. Diagnosis and treatment of overactive bladder (non-neurogenic) in adults: AUA/SUFU guideline. J Urol. 2012;188(6 Suppl):2455–63.
11. Dray E, Cameron AP, Clemens JQ, Qin Y, Covalschi D, Stoffel J. Does post-void residual volume predict worsening urological symptoms in patients with multiple sclerosis? J Urol. 2018;200(4):868–74.

12. Ginsberg D, Gousse A, Keppenne V, Sievert K-D, Thompson C, Lam W, et al. Phase 3 efficacy and tolerability study of onabotulinumtoxinA for urinary incontinence from neurogenic detrusor overactivity. J Urol. 2012;187(6): 2131–9.
13. Puccini F, Bhide A, Elneil S, Digesu GA. Sacral Neuromodulation: an effective treatment for lower urinary tract symptoms in multiple sclerosis. Obstet Gynecol Surv. 2016;71(7):401.
14. Information for Prescribers. Medtronic; 2018. Available from: http://manuals.medtronic.com/content/dam/emanuals/neuro/M976705A_a_001_view.pdf.
15. Peters KM, Carrico DJ, Perez-Marrero RA, Khan AU, Wooldridge LS, Davis GL, et al. Randomized trial of percutaneous tibial nerve stimulation versus sham efficacy in the treatment of overactive bladder syndrome: results from the SUmiT trial. J Urol. 2010;183(4):1438–43.
16. Fjorback MV, van Rey FS, van der Pal F, Rijkhoff NJM, Petersen T, Heesakkers JP. Acute urodynamic effects of posterior tibial nerve stimulation on neurogenic detrusor overactivity in patients with MS. Eur Urol. 2007;51(2): 464–70 discussion 471–2.
17. Kabay SC, Yucel M, Kabay S. Acute effect of posterior tibial nerve stimulation on neurogenic detrusor overactivity in patients with multiple sclerosis: urodynamic study. Urology. 2008;71(4):641–5.
18. Kabay S, Kabay SC, Yucel M, Ozden H, Yilmaz Z, Aras O, et al. The clinical and urodynamic results of a 3-month percutaneous posterior tibial nerve stimulation treatment in patients with multiple sclerosis-related neurogenic bladder dysfunction. Neurourol Urodyn. 2009;28(8):964–8.
19. Gobbi C, Digesu GA, Khullar V, El Neil S, Caccia G, Zecca C. Percutaneous posterior tibial nerve stimulation as an effective treatment of refractory lower urinary tract symptoms in patients with multiple sclerosis: preliminary data from a multicentre, prospective, open label trial. Mult Scler. 2011; 17(12):1514–9.
20. Zecca C, Digesu GA, Robshaw P, Singh A, Elneil S, Gobbi C. Maintenance percutaneous posterior nerve stimulation for refractory lower urinary tract symptoms in patients with multiple sclerosis: an open label, multicenter, prospective study. J Urol. 2014;191(3):697–702.
21. Zecca C, Digesu GA, Robshaw P, Puccini F, Khullar V, Tubaro A, et al. Motor and sensory responses after percutaneous tibial nerve stimulation in multiple sclerosis patients with lower urinary tract symptoms treated in daily practice. Eur J Neurol. 2014;21(3):506–11.
22. Canbaz Kabay S, Kabay S, Mestan E, Cetiner M, Ayas S, Sevim M, et al. Long term sustained therapeutic effects of percutaneous posterior tibial nerve stimulation treatment of neurogenic overactive bladder in multiple sclerosis patients: 12-months results. Neurourol Urodyn. 2017;36(1):104–10.
23. Cox L, Cameron AP, Wittman D, Papin JE, Stoffel JT. Analysis Of Urinary Symptoms And Urodynamic Findings In Multiple Sclerosis Patients By Gender And Disease Subtype. J Neurol Neurobiol. 2015; 1(2). Available from: https://www.researchgate.net/publication/276961511_Analysis_Of_Urinary_Symptoms_And_Urodynamic_Findings_In_Multiple_Sclerosis_Patients_By_Gender_And_Disease_Subtype. Cited 2019 Apr 8.
24. Sanagapalli S, Neilan L, Lo JYT, Anandan L, Liwanag J, Raeburn A, et al. Efficacy of percutaneous posterior Tibial nerve stimulation for the Management of Fecal Incontinence in multiple sclerosis: a pilot study: PTNS for fecal incontinence in multiple sclerosis. Neuromodulation. 2018;21(7): 682–7.
25. Harris PA, Taylor R, Thielke R, Payne J, Gonzalez N, Conde JG. Research electronic data capture (REDCap)--a metadata-driven methodology and workflow process for providing translational research informatics support. J Biomed Inform. 2009;42(2):377–81.
26. Groen J, Pannek J, Castro Diaz D, Del Popolo G, Gross T, Hamid R, et al. Summary of European Association of Urology (EAU) guidelines on Neuro-urology. Eur Urol. 2016;69(2):324–33.
27. Bright E, Drake MJ, Abrams P. Urinary diaries: evidence for the development and validation of diary content, format, and duration. Neurourol Urodyn. 2011;30(3):348–52.
28. Barry MJ, Fowler FJ Jr, O'Leary MP, Bruskewitz RC, Holtgrewe HL, Mebust WK, et al. The American urological association symptom index for benign prostatic hyperplasia. The measurement Committee of the American Urological Association. J Urol. 1992;148(5):1549–57 discussion 1564.
29. Weissbart SJ, Pechersky D, Malykhina A, Bavaria T, Parrillo L, Arya LA, et al. The impact of pontine disease on lower urinary tract symptoms in patients with multiple sclerosis. Neurourol Urodyn. 2017;36(2):453–6.
30. Suskind AM, Dunn RL, Morgan DM, DeLancey JOL, McGuire EJ, Wei JT. The Michigan incontinence symptom index (M-ISI): a clinical measure for type, severity, and bother related to urinary incontinence. Neurourol Urodyn. 2014;33(7):1128–34.
31. Welk B, Morrow S, Madarasz W, Baverstock R, Macnab J, Sequeira K. The validity and reliability of the neurogenic bladder symptom score. J Urol. 2014;192(2):452–7.
32. Marrie RA, Miller DM, Chelune GJ, Cohen JA. Validity and reliability of the MSQLI in cognitively impaired patients with multiple sclerosis. Mult Scler. 2003;9(6):621–6.
33. Guidebook - MSQLI Manual and Forms (.pdf). Available from: https://www.nationalmssociety.org/NationalMSSociety/media/MSNationalFiles/Brochures/MSQLI_-A-User-s-Manual.pdf.
34. Ware J Jr, Kosinski M, Keller SD. A 12-item short-form health survey: construction of scales and preliminary tests of reliability and validity. Med Care. 1996;34(3):220–33.
35. Nortvedt MW, Riise T, Myhr KM, Nyland HI. Performance of the SF-36, SF-12, and RAND-36 summary scales in a multiple sclerosis population. Med Care. 2000;38(10):1022–8.
36. Kurtzke JF. Rating neurologic impairment in multiple sclerosis: an expanded disability status scale (EDSS). Neurology. 1983;33(11):1444–52.
37. Society of Urodynamics, Female Pelvic Medicine and Urogenital Reconstruction 3 day voiding Diary. SUFU 3 day voiding diary. Available from: https://sufuorg.com/docs/guidelines/sufu-voiding-diary-faq.aspx. Cited 2019 Apr 5.
38. de Sèze M, Raibaut P, Gallien P, Even-Schneider A, Denys P, Bonniaud V, et al. Transcutaneous posterior tibial nerve stimulation for treatment of the overactive bladder syndrome in multiple sclerosis: results of a multicenter prospective study. Neurourol Urodyn. 2011;30(3):306–11.

# Permissions

All chapters in this book were first published by BioMed Central; hereby published with permission under the Creative Commons Attribution License or equivalent. Every chapter published in this book has been scrutinized by our experts. Their significance has been extensively debated. The topics covered herein carry significant findings which will fuel the growth of the discipline. They may even be implemented as practical applications or may be referred to as a beginning point for another development.

The contributors of this book come from diverse backgrounds, making this book a truly international effort. This book will bring forth new frontiers with its revolutionizing research information and detailed analysis of the nascent developments around the world.

We would like to thank all the contributing authors for lending their expertise to make the book truly unique. They have played a crucial role in the development of this book. Without their invaluable contributions this book wouldn't have been possible. They have made vital efforts to compile up to date information on the varied aspects of this subject to make this book a valuable addition to the collection of many professionals and students.

This book was conceptualized with the vision of imparting up-to-date information and advanced data in this field. To ensure the same, a matchless editorial board was set up. Every individual on the board went through rigorous rounds of assessment to prove their worth. After which they invested a large part of their time researching and compiling the most relevant data for our readers.

The editorial board has been involved in producing this book since its inception. They have spent rigorous hours researching and exploring the diverse topics which have resulted in the successful publishing of this book. They have passed on their knowledge of decades through this book. To expedite this challenging task, the publisher supported the team at every step. A small team of assistant editors was also appointed to further simplify the editing procedure and attain best results for the readers.

Apart from the editorial board, the designing team has also invested a significant amount of their time in understanding the subject and creating the most relevant covers. They scrutinized every image to scout for the most suitable representation of the subject and create an appropriate cover for the book.

The publishing team has been an ardent support to the editorial, designing and production team. Their endless efforts to recruit the best for this project, has resulted in the accomplishment of this book. They are a veteran in the field of academics and their pool of knowledge is as vast as their experience in printing. Their expertise and guidance has proved useful at every step. Their uncompromising quality standards have made this book an exceptional effort. Their encouragement from time to time has been an inspiration for everyone.

The publisher and the editorial board hope that this book will prove to be a valuable piece of knowledge for researchers, students, practitioners and scholars across the globe.

# List of Contributors

**Christopher El Mouhayyar, Haoyang Wang, Laith Hattar, Fang-Yu Liu, Karen Feghali and Vaidyanathapuram Balakrishnan**
Department of Medicine, St. Elizabeth's Medical Center, Boston, MA, USA
Department of Medicine, Tufts University School of Medicine, Boston, MA, USA

**Chen Hu, Yu Bai, Jun Li, Guoyin Zhang, Libo Yang, Chengwei Bi, Bin Zhao, Yong Yang, Ruiqian Li, Hongyi Wu, Qilin Wang and Yang Qin**
Department of Urology, Yunnan Cancer Hospital, The Third Affiliated Hospital of Kunming Medical University, Kunming 650118, Yunnan, China

**Shota Omura, Satoru Taguchi, Shogo Miyagawa, Ryuki Matsumoto, Mio Samejima, Naoki Ninomiya, Kazuki Masuda, Yu Nakamura, Tsuyoshi Yamaguchi, Manami Kinjo, Mitsuhiro Tambo, Takatsugu Okegawa and Hiroshi Fukuhara**
Department of Urology, Kyorin University School of Medicine, 6-20-2 Shinkawa, Mitaka, Tokyo 181-8611, Japan

**Eiji Higashihara**
Department of ADPKD Research, Kyorin University School of Medicine, 6-20-2 Shinkawa, Mitaka, Tokyo 181-8611, Japan

**Francine Toye and Karen L. Barker**
Nuffield Orthopaedic Centre, Oxford University Hospitals NHS Foundation Trust, Windmill Road, Oxford OX3 7HE, UK
Nuffield Department of Orthopaedics, Rheumatology and Musculoskeletal Sciences (NDORMS), University of Oxford, Oxford, UK

**Yuzhi Zuo, Zhenyu Zhang, Bingbing Shi, Zhigang Ji and Zhongming Huang**
Department of Urology, Peking Union Medical College Hospital, Peking Union Medical College and Chinese Academy of Medical Sciences, No.1 Shuaifuyuan, Beijing 100730, P.R. China

**Kazumasa Torimoto, Makito Miyake, Yasushi Nakai, Katsuya Aoki, Nobumichi Tanaka and Kiyohide Fujimoto**
Department of Urology, Nara Medical University, 840 Shijocho, Kashihara, Nara 634-8522, Japan

**Telma Zahirian Moghadam and Hamed Zandian**
Social Determinants of Health Research Center, Ardabil University of Medical Sciences, Ardabil, Iran

**Hamed Mohseni Rad and Ali Hosseinkhani**
Department of Surgery, School of Medicine and Allied Medical Sciences, Imam Reza Hospital, Ardabil University of Medical Sciences, Ardabil, Iran

**Yi-Kai Chang and Hong-Chiang Chang**
Department of Urology, National Taiwan University Hospital and National Taiwan University College of Medicine, No.1, Changde St., Zhongzheng Dist, Taipei City 10048, Taiwan

**Yu-An Chen**
Department of Urology, National Taiwan University Hospital and National Taiwan University College of Medicine, No.1, Changde St., Zhongzheng Dist, Taipei City 10048, Taiwan
Department of Urology, Cardinal Tien Hospital, School of Medicine Fu-Jen Catholic University, No.362, Zhongzheng Rd., Xindian Dist, New Taipei City 231, Taiwan

**Yann-Rong Su**
Department of Urology, National Taiwan University Hospital Hsin-Chu Branch, NO.25, Lane 442, Sec.1, Jingguo Rd, Hsinchu City 300, Taiwan

**Ai-Ling Shen and Yuan-Fu Tseng**
Department of Neurology, Sijhih Cathay General Hospital, No.2, Ln. 59, Jiancheng Rd., Sijhih Dist, New Taipei City 221, Taiwan

**Hsiu-Li Lin**
Department of Neurology, Sijhih Cathay General Hospital, No.2, Ln. 59, Jiancheng Rd., Sijhih Dist, New Taipei City 221, Taiwan
Graduate Institute of Biomedical Informatics, Taipei Medical University, No. 252, Wu-Xing Street, Taipei 110, Taiwan

**Hsiu-Chen Lin**
Department of Pediatrics, School of Medicine, College of Medicine, Taipei Medical University, No. 252, Wu-Xing Street, Taipei 110, Taiwan
Department of Laboratory Medicine, Taipei Medical University Hospital, No. 252, Wu-Xing Street, Taipei 110, Taiwan

**Chien-Yeh Hsu**
Graduate Institute of Biomedical Informatics, Taipei Medical University, No. 252, Wu-Xing Street, Taipei 110, Taiwan
Department of Information Management, National Taipei University of Nursing and Health Science, No. 365, Mingde Rd, Taipei 112, Taiwan

**Che-Yi Chou**
Division of Nephrology, Asia University Hospital, NO 222, Fuxin Rd, Wufeng Dist, Taichung 413, Taiwan
Department of Post-baccalaureate Veterinary Medicine, Asia University, NO 222, Fuxin Rd, Wufeng Dist, Taichung 413, Taiwan
Division of Nephrology, China Medical University Hospital, Tacihung, Taiwan

**Agustina Bessa, Fidelma Cahill, Harriet Wylie, Anna Haire, Saran Green and Mieke Van Hemelrijck**
King's College London, School of Cancer and Pharmaceutical Studies, Translational Oncology & Urology Research (TOUR), TOUR, Guy's Hospital, 3rd Floor Bermondsey Wing, London SE1 9RT, UK

**Rebecca Martin and Pardeep Kumar**
The Royal Marsden, Department Urology, London, UK

**Christel Häggström**
King's College London, School of Cancer and Pharmaceutical Studies, Translational Oncology & Urology Research (TOUR), TOUR, Guy's Hospital, 3rd Floor Bermondsey Wing, London SE1 9RT, UK
Department of Surgical Sciences, Uppsala University, Uppsala, Sweden
Department of Biobank Research, Umeå University, Umeå, Sweden

**Deborah Enting**
King's College London, School of Cancer and Pharmaceutical Studies, Translational Oncology & Urology Research (TOUR), TOUR, Guy's Hospital, 3rd Floor Bermondsey Wing, London SE1 9RT, UK
Department of Oncology, Guy's and St Thomas' NHS Foundation Trust, London, UK

**Suzanne Amery, Muhammad Shamim Khan, Samantha Broadhead, Kathryn Chatterton, Sachin Malde, Rajesh Nair, Ramesh Thurairaja, Margaret Northover and Karen Briggs**
Department of Urology, Guy's and St Thomas' NHS Foundation Trust, London, UK

**Laurent Alexandre**
Pelvipharm, Montigny-le-Bretonneux, France

**Rana Assaly, Julie Faugeroux, Miguel Laurin, Sandrine Compagnie and Delphine Behr-Roussel**
Pelvipharm, Montigny-le-Bretonneux, France
Université Paris-Saclay, UVSQ, Inserm, END-ICAP, Versailles, France

**François Giuliano**
Pelvipharm, Montigny-le-Bretonneux, France
Université Paris-Saclay, UVSQ, Inserm, END-ICAP, Versailles, France
AP-HP, Neuro-Uro-Andrology, Department of Physical Medicine and Rehabilitation, Raymond Poincaré Hospital, Garches, France

**Lauren Folgosa Cooley, Mary Kate Keeter, Isaac Lam and Nelson Bennett**
Department of Urology, Northwestern University Feinberg School of Medicine, 676 N. St. Clair St. Arkes 23-015, Chicago, IL 60611, USA

**Zhaohua Ye, Qiwu Mi, Daosheng Luo, Zhixiong Li and Jiexin Luo**
Department of Urology, Dongguan People's Hospital, Dongguan 523000, China

**Birgitt Schoenfisch, Sara Yvonne Brucker and Christl Reisenauer**
Department of Obstetrics and Gynecology, University Hospital Tübingen, Calwerstrasse 7, 72076 Tübingen, Germany

**Tilemachos Kavvadias**
Department of Obstetrics and Gynecology, University Hospital Tübingen, Calwerstrasse 7, 72076 Tübingen, Germany
Department of Gynecology and Obstetrics, University Hospital Basel, Spitalstrasse 21, 4031 Basel, Switzerland

**Zongchen Li**
National University Hospital, Singapore, Singapore

**Joey Chan Yiing Beh**
Ng Teng Fong General Hospital, Singapore, Singapore

**Qiong Xu and Yu Zou**
Department of Radiology, Women's Hospital School of Medicine Zhejiang University, Hangzhou 310006, Zhejiang province, China

**Ikenna I. Nnabugwu**
Department of Surgery, College of Medicine, University of Nigeria Ituku-Ozalla, Enugu PMB 01129, Nigeria

**Ijeoma L. Okoronkwo and Chinwe A. Nnabugwu**
Department of Health Administration and Management, Faculty of Health Sciences and Technology, University of Nigeria Enugu Campus, Enugu, Nigeria

**Mostafa Kotb, Ahmed Hassan and Mohamed Abouheba**
Pediatric Surgery, Alexandria Faculty of Medicine, Alexandria, Egypt

**Yu Fu**
Leeds Institute of Health Sciences, University of Leeds, Leeds LS2 9NL, UK

**E. Andrea Nelson**
School of Health and Life Sciences, Glasgow Caledonian University, Glasgow, UK.

**Linda McGowan**
School of Healthcare, University of Leeds, Leeds, UK

**Zao-Ming Huang, Yan-Feng Li, Yong Zhang, Yong Luo, Zhi-Lin Nie, Ke Li, Qing-Xing Feng and Xu-Dong Liu**
Department of Urology, Daping Hospital, Army Medical University, No.10, Daping Changjiangzhilu, Yuzhong District, Chongqing 400042, China

**Qi Wang**
Department of Urology, Chongqing Renji Hospital, University of Chinese Academy of Sciences, Chongqing 400062, China

**Jing Peng, Dong Fang, Huixi Li, Yuan Tang, Yiming Yuan, Wanshou Cui, Bing Gao and Zhichao Zhang**
Andrology Center, Department of Urology, Peking University First Hospital, Institute of Urology, Peking University, No. 59A, Di'anmen West St., Xicheng District, Beijing 100034, China

**Hongjun Li**
Department of Urology, Peking Union Medical College Hospital, Peking Union Medical College, Chinese Academy of Medical Sciences, No. 1 Shuaifuyuan, Dongcheng District, Beijing 100730, China

**Wout Devlies**
Faculty of Medicine, KU Leuven, Leuven, Belgium
Department of Urology, Regional hospital St. Franciskus, Heusden-Zolder, Belgium

**Kurt Dilen**
Department of Urology, Regional hospital St. Franciskus, Heusden-Zolder, Belgium

**Mattias Seghers**
Department of Radiology, Regional hospital St. Franciskus, Heusden-Zolder, Belgium

**Samuel L. Washington III, Sima P. Porten and Maxwell V. Meng**
Department of Urology, University of California, San Francisco, 550 16th Street, 6th Floor, San Francisco, CA 94158, USA

**Kyle B. Zuniga**
Department of Urology, University of California, San Francisco, 550 16th Street, 6th Floor, San Francisco, CA 94158, USA
Osher Center for Integrative Medicine, University of California, San Francisco, 1545 Divisadero Street, Suite 301, San Francisco, CA 94143, USA
Vagelos College of Physicians and Surgeons, Columbia University Medical Center, 630 West 168th Street, New York, NY 10032, USA

**Saadat Mehrabi, Mohammad Javad Yavari Barhaghtalab and Mehdi Babapour**
Department of General Surgery, Shahid Beheshti Hospital, Yasuj University of Medical Sciences, Yasuj, Iran

**Wei-Jen Chen and Eric Yi-Hsiu Huang**
Department of Urology, School of Medicine, National Yang-Ming University, Taipei, Taiwan
Department of Urology, Taipei Veterans General Hospital, No 201, Section 2, Shipai Rd, Taipei 112, Taiwan, Republic of China
Department of Urology, School of Medicine, Shu-Tien Urological Research Center, National Yang-Ming University, Taipei, Taiwan

**I-Shen Huang and William J. Huang**
Department of Physiology, School of Medicine, National Yang-Ming University, Taipei, Taiwan
Department of Urology, School of Medicine, National Yang-Ming University, Taipei, Taiwan
Department of Urology, Taipei Veterans General Hospital, No 201, Section 2, Shipai Rd, Taipei 112, Taiwan, Republic of China
Department of Urology, School of Medicine, Shu-Tien Urological Research Center, National Yang-Ming University, Taipei, Taiwan

**Richard J. Fantus**
Section of Urology, Department of Surgery, University of Chicago Medicine, 5841 S. Maryland Avenue, Chicago, IL 60637, USA

**Nelson E. Bennett, Robert E. Brannigan and James Wren**
Division of Male Reproductive Surgery and Men's Health, Department of Urology, Northwestern University Feinberg School of Medicine, NMH/Arkes Family Pavilion Suite 2300, 676 N Saint Clair, Chicago, IL 60611, USA

**Wei-Tang Kao**
Department of Urology, Shuang Ho Hospital, Taipei Medical University, No.291, Zhongzheng Rd., Zhonghe District, New Taipei City 23561, Taiwan
Graduate Institute of Clinical Medicine, Taipei Medical University, New Taipei City, Taiwan

**Christian Tiburtius and Ralf Böthig**
Centre for Spinal Injuries, Department Neuro-Urology, BG Trauma Hospital Hamburg, Bergedorfer Str. 10 Germany, 21033 Hamburg, Germany

**Birgitt Kowald**
Biomechanical Laboratory, BG Trauma Hospital Hamburg, Hamburg, Germany

**Sven Hirschfeld and Roland Thietje**
Centre for Spinal Injuries, BG Trauma Hospital Hamburg, Hamburg, Germany

**Carlos Martínez-Figueroa, Karen Cortés-Sarabia, Luz del Carmen Alarcón-Romero and Amalia Vences-Velázquez**
Laboratorio de Inmunobiología y Diagnóstico Molecular, Facultad de Ciencias Químico Biológicas, Universidad Autónoma de Guerrero, Av. Lázaro Cárdenas s/n, University City, C.P.39090 Chilpancingo, Guerrero, Mexico

**Hilda Guadalupe Catalán-Nájera and Micaela Martínez-Alarcón**
Servicio de urgencias, Laboratorio clínico, Clínica Hospital ISSSTE, Iguala, Guerrero, Mexico

**Ulrich Biber, Ovidiu Jurjut and Markus D. Enderle**
Erbe Elektromedizin GmbH, Waldhoernlestrasse 17, 72072 Tuebingen, Germany

**Wilhelm K. Aicher**
Department of Urology, University Hospital Tuebingen, Tuebingen, Germany

**Giulia I. Lane, Paholo Barboglio-Romo, J. Quentin Clemens, Priyanka Gupta, Rod Dunn, Yongmei Qin, Anne P. Cameron and John T. Stoffel**
Department of Urology, University of Michigan, 1500 East Medical Drive, Taubman Center 3875, Ann Arbor, MI 48109, USA

**Yang Mao-Draayer**
Department of Neurology, University of Michigan, Ann Arbor, MI, USA

# Index

www.ingramcontent.com/pod-product-compliance
Lightning Source LLC
LaVergne TN
LVHW060057220926
848484LV00008BA/2054
* 9 7 9 8 8 8 7 4 0 0 0 6 8 *